MUSCLE RELAXANTS IN CLINICAL ANESTHESIA

The first administration of "Curare" (Intocostrin) drug anesthesia. Anesthesia record of 20-year-old patient with appendicitis who received an intravenous injection of "Curare" (Intocostrin) during cyclopropane anesthesia in 1942. (Courtesy of Queen Elizabeth Hospital, Montreal.)

Muscle Relaxants in Clinical Anesthesia

David R. Bevan, M.B.
Professor of Anesthesia
McGill University
Anesthetist-in-Chief
Royal Victoria Hospital
Montreal, Quebec, Canada

Joan C. Bevan, M.D.
Associate Professor of Anesthesia
McGill University
Montreal, Quebec, Canada

François Donati, M.D.
Assistant Professor of Anesthesia
McGill University
Montreal, Quebec, Canada

YEAR BOOK MEDICAL PUBLISHERS, INC.
CHICAGO • LONDON • BOCA RATON

1 2 3 4 5 6 7 8 9 0 K R 92 91 90 89 88

Library of Congress Cataloging-in-Publication Data

Bevan, David R.
  Muscle relaxants in clinical anesthesia.

  Includes bibliographies and index.
  1. Malignant hyperthermia—Chemotherapy. 2. Muscle
relaxants. 3. Anesthesia—Complications and sequelae.
I. Bevan, Joan C. II. Donati, François. III. Title.
[DNLM: 1. Anesthesia—methods. 2. Muscle Relaxants,
Central—pharmacodynamics. WO 297 B571m]
RD82.7.M48 1988   617'.96   87-25451
ISBN 0-8151-0734-X

Sponsoring Editor: David K. Marshall
Associate Managing Editor, Manuscript Services: Deborah Thorp
Copyeditor: Sally J. Jansen
Production Project Manager: Nancy Baker
Proofroom Supervisor: Shirley E. Taylor

PREFACE

During the last 10 years, there has been an explosion of new information concerning muscular relaxation during anesthesia. In part, this has resulted from the development of new neuromuscular blocking drugs and a reevaluation of drugs used for their reversal. These new agents encouraged the search for sensitive assays to examine their pharmacokinetic profile and to relate these changes to the action of the drugs. This, in turn, encouraged a standardized system of measuring neuromuscular activity, which led to closer evaluation of the action of the agents at different muscle groups. Standardized measurement also allowed improved evaluation of drug interactions, and defined the behavior of the relaxants and their reversal agents at the extremes of age and in states of major organ dysfunction. Simultaneously, many refinements in electrophysiologic and histochemical techniques have allowed greater understanding of the morphology and function of the acetylcholine receptor.

Several questions remain. For example, which are the sites of action of the relaxant drugs? Will it be possible to develop a short-acting relaxant without undesirable side effects? Is reversal of neuromuscular blockade always necessary? The purpose of the present text is to review the current state of knowledge of neuromuscular physiology and pharmacology for the clinician. In particular, attempts have been made to provide an extensive bibliography and to include much of the factual details in a graphical format. The drugs that have been discussed are those currently available in the Western world.

It seemed appropriate to produce a text by a group of anesthesiologists who enjoy clinical investigation from a city, Montreal, that was influential in the introduction of muscle relaxants into clinical anesthetic practice.

David R. Bevan, M.B.
Joan C. Bevan, M.D.
François Donati, M.D.

v

CONTENTS

Preface   *v*

1 / The Arrival of Curare in Montreal   *1*
  Bernard-Sibson-Sayre   *1*
  Boehm-Lawen   *2*
  Ranyard West—Sherrington   *2*
  Amazon, Orinoco, and the Royal Botanical Gardens   *2*
  Harold King and the British Museum   *3*
  Richard Gill   *3*
  Multiple Sclerosis—Walter Freeman   *4*
  Merck—Squibb—Ecuador   *4*
  Burman—Bennett—McIntyre   *4*
  Holaday—Dutcher—Wintersteiner   *5*
  Wright—Rovenstine—Papper—Cullen   *5*
  Harold Griffith—Montreal Homeopathic Hospital   *6*
  Columbus—Martyr—Keynes—Raleigh   *7*
  Treaty of Tordessiles   *7*
  Condamine—Bancroft—Abée Fontana—Von Humboldt   *7*
  Brodie—Waterton—"Wouralia"   *8*
  Schomburgk—Bernard   *8*
  Gray—Halton   *8*
  Beecher and Todd   *9*
  Polio—Intensive Care Units—Intermittent Positive-Pressure Ventilation   *9*
  Scientific Basis of Anesthesia   *10*
  Synthetic Relaxants   *10*
  Atracurium and Vecuronium   *11*
  Our Heritage   *11*

2 / The Neuromuscular Junction: Structure and Function   *13*
  Nerve and Muscle   *14*
  Physiology of Excitable Cells   *19*
  Acetylcholine Production and Release   *26*
  Acetylcholine Receptor   *32*
  Antagonist Action   *37*
  Relaxant Antagonism   *40*
  Conclusion   *42*

3 / Clinical Measurement   *49*
  Clinical Assessment   *49*
  Nerve Stimulation   *50*

Clinical Measurement   57
Applications   61
Conclusion   65

4 / Pharmacodynamic Principles   71
Agonist-Receptor Interactions   72
Effects of Antagonists   78
Nerve Stimulation   80
Other Types of Receptors and Interactions   83
Onset and Offset of Neuromuscular Blockade   86
Plasma Concentrations   90
Dose-Response Relationships   91
Factors Affecting Dose-Response Relationships   93

5 / Pharmacokinetic Principles   100
Compartmental Analysis   101
Pharmacokinetics of Relaxants and Their Antagonists   106
Relationship of Concentration to Effect   116
Pharmacokinetic Alterations   123

6 / Nondepolarizing Relaxants   133
Alcuronium   133
Atracurium   138
Fazadinium   155
Gallamine   160
Metocurine   168
Pancuronium   176
d-Tubocurarine   192
Vecuronium   204

7 / Depolarizing Agents: Succinylcholine   247
Structure   247
Metabolism   248
Reduced Plasma Cholinesterase Activity   248
Increased Plasma Cholinesterase Activity   251
Physiologic Role of Plasma Cholinesterase   251
Pharmacokinetics   254
Neuromuscular Blockade   254
Cardiovascular Effects   258
Complications of Initial Stimulation   259
Drug Interactions   263
Mode of Administration   265
Other Uses   266
Conclusion   266

8 / Malignant Hyperthermia   278
    Epidemiology, Incidence, and Mortality   278
    Triggering Agents   279
    Pathophysiology   279
    Identification of Malignant Hyperthermia Susceptibility   280
    Clinical Features   281
    Pathophysiologic Tests   282
    Masseter Spasm   283
    Management of an Acute Malignant Hyperthermic Reaction   284
    Dantrolene   285
    Subsequent Management of Malignant Hyperthermia-Susceptible Patients   287

9 / Pharmacology: Antagonists   293
    Anticholinesterases   293
    4-Aminopyridine   308
    Germine Monoacetate   308
    The Adequacy of Reversal   308

10 / Renal and Hepatic Disease   317
    Renal Failure   317
    Hepatic Disease   328
    Electrolytes and Acid-Base Disturbances   333

11 / Age and the Neuromuscular Junction   345
    Pediatric Responses   345
    Geriatric Responses   375

12 / Drug Interactions   389
    Analgesics   389
    Anesthetic Agents   393
    Antiarrhythmic Agents   395
    Antibiotics   397
    Anticonvulsants   399
    Corticosteroids   400
    Diuretics   400
    Electrolytes   401
    Enzyme Inhibitors   401
    Immunosuppressants and Anticancer Therapy   402
    Muscle Relaxants   402
    Phosphodiesterase Inhibitors   403
    Prostaglandin Inhibitors   403
    Psychotropic Drugs   403

x   Contents

13 / Neuromuscular Diseases   414
        Myasthenia Gravis   414
        Myotonia   419
        Muscular Dystrophy   421
        Upper Motor Neuron Lesions   422
        Miscellaneous   423

Index   431

1

The Arrival of Curare in Montreal

> We have been so much impressed by the dramatic effect produced in every one of our patients that we believe this investigation should be continued.
>
> H.R. Griffith and G.E. Johnson, 1942[1]

This modest conclusion by Griffith and Johnson revolutionized anesthetic practice. Very quickly, the use of muscle relaxants during anesthesia spread from Montreal around the world. However, many others were involved in transferring the lethal poison from the arrow tips of the South American jungle to the operating room. Medieval explorers, scientists, and medical pioneers of the 19th century were all entranced by the mystique of curare. The purpose of this chapter is to summarize those achievements that culminated in Griffith's success.

BERNARD–SIBSON–SAYRE

Medical uses for curare have been suggested since the mid-1800s. Claude Bernard showed that it produced paralysis only after injection into the bloodstream and by a selective action at the neuromuscular junction. In 1839, Dr. Francis Sibson in Nottingham, England, attempted to treat rabies with crude curare extract, and by 1857 Dr. Lewis Albert Sayre in New York had advocated the use of the drug to relieve the spasms of tetanus. Until the end of the 19th century, curare was used primarily to produce immobility in animals for physiologic experiments.

BOEHM–LAWEN

It was recognized that the crude curare extract varied in quality. From 1895 to 1897, Rudolf Boehm classified the curare extract as calabash, tube, or pot curare according to the native containers in which it reached Europe. In 1912, he gave Arthur Läwen, a surgeon of Leipzig, some of the curarine extracted from calabash curare. This was injected during surgery to produce relaxation for abdominal closure, while avoiding deep anesthesia.[2] The work went unnoticed for the next 30 years. It needed the enthusiasm of neurophysiologists and psychiatrists to suggest the first practical application for curare; a determined explorer to bring back large quantities from the South American jungle; and careful pharmacologic studies before a purified standardized preparation was available for clinical use. Experience with curare in electroconvulsive therapy encouraged others to suggest a place for it in anesthesia.

RANYARD WEST—SHERRINGTON

In the early 1930s, Dr. Ranyard West of Scotland, at the suggestion of Dr. Hamilton Hartridge, professor of physiology in London, attempted to use curare for its selective relaxing or lissive effect in the investigation of tetany and treatment of neurologic spasticities.[3] However, their supplies of curare were as uncertain as the pharmacologic effects. The curare extracts originated from an unknown source supplied to Burroughs Wellcome Co. from France and some pot curare from the Orinoco region that was a gift from Sir Charles Sherrington at Oxford. Clearly, several groups wished to investigate the properties of curare, but material was scarce.

AMAZON, ORINOCO, AND THE ROYAL BOTANICAL GARDENS

The Amazon basin was the site of a number of expeditions, but none of the treks was successful in obtaining adequate supplies. Eventually, links with Indians in the Orinoco region were made through the forestry service in the British colony of Guiana. In 1932, T. A. Warren Davis, the conservator of the forests, collected rare plants from the Mayarum River. These included *Strychnos toxifera, cogens,* and *pedunculata,* which were used by the natives in the preparation of curare arrow poison: "the flying death." The botanical specimens were authenticated by N. Y. Sandwich of the Royal Botanical Gardens at Kew.

HAROLD KING AND THE BRITISH MUSEUM

Chemical analysis was delayed while Burroughs Wellcome Co. awaited supplies of the plants. So, Ranyard West sought help from Dr. J. H. Daly of the Medical Research Council, a physiologist investigating the action of acetylcholine in neuromuscular transmission. In Daly's laboratory, Harold King, a chemist who studied alkaloids, was interested in "the flying death" and knew that curare interfered in some way with the action of acetylcholine. In the British Museum, a bamboo tube labeled "Ucayali River, 1871," containing 25 gm of tube curare was found, from which Harold King isolated pure d-tubocurarine chloride in 1935.[4] Later King extracted considerable supplies of crude curarine from the abundant supplies of bark of the *Strychnos toxifera* tree from Guiana. These extracts often produced bronchospasm. At this time, although the chemistry and pharmacology of curare had been determined, the botanically identifiable source remained elusive.

RICHARD GILL

Eventually large supplies of the plants used in curare making by the Indians in Ecuador[5] were obtained by Richard C. Gill. This allowed the first authenticated variety of curare to become commercially available. Born in 1901, the son of a Washington physician, Gill adopted an unconventional life-style. He abandoned medical studies to teach English, and then, in 1927, he followed his love of the wilderness to become a salesman for the American Rubber Company in Lima, Peru. Leaving the business life, he bought land on the eastern slopes of the Andes in the valley of the Rio Pastaza, a tributary of the Marañón and Amazon rivers. Here, he and his wife, Ruth, built a ranch, cultivated coffee, and learned the ways of the jungle.

MULTIPLE SCLEROSIS—WALTER FREEMAN

In 1932 the Gills returned to Maine on vacation. A few days before leaving, Gill was thrown from a horse, a fall which later he blamed for the development of bizarre symptoms of numbness, tingling, and clumsiness. He became paralyzed, and the illness, which was diagnosed as multiple sclerosis by the New York neurologist Dr. Walter Freeman, confined him to Washington for the next 4 years. As his health improved, he became obsessed with this doctor's notion that curare might relieve some of the symptoms of his spastic neurologic disease. He was determined to return to Ecuador where he knew he could locate supplies of curare.

MERCK—SQUIBB—ECUADOR

Gill approached the pharmaceutical firm, Merck & Co., Inc., which had shown an interest previously in collecting plants in South America. Their botanist, Dr. Boris A. Krukoff, taught him how to identify, collect, and preserve botanical specimens. Financial backing for his expedition was offered by a Massachusetts businessman, Sayre Merrill, who was impressed by Gill's jungle tales. Gill returned to Ecuador in 1938 during a remission of his disease, after organizing a 5-month jungle expedition. He became a jungle "brujo," or medicine man, learned the secrets of native manufacture of curare, and observed its use in blowguns to kill birds and small animals. He collected lianas from which he extracted the sticky tar-like, crude curare and returned to the United States later the same year with 25 lb of the substance. Unfortunately, Merck had turned its attention to the investigation of a different plant with curariform properties that yielded the alkaloid erythroidine. However, with characteristic persistence, Gill persuaded another pharmaceutical company, E. R. Squibb & Sons, Inc., to buy his supplies in 1939.

BURMAN—BENNETT—McINTYRE

Meanwhile, Michael Burman, an orthopedic surgeon, influenced by Ranyard West's work, attempted to relieve spastic paralysis with curare and erythroidine and found the responses promising but unpredictable.[6] This encouraged A. E. Bennett, a neuropsychiatrist in Omaha, Nebraska, to use curarization to prevent the fractures and dislocations associated with convulsive shock therapy. Bennett, a colleague of Dr. Walter Freeman, had learned of Gill's successful expedition and obtained supplies of curare from him. The drug was standardized by A. R. McIntyre, chairman of pharmacology at the University of Nebraska, by traditional methods using frog muscle and mice. First, Bennett repeated Burman's work on spastic children and then applied curarization successfully to convulsive shock therapy. The incidence of extremity fractures and vertebral dislocations associated with unmodified treatment was drastically reduced from 40% to 50% to less than 1%.[7]

HOLADAY—DUTCHER—WINTERSTEINER

The active principle of the purified curare had not yet been isolated, but the plant source was identified as *Chondodendron tomentosum* by Squibb's chemist, Horace Holaday. He devised an accurate biologic assay, the rabbit head-drop test,[8] to assess the potency of the new drug Intocostrin. Supplies were sent to McIntyre, who held a research grant from Squibb, and Bennett. They found that its action was uniform and predictable in 1,500 psychiatric patients, which encouraged its widespread use by other psychiatrists. Squibb then distributed ampules of Intocostrin to selected doctors and sought Food and Drug Administration permission for its sale. This approval was not forthcoming until 1945.[9] In 1942 James Dutcher and Oskar Wintersteiner, working with Gill's supplies, established with certainty that the origin of the d-tubocurarine chloride, previously isolated by King from a 65-year-old museum specimen, was *Chondodendron tomentosum*.[10]

WRIGHT—ROVENSTINE—PAPPER—CULLEN

The idea to use curare in anesthesia originated with Lewis H. Wright, who had used curare in the physiology laboratory, practiced as an obstetrician, and then joined Squibb to advise in anesthesia. At the 91st annual meeting of the American Medical Association held in New York in 1940, he watched a film on the use of Intocostrin in shock therapy by Drs. A. E. Bennett and A. R. McIntyre. It seemed logical to him to extrapolate this method of relaxation to supplement the action of the newer anesthetic agents that he promoted. Usually his suggestions were greeted with ridicule, but two anesthetists, Dr. Emery A. Rovenstine and Dr. Stuart C. Cullen, left that meeting to return to New York and Iowa with several ampules of Intocostrin, while Dr. Griffith left for

Montreal with only his thoughts. Rovenstine's research assistant, Dr. E. M. Papper, experimented with the drug in etherized cats, and it provoked severe, sometimes fatal bronchospasm. Following the injection of a dose, thought to be safe, to two patients, he was horrified to have to resuscitate them overnight. Cullen fared no better with his attempts to use the drug in dogs and categorically asserted that there was no possibility of introducing Intocostrin into anesthesia.[11]

HAROLD GRIFFITH—MONTREAL HOMEOPATHIC HOSPITAL

When Harold Griffith next met Wright at a meeting in Montreal in 1941, he learned the outcome of Papper and Cullen's efforts. However, his certainty that Intocostrin could be used safely, as a result of Bennett's work in psychiatry, persisted. Griffith decided to try it. Harold Griffith was well established as an anesthetist practicing in Montreal at the Homeopathic Hospital (now the Queen Elizabeth Hospital) where his father had been its first medical director and his brother was chief surgeon. His interest in anesthesia began as a medical student and lasted through years of general practice and war service. He was influenced by the principles of homeopathy and believed in the use of the smallest effective dose of any drug. He wanted to use less toxic amounts of anesthetic agents and curare might allow him to do this. Unlike Papper and Cullen, he was familiar with cyclopropane, a drug which he saw used by Ralph Waters in Wisconsin in 1933 and he introduced it into Canada that same year. Unlike ether, cyclopropane had no hypotensive effect or marked peripheral muscle relaxant action and so lacked synergism with curare. Moreover, Griffith remembered that one of his patients had died from laryngeal spasm in 1925 and was conscious of the possible need for endotracheal intubation and artificial ventilation in an anesthetized patient. When he first gave an intravenous injection of 5 ml of Intocostrin, an unauthenticated extract of curare, to a 20-year-old plumber during cyclopropane anesthesia for appendectomy (see Frontispiece), it was as a caring doctor rather than as a controversial medical pioneer. Griffith was satisfied.

Harold Griffith's report of the administration of curare to 25 patients under cyclopropane anesthesia was published in July 1942.[1] Without the constraints of ethics committees and peer reviews, this information was disseminated to an eager readership of clinical anesthetists within 6 months of its first clinical trial!

COLUMBUS—MARTYR—KEYNES—RALEIGH

Griffith knew nothing of Lawen's earlier use of curare for abdominal relaxation. Curare's reputation as a poison, surrounded by superstition and mythology, was centuries old and could not be dispelled prematurely. Soon after Columbus's explorations of South America in 1498, stories were brought back to Europe of travelers killed by poison arrows. These accounts and descriptions of the preparation of curare were collected by Pieter Martyr, an Italian who lived in Spain, in a book *De Orbe Novo*. Sir Walter Raleigh's expeditions took him to the same region, the Orinoco River in present day Venezuela, in 1554. One of his lieutenants, Lawrence Keynes, described the tribes of Indians they encountered and first used the word "ourari." It is probable that this meant "bird-killer," and variations include urari, woorara, oorali, cururu, ticunas and wourali, as well as the now familiar curare.[12]

TREATY OF TORDESSILES

The wars between the English and Spanish had resulted in the Treaty of Tordessiles in 1494, which gave Portugal sovereignty over part of Brazil and Africa, and Spain took all the lands west of Brazil. This effectively barred travel between Guiana and parts of Brazil in the east and Venezuela, Colombia, Ecuador, and Peru in the west for more than three centuries.

CONDAMINE—BANCROFT—ABEE FONTANA—Von HUMBOLDT

Charles Marie de la Condamine led an expedition to Ecuador in 1735 where he spent 10 years. As a scientist, he was interested in the configuration of the equator and North and South Poles, but he also wrote about a tribe called the Yameos who hunted with blow darts. He noticed that it was not dangerous to eat the meat that they killed. He took the first samples of curare back to Europe, where he demonstrated its lethal effect on chickens. Early investigators of the 18th century, Roger Herrisant, Richard Brockelsby, and the better-known Edward Bancroft, Abee Felix Fontana, and Friedrich von Humboldt also contributed to an understanding of the actions of curare.

BRODIE—WATERTON—"WOURALIA"

Bancroft's son, a physician, later supplied Benjamin Collins Brodie with the curare that Brodie used in 1812 to show that a curarized cat could be kept alive by artificial respiration through a tracheostomy. The eccentric Charles Waterton, Squire of Walton Hall, left England to manage his family's sugar plantation in Guiana. His stories of Indians killing birds with blowpipes and poison arrows, and descriptions of plants, including *Chondrodendron tomentosum,* were told in his book *Wanderings in South America.* When he returned to England in 1812, he took with him supplies of curare sufficient to repeat Brodie's experiments on a larger animal, a donkey, thereafter named Wouralia.[13]

SCHOMBURGK—BERNARD

The mechanism of action of curare, as well as the plants from which it came, remained unknown. Twenty years after Waterton's exploration, the Schomburgk brothers, Robert and Richard, saw the "urari" plant in the same area and described the apples and stems of *Strychnos toxifera.* It was later found that the curare plants from the eastern Amazon region have *Strychnos toxifera* as their chief ingredient. Despite these tentative scientific advances, Claude Bernard's experiments of the 1840s repeating those of Fontana, were needed to allow curare to move out of the laboratory and into clinical use. Perhaps Lawen failed to get acceptance for the paralyzing properties of curare for therapeutic uses only because the active ingredient had not been isolated, and the drug was not yet standardized.

GRAY—HALTON

Although the introduction of curare into clinical anesthesia required a long time, its subsequent acceptance was rapid. Cullen[14] followed Griffith's lead enthusiastically and reported more than 1,000 successful cases in which Intocostrin was used by 1945 removing any remaining impediment to its acceptance. Despite delays due to wartime difficulties in obtaining supplies, the next advances came from England. As a result of King's isolation of d-tubocurarine chloride and of its availability from Gill's supplies of *Chondodendron tomentosum,* Gray and Halton introduced this authenticated extract of curare (3 mg of d-tubocurarine was equivalent to 1 ml of Intocostrin) clinically. Their

1946 account of its use in 1,000 patients was aptly entitled "A Milestone in Anaesthesia?"[15] More importantly, they dispelled the belief that low doses were necessary so that spontaneous respiration was preserved and they deliberately paralyzed their patients with large doses, necessitating the use of controlled artificial ventilation. Thus, the technique of balanced anesthesia was developed, using minimal doses of drugs to provide unconsciousness, analgesia, and relaxation, the components of the "triad of anesthesia."[16]

BEECHER AND TODD

Inevitably doubts arose. The most damaging to curare's reputation was Beecher and Todd's 1954 report on deaths associated with anesthesia, suggesting a sixfold increase in mortality when curare was used.[17] An inherent toxic effect of curare was refuted, and Dripps,[18] in a critical review of these findings, drew attention to the role of inadequate reversal of paralysis in these deaths. While the need for ventilatory assistance during surgery was apparent, the use of pharmacologic reversal of paralysis at the end of surgery was not widespread. Clinical criteria were subjective, leaving uncertainties about residual curarization.

POLIO—INTENSIVE CARE UNITS—INTERMITTENT POSITIVE-PRESSURE VENTILATION

During these early years, manual compression of the reservoir bag served as a means of artificial ventilation. Satisfactory mechanical ventilators were not available until experience in the poliomyelitis epidemic in Denmark in 1952 necessitated their development. Body respirators were found to be ineffective in severe cases. Ibson instituted the technique of endotracheal intubation and intermittent positive pressure ventilation. Initially it was applied manually and later by mechanical respirators.[19] Once measurements of acid-base state became easier, with the introduction of electrodes to measure blood oxygen and carbon dioxide tensions,[20] control of ventilatory parameters was possible. Respiratory support could then be guaranteed, and curarization became a technique of choice in anesthesia.

The acceptance of muscle relaxants in anesthesia allowed interactions with developments in medicine and surgery and facilitated the treatment of thoracic, cardiac, and neurosurgical conditions previously considered inoperable. By extrapolation to the management of respiratory failure, the outcome of such conditions as tetanus and botulism was improved. These improved outcomes encouraged the growth of intensive care units to centralize the care of critically ill patients.

SCIENTIFIC BASIS OF ANESTHESIA

Curiously, the introduction of curare into anesthesia resulted not only in technical achievements, but changed the basic philosophy of anesthesia. It was the single event that appeared to stimulate the organization of the specialty. Hitherto, two recorded groups of physicians existed who practiced anesthesia met as the London Society of Anaesthetists (from 1893) and the Long Island Society of Anesthetists (from 1905). Publications in the specialty were limited to *Current Researches in Anesthesia and Analgesia,* which appeared in 1922, and the *British Journal of Anaesthesia,* which followed a year later. With increased interest in the scientific basis of anesthesia, the two decades after curare's introduction saw the founding of university departments devoted to the teaching of anesthesia, the institution of specialist examinations, and the promotion of research activities. Professional associations flourished, and their meetings provided the necessary forum for national and international exchange.

SYNTHETIC RELAXANTS

The rational use of muscle relaxants became an issue of debate.[21] Not simply whether a low- or high-dose technique was desirable, but whether some ideal muscle relaxant could be found. The awareness of the relationship of chemical structure to action enabled a series of muscle relaxants to be synthesized, most chemically unrelated to each other, but all claiming an advantage over the naturally occurring alkaloids. The most successful of these were succinylcholine, a short-acting depolarizing drug with a rapid onset of action, introduced into clinical practice in 1949,[22] and pancuronium bromide, a steroidal nondepolarizing drug introduced in 1967.[23] The ideal muscle relaxant would seem to be a curariform drug with the potency, rapidity of onset, and short duration of action of succinylcholine, the mode of action and reversibility of pancuronium bromide, but lacking unwanted side effects.

ATRACURIUM AND VECURONIUM

The most recently introduced synthetic drugs, atracurium[24] and vecuronium,[25] held promise as the ultimate neuromuscular blockers. Although this distinction has eluded them, they have been introduced into a climate of opinion vastly different than the one that received curare. Current scientific methods have replaced clinical observations and their inherent biases on which earlier studies depended. The commonly used inhalational agents, halothane, enflurane, and isoflurane potentiate the neuromuscular blocking drugs in a predictable manner. New drugs have been evaluated in the laboratory and under controlled clinical conditions, while older drugs have been reappraised. The ability to monitor the neuromuscular junction clinically has removed the physician's fear of admixtures of drugs, the use of priming doses and infusions, and the specter of residual postoperative paralysis.

OUR HERITAGE

Despite the progress made since curare was first used in anesthesia, much remains to be learned. There is still a need to understand the modes of action of neuromuscular blocking drugs and their reversal agents, the mechanisms involved in their interactions with other drugs, and the modifications of their actions with age and pathologic conditions. In Montreal the investigation begun by Griffith continues.

REFERENCES

1. Griffith HR, Johnson GE: The use of curare in general anesthesia. *Anesthesiology* 1942; 3:418−420.
2. Lawen A: Ueber die Verbindung der Lokalanasthesie mit der Narkose, über hohe Extraduralanasthesie und epidurale Injektionen Anasthesia render Losungen bei tabischen Magenkrisen. *Beitr Klin Chir* 1912; 80:168−189.
3. West R: An excursion into pharmacology: Curare in medicine. *Med Hist* 1984; 28:391−405.
4. King HF: Curare. *Nature* 1935; 135:469−470.
5. Gill RC: *White Water and Black Magic.* New York, H. Holt & Co, Inc, 1940.
6. Burman MS: Therapeutic use of curare and erythroidine hydrochloride for spastic and dystonic states. *Arch Neurol Psychiatry* 1939; 41:307−327.

7. Bennett AE: Curare: A preventive of traumatic complications in convulsive shock therapy. *Am J Psychiatry* 1941; 97:1040–1060.

8. McIntyre AR: Historical background, early use and development of muscle relaxants. *Anesthesiology* 1959; 20:409–415.

9. Council on Pharmacy and Chemistry: New and nonofficial remedies: Intocostrin. *JAMA* 1943; 129:517.

10. Wintersteiner O, Dutcher JD: Curare alkaloids from *Chondodendron tomentosum. Science* 1943; 97:467–470.

11. Betcher AM: The civilizing of curare: A history of its development and introduction into anesthesiology. *Anesth Analg* 1977; 56:305–319.

12. Thomas KB: *Curare: Its History and Usage.* London, Pitman Medical Publishing Co, Ltd, 1964, pp 21–22.

13. Smith P: *Arrows of Mercy.* New York, Doubleday & Co, Inc, 1969, pp 77–87.

14. Cullen SC: Curare in anesthesia. *Surgery* 1945; 18:45–47.

15. Gray TC, Halton J: A milestone in anaesthesia? (d-tubocurarine chloride). *Proc R Soc Med* 1946; 39:400–410.

16. Gray TC, Halton J: Technique for the use of d-tubocurarine chloride with balanced anaesthesia. *Br Med J* 1946; 2:293–295.

17. Beecher HK, Todd DP: Study of deaths associated with anesthesia and surgery based on a study of 599,548 anesthesias in 10 institutions 1948–1952 inclusive. *Ann Surg* 1954; 140:2–35.

18. Dripps RD: The role of muscle relaxants in anesthesia deaths. *Anesthesiology* 1959; 20:542–545.

19. Engstrom CG: Experience of prolonged controlled ventilation in poliomyelitis. *Acta Anaesthesiol Scand* 1963; 13(suppl):31–33.

20. Severinghaus JW, Bradley AF: Electrodes for blood PO_2 and pCO_2 determination. *J Appl Physiol* 1958; 13:515–520.

21. Scurr CF: A comparative review of the relaxants. *Br J Anaesth* 1951; 23:103–116.

22. Mayrhofer OK: Self-experiments with succinylcholine chloride: A new ultra-short-acting muscle relaxant. *Br Med J* 1952; 2:1332–1334.

23. Baird WLM, Reid AM: The neuromuscular blocking properties of a new steroid compound, pancuronium bromide. *Br J Anaesth* 1967; 39:775–789.

24. Basta SJ, Ali HH, Savarese JJ, et al: Clinical pharmacology of atracurium besylate (BW 33A): A new non-depolarizing muscle relaxant. *Anesth Analg* 1982; 61:723–729.

25. Marshall IG, Agoston S, Booij J, et al: Pharmacology of ORG NC45 compared with other nondepolarizing neuromuscular blocking drugs. *Br. J Anaesth* 1980; 52:11S–19S.

2

The Neuromuscular Junction: Structure and Function

Both nerve and muscle tissue contain excitable cells that respond to and transmit electrical stimuli. Such stimuli are carried from one end of the cell to the other by propagation of an electrical signal called the action potential. Thus, information can travel over distances that are, at the cellular level, relatively long. In the transmission of information from nerve to muscle, electrical changes in the nerve allow the release of a chemical mediator, acetylcholine, which in turn triggers the generation of an action potential in the muscle cell. The chemical event involves a much shorter distance than the electrical events but has an important role in the modulation of information. Neuromuscular relaxants and their antagonists have their major effects at this chemical hinge, the neuromuscular junction, between peripheral nerve and skeletal muscle.

Knowledge of the function of the neuromuscular junction has emerged from many avenues. The electrical organ of the eel consists of a large number of excitable cells, stacked in layers on top of each other, that respond to acetylcholine. It is nature's largest factory of acetylcholine and acetylcholine receptor and thus is particularly well suited for chemical studies. Synaptic interactions can be studied relatively easily in the squid given the large size of its axons and nerve terminals. On the other hand, the electrical response of muscle to acetylcholine and its agonists and antagonists has been studied especially in the frog, which has elongated neuromuscular junctions and large muscle cells. These features make the insertion of electrodes relatively

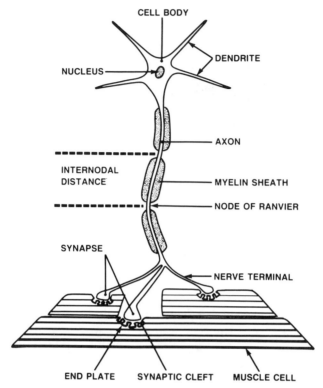

CELL BODY

DENDRITE

NUCLEUS

AXON

INTERNODAL
DISTANCE

MYELIN SHEATH

NODE OF RANVIER

SYNAPSE

NERVE TERMINAL

END PLATE   SYNAPTIC CLEFT   MUSCLE CELL

FIG 2–1.

Functional organization of a motor neuron (not drawn to scale). (From Katz B: *Nerve, Muscle and Synapse.* New York, McGraw-Hill Book Co, 1966, p 4. Used by permission.)

easy. Unfortunately, the information derived from mammalian neuromuscular junctions is more limited. Although the basic mechanisms appear to be similar in all acetylcholine receptors, direct extrapolation of animal data to the human neuromuscular junction should be made with caution.

NERVE AND MUSCLE

Peripheral Nerves

The nerve cells, or neurons, supplying skeletal muscle constitute a one-cell link between the central nervous system and the effector organ. They consist of a cell body with several fine appendages, known as the dendrites, and a long cylindrical extension, called the axon[1, 2] (Fig 2–1). The cell body of motor neurons lies within the spinal cord and contains the nucleus, which holds the genetic information necessary for the manufacture of enzymes and proteins.[2, 3] The cell body is also the site of integration of information coming from the dendrites and the other nerve cells synapsing with the cell body.[1] The information is transmitted down the axon to the periphery over distances of up to 1 m.[1, 2, 4] Conduction velocities of 40 to 70 m/second have been measured in human motor neurons.[5] Such relatively rapid conduction velocities can be achieved because of the large axonal diameter, which can reach 20 μm, and the existence of an electrically insulating myelin sheath, consisting of as many as 100 layers of membrane manufactured by specialized cells called Schwann cells.[6] The myelin sheath is interrupted periodically, leaving the axonal membrane in direct contact with the extracellular environment. These gaps, called nodes of Ranvier, are only 0.5 to 1 μm in length but are necessary for the propagation of the action potential because they are the only excitable portion of the axon.

Each nerve cell supplies many muscle fibers a short distance after branching into small terminals and losing its myelin sheath. The nerve cell and the muscle fibers it innervates is called the "motor unit." Although motor units are restricted to a given geographic area, they overlap to a certain extent.[7] A motor unit is the smallest contractile unit under normal circumstances, and gradation of muscular tension is possible to the extent that the force developed by a single motor unit is small compared with that generated by the whole muscle. It is therefore not surprising that muscles that are designed for fine, delicate movements have smaller units than strong muscles. For example, a mean of 13 and 1,700 muscle fibers per motor unit have been estimated in the human external rectus of the eye and gastrocnemius muscles, respectively.[8]

The axon terminates as a specialized structure designed to transmit information to the muscle (Fig 2–2). In mammals, the synapse has an oval shape. Its size depends on the size of the corresponding muscle fiber[9] and is typically 40 to 60 μm in length and 32 μm in width.[3] It is in close apposition to the muscle fiber, being separated from it by a synaptic cleft of 20 to 50 nm (.02 to .05 μm). It contains the acetylcholine that is released to trigger muscular contraction. However, a Schwann cell sheath invests these structures and is thought to provide structural stability to the neuromuscular junction. Opposite the nerve synapse, the cell membrane of the muscle forms a depression, the synaptic gutter, which matches the shape of the synapse (Fig 2–3).

In most cases, the human skeletal muscle is supplied by only one synapse (en plaque ending), which usually lies in its midportion.[9] How-

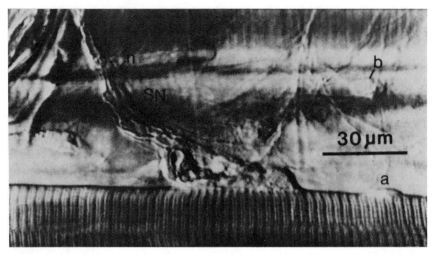

FIG 2–2.
Guinea pig nerve terminal and motor end-plate viewed using the Nomarski-interference microscope. Note the nerve fiber *(n)* expanding into the nerve synapse, Schwann cell nucleus *(SN),* and muscle fiber with cross-striations corresponding to light *(l)* and dark *(A)* bands. (From Dreyer F, Muller KD, Peper K, et al: The M. omohyoideus of the mouse as a convenient mammalian muscle preparation. *Pflugers Arch* 1976; 367:115–122. Used by permission.)

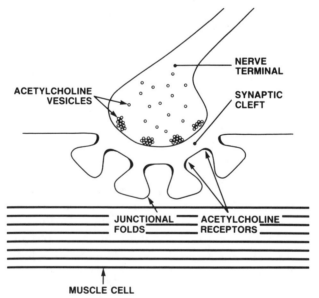

FIG 2–3.
Schematic diagram of the neuromuscular junction.

ever, some muscles contain fibers that are supplied by many nerve terminals (*en grappe* endings). In humans, such exceptions include fibers in the extraocular muscles, intrinsic laryngeal muscles, and facial muscles.[7]

Skeletal Muscle

Skeletal muscle makes up 30% to 40% of total body mass in humans, and most if not all our activities depend on its proper functioning. In particular, such vital functions as respiration and posture are made possible through muscle, which contains cells with contractile properties designed to produce force and movement. These multinucleated, elongated cells, 30 to 150 μm in diameter, contain filaments that slide over each other. These myofilaments appear as alternate dark (A) and light (I) bands under the microscope (see Fig 2–2). The bands correspond to the location of the proteins myosin and actin, respectively.[10, 11] The I band also contains tropomyosin and troponin, which have a regulatory role.[10, 12] Myofilaments are grouped into larger longitudinal structures called myofibrils. The cell membrane, or sarcolemma, has many invaginations called transverse tubules that extend into the core of the muscle cell. There they come into close proximity to the sarcoplasmic reticulum, a membrane-bound structure that acts as a reservoir for calcium. The sarcoplasmic reticulum lies between myofibrils, and comes into close contact with the transverse tubule at the center of the light (I) band. Such a system is designed to propagate the membrane potential changes far into the cell[13] to release calcium from the sarcoplasmic reticulum into the myofibril.[10]

Muscle cells have been classified according to their biochemical, morphological, and functional characteristics. The classification has led to some confusion because of the proliferation of synonyms,[14] the lack of correspondence between anatomical and physiologic characteristics, and finally the existence of intermediate types.[7, 15] Although it is impossible to propose a simple classification that accounts for all muscle descriptions in the literature, it is useful to group muscle types into categories. First, there are tonic, or slow, fibers, which are very common in submammalian vertebrates.[15] They are characterized by the existence of more than one end-plate, the absence of a propagated action potential in response to end-plate depolarization, and the production of a slow, graded, sustained contraction.[14, 15] This type of muscle is rare in humans and is probably restricted to extraocular muscles, intrinsic muscles of the ear, and laryngeal muscles.[7, 14, 15]

Twitch, or fast, fibers are usually innervated by a single nerve terminal, can propagate an action potential, and respond to the action potential in an all-or-none fashion with a rapid contraction. Of this common type of muscle, three subtypes can be identified. Type I (slow-twitch) fibers are rich in myoglobin and mitochondria and have poor glycolytic capacities and low contraction and relaxation speeds. Their high myoglobin content gives them a red appearance. Their resistance to fatigue makes them well suited for long, steady work. Type IIA (intermediate) fibers combine high glycolytic capacity and fast contraction speed with an abundance of mitochondria and resistance to fatigue. Type IIB fibers are usually large, have few mitochondria and little sarcoplasmic reticulum, and rely on glycogen for energy production. They have high contraction speeds but are not suited for sustained work.

It appears that the type of muscle is determined by its nerve supply. Conversion of a muscle fiber from one type to another is possible by cross innervation.[16] It also follows that all muscle fibers belonging to the same unit are of the same type.[7] Differentiation into fast- and slow-twitch muscles occurs late in fetal life or early in postnatal life. For example, fewer type I (slow-twitch) fibers exist in the human diaphragm and intercostal muscles of premature infants than in the same muscles of individuals older than 2 years[17] (Fig 2–4). The proportion of type I

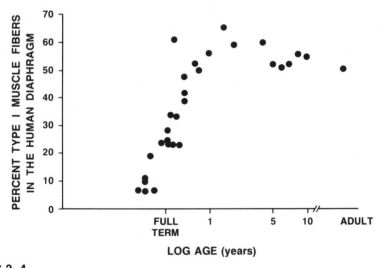

FIG 2–4.
Proportion of type I (slow twitch, high oxidative, fatigue-resistant) fibers in human diaphragm muscle as a function of age. (From Keens TG, Bryan AC, Levison H: Developmental pattern of muscle fiber types in human ventilatory muscles. *J Appl Physiol* 1978; 44:909–913. Used by permission).

fibers varies from muscle to muscle. Adult respiratory muscles contain an approximately equal mixture of type I and type II muscles,[17] whereas the commonly monitored adductor pollicis muscle is predominantly a slow (type I) muscle.[18]

Muscle also contains spindles that consist of specialized cells, the intrafusal fibers, which are not designed to provide force but are part of a delicate control system. These fibers contain sensory endings that respond either to velocity or to velocity and length.[4] These endings are activated as a result of stretching, such as when deep tendon reflexes are tested. An efferent system, which involves the gamma motor fibers, produces contraction in the intrafusal fibers to modulate the input from the sensory endings.

The Neuromuscular Junction

The nerve terminal is the site of high metabolic activity as revealed morphologically by the large number of mitochondria it contains. Microtubules are also conspicuous, suggesting the importance of the transport of enzymes. In addition, numerous acetylcholine-containing vesicles can be observed to congregate on the junctional side (Fig 2–5). In the frog, which has elongated instead of oval-shaped nerve terminals, the vesicles all line up in longitudinal bands called "active zones."[19] In oval-shaped mammalian junctions, such an arrangement is less obvious, but the geometry of the system tends to minimize the distance between the vesicles and the acetylcholine receptor[20] (Fig 2–6).

The nerve synapse lies opposite a specialized area of muscle fiber. The muscle membrane exhibits many folds that were thought to increase the surface area for, and thus the number of, acetylcholine receptors. However, it appears that most of the receptors lie near the crests, so that the function of these folds is unclear.[19]

PHYSIOLOGY OF EXCITABLE CELLS

Ionic Gradients

The properties of electrically excitable tissue in nerve and muscle depend on the distribution of ions across the cell membrane. The extracellular environment is rich in sodium (Na^+) and poor in potassium (K^+). However, the inside of the cell contains more potassium than sodium. Chloride (Cl^-) is the main anion on both sides of the plasma membrane, and it contributes very little to the excitation processes. The cell, or plasma, membrane consists of a double layer of phospholipids

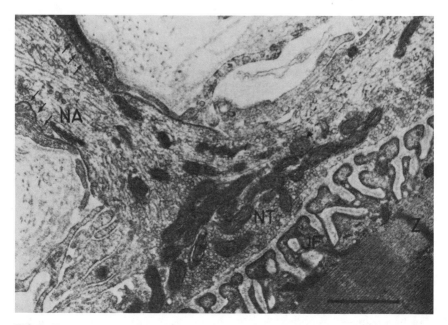

FIG 2–5.
Electron micrograph of the rat neuromuscular junction. *NA* = nerve axon. Note the vesicle-rich nerve terminal *(NT)*, separated by a synaptic cleft from junctional folds *(JF)*. Muscle striations *(Z)* can be seen at right; ×20,000. (From Ellisman MH, Rash JE, Staehelin A, et al: Studies of excitable membranes: II. A comparison of specializations at neuromuscular junctions and nonjunctional sarcolemmas of mammalian fast and slow twitch muscle fibers. *J Cell Biol* 1976; 86:752–774. Used by permission.)

in which are embedded many proteins (Fig 2–7). It is normally more permeable to potassium than to sodium. Therefore, potassium moves down its concentration gradient from the inside to the outside of the cell. This creates a minute excess of positive ions on the outside, which establishes a potential difference across the membrane, the inside of the cell being negative. This electrical potential tends to pull positively charged potassium ions back into the cell. An equilibrium is reached when the potential difference across the membrane is such that the electrostatic force that tends to pull the ions back into the cell counterbalances the tendency of potassium to move down its concentration gradient. This potential, called resting potential, is proportional to the natural logarithm of the ratio of inside to outside potassium concentrations.[1, 14, 21] It is about −90 mV in most cells.

Passive Electrical Properties

A nerve or muscle fiber is an elongated structure that behaves electrically as a conductive core surrounded by an insulating membrane bathing in another conductive medium. It is analogous to a shielded electrical cable, which is ideally suited for the transmission of electrical signals. If the insulating material is perfect and the core an ideal conductor, any electrical signal will be transmitted without attenuation. Biologic cells are not so efficient, and a potential change at one point will decrease exponentially with distance, the length constant being a few millimeters in most cells.[1, 22] If only passive transmission occurred,

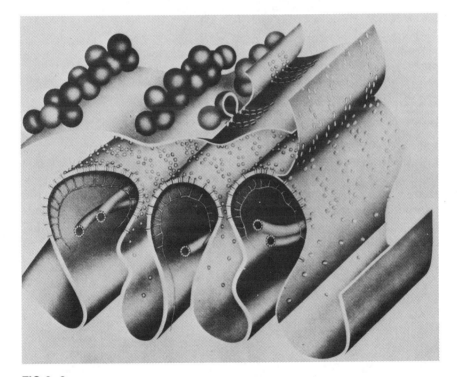

FIG 2–6.
Diagram consistent with the morphological features of the mammalian neuromuscular junction. A double row of vesicles lies near the prejunctional membrane (*top*), opposite the crests of the junctional folds of the postsynaptic membrane, where the vast majority of acetylcholine receptors can be found (small dots). Underneath the folds, filaments and microtubules can be identified. (From Ellisman MH, Rash JE, Staehelin A, et al: Studies of excitable membranes: II. A comparison of specializations at neuromuscular junctions and nonjunctional sarcolemmas of mammalian fast and slow twitch muscle fibers. *J Cell Biol* 1976; 68:752–774. Used by permission.)

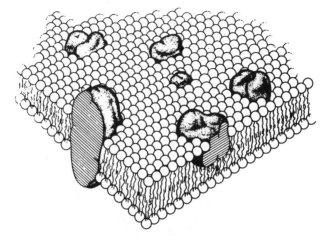

FIG 2–7.
Three-dimensional representation of biological membrane, showing the double phospholipid layer and the proteins. (From Buller AJ: The mechanism of skeletal muscle contraction, in Scurr C, Feldman S (eds): *Scientific Foundations of Anesthesia,* ed 2. Chicago, Year Book Medical Publishers, 1982, p 765. Used by permission.)

action potentials could not be propagated beyond distances greater than a few millimeters. The presence of excitable tissue in nerve and muscle allows the regeneration of electrical impulses. In the nerve, this regeneration takes place at nodes of Ranvier only, which implies that the internodal distance is short enough for passive transmission to occur with little attenuation. Also, the nerve terminal is thought to be invaded passively because of the absence of sodium channels distal to the last node of Ranvier.[6, 23]

Generation of the Action Potential

Excitable membranes allow electrical impulses to be generated and propagated. When the potential inside an excitable cell is made less negative (depolarization), a self-perpetuating chain of events is triggered. The membrane permeability to sodium is increased by activation of a channel that is specific for sodium.[24, 25] Then sodium moves down its chemical and electrical gradients into the cell, making the inside more and more positive. This potential change, called action potential, is rapidly transmitted to a neighboring area of membrane, which causes the sodium channels in that area to be activated, and the sequence is repeated until the end of the cell is reached. The process terminates by inactivation of sodium channels and activation of potassium channels, both of which tend to bring the potential back to resting values.[24, 25]

The nerve action potential lasts less than 1 msec (Fig 2–8). In skeletal muscle, it is slightly longer. In cardiac muscle, the electrical events are qualitatively the same, except that potassium channels are activated very late, making the duration of the action potential much longer—of the order of a few hundred milliseconds.

The conduction velocity of the action potential in an axon depends on many factors, such as its size and the degree of electrical insulation provided by the axonal membrane and surrounding tissue. The presence of a myelin sheath increases the efficiency of nerve axons as impulse-conducting structures.[6] However, this sheath, which consists of many layers of membrane, makes the axon membrane inexcitable. This sheath is interrupted by short gaps of excitable tissue, the nodes of Ranvier, to make possible the regeneration and propagation of the action potential. In large human myelinated fibers, conduction velocity reaches 40 to 70 m/second.[5] In muscle, conduction velocity is only 3 to 5 m/second[26] because of the lack of myelination and the numerous invaginations of the membrane.

The action potential generated at one point along the length of a cell propagates in both directions. This occurs physiologically in muscle after acetylcholine has depolarized the end-plate. In nerve, the site of generation of action potentials is normally at one end of the cell, and this favors propagation in only one direction, called orthodromic.

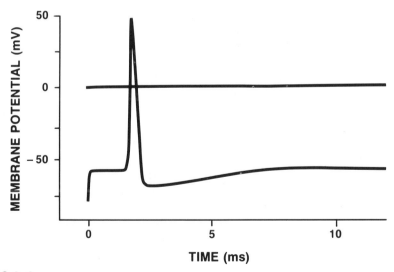

FIG 2–8.
Action potential recorded from the inside of a squid nerve axon.

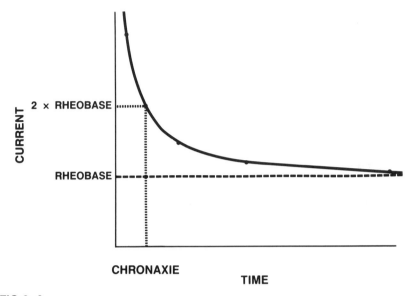

FIG 2–9.
Strength-duration curve, showing rheobase and chronaxie.

However, action potentials may travel in the opposite direction (anti-dromic) under artificial conditions, such as when a nerve stimulator is applied during anesthesia.

When stimulated electrically, excitable membranes require a minimum voltage called rheobase to reach threshold and propagate an action potential. A voltage smaller than the rheobase, even applied for a long time, would not cause the membrane to fire.[4, 22] Chronaxie is the smallest duration of a stimulus with a voltage twice rheobase that can elicit an action potential (Fig 2–9).

After an action potential, the nerve or muscle is refractory to further stimulation for a short period of time. This concept of a refractory period applies to electrical as well as chemical events. For example, the refractory period of human motor nerves stimulated during anesthesia is of the order of 1 msec or less.[27] When stimulated by nerve impulses separated by less than 2 to 3 msec, muscle may not respond to the second impulse.[27, 28] Thus the refractory period of the neuromuscular junction, which involves chemical transmission, is 2 to 3 msec.

Contractile Properties of Muscle

The spread of the action potential throughout the length of the muscle fiber causes an influx of calcium, which is normally sequestered in the sarcoplasmic reticulum. This calcium current is a passive process because the inside of the muscle cell has a much smaller calcium concentration than either the extracellular fluid or the sarcoplasmic reticulum. The presence of intracellular calcium allows actin and myosin to slide over each other, thereby producing a shortening of the muscle fiber.[10, 11] Threshold intracellular calcium concentrations to initiate contraction are of the order of 10^{-7}M and maximum contractile response is obtained at values of approximately 10^{-6}M.[10] Relaxation occurs with reuptake of calcium into the sarcoplasmic reticulum, and this process requires energy.

The contraction produced by a single action potential can be modified by external factors. An isotonic contraction occurs when a constant force, or load, is applied to the contracting muscle. The initial velocity of contraction and the maximum shortening are inversely related to the load applied to the muscle.[11] An isometric contraction takes place when the length of the muscle is held constant, and the force generated depends on the degree of stretch experienced by the muscle. With maximal stretching, there is little overlap between actin and myosin filaments, and the force generated is small. With no stretching, the filaments overlap already, so little force is generated. Between these two extremes, there is an optimal degree of stretching corresponding to a degree of overlap that produces maximal contractile force (Fig 2–10). During neuromuscular monitoring of the force of contraction of the adductor pollicis muscle, isometric work is accomplished by the muscle. A resting tension of 200 to 300 gm has been found to result in larger evoked force of contraction than smaller loads,[29] probably because the optimal length of muscle is not reached until a certain tension is applied.

In muscle, electrical and mechanical events are not simultaneous. The duration of the action potential is only a few milliseconds, after which there is a delay before the contraction starts (Fig 2–11). The twitch tension, when plotted against time, has a rapid upstroke, followed by a slower relaxation phase. The whole event lasts about 100 msec. If a second action potential is generated within 100 msec of the first one, the second twitch will be superimposed on the first one. If the rate of stimulation is sufficiently rapid, the successive twitches will add to the upstroke of the preceding one, leading to a smooth, strong contraction (Fig 2–12).

ACETYLCHOLINE PRODUCTION AND RELEASE

Electrical impulses are well suited for the transmission of information within cells because the cell interior is a good electrical conductor. However, they are not well suited for transmission from one cell to another because the impulse attenuates considerably when cross-

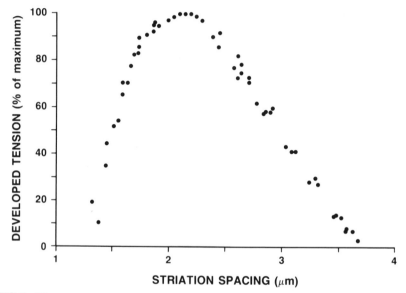

FIG 2–10.
Relationship between maximum contractile force developed by frog muscle and sarcomere length, or distance between two adjacent *Z* lines. (From Floyd K: The physiology of striated muscle. *Br J Anaesth* 1980; 52:111–121. Used by permission.)

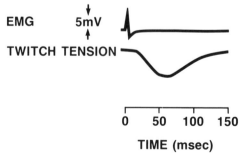

FIG 2–11.
Electromyographic and twitch measurements recorded from the human adductor pollicis.

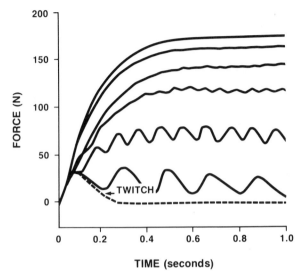

FIG 2–12.
Effect of stimulus frequency on the tension developed by the quadriceps in humans. (From Edwards RHT, Young A, Hosking GP, et al: Human skeletal muscle function: Description of tests and normal valves. *Clin Sci* 1977; 52:283–290. Used by permission.)

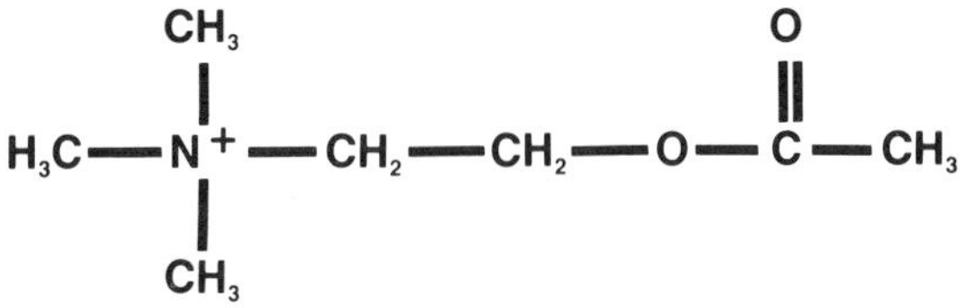

FIG 2–13.
Chemical structure of the acetylcholine molecule.

ing electrically insulating biologic membranes.[1] Thus, chemical mediators have evolved in response to the need to carry messages from one cell to the other.[1]

Chemical Transmission

Acetylcholine is the neurotransmitter present at the neuromuscular junction. It is also found in certain synapses of the central nervous system, the autonomic ganglia, and the postganglionic parasympathetic nerve endings.[30] This simple molecule (Fig 2–13) is synthesized from choline and acetate and stored in the nerve terminal. Acetylcholine release is triggered by depolarization of the nerve terminal, and very small quantities of the neurotransmitter, of the order of 10^{-17} moles,[31] are required to depolarize the adjacent muscle cell.

Production of Acetylcholine

The uptake of choline from the extracellular fluid into the nerve terminal seems to be carrier-mediated[32] and linked with the simultaneous entry of sodium.[33, 34] The acetate part of the acetylcholine molecule comes from acetylcoenzyme A, which is provided by the mitochondria within the nerve terminal.[23, 34] The enzyme choline acetyltransferase, manufactured in the cell body of the nerve and transported intracellularly to the nerve terminal, catalyzes the synthesis of acetylcholine.

Quantal Release

The postsynaptic membrane is very sensitive to acetylcholine, and it is not surprising that its electrophysiologic behavior was the first clue to the nature of acetylcholine release. When intracellular recordings are made at the end-plate of a muscle whose nerve is unstimulated, small changes in resting potential are observed.[35] These changes are uniform in size (about 0.5 mV) and duration (a few msec) and occur randomly at a frequency of about 1/second. It has been suggested that such miniature end-plate potentials (MEPPs) were produced by the random release of a quantum or packet of acetylcholine.[35, 37] The MEPP is too small to produce a contraction because it does not bring the end-plate potential to the threshold required to generate an action potential. Clearly, a concerted release of many quanta of acetylcholine is therefore needed to bring the end-plate potential (EPP) above threshold.[46] This occurs when a nerve action potential produces depolarization of the synaptic area.[36, 37] The number of quanta normally released by a nerve action potential has been estimated at 200 to 400.[38-40] Acetylcholine is the chemical mediator producing these changes because the direct application of acetylcholine by means of a microelectrode (iontophoretic application) produces similar changes on the end-plate (Fig 2–14). The number of acetylcholine molecules per quantum has been calculated to be as little as 1,000 and as high as 60,000 with most estimates in the 5,000 to 10,000 range.[19, 38, 47, 55, 56] Thus, nerve stimulation causes the release of 1 to 4 million acetylcholine molecules.

Calcium is essential in the release process, and the number of released quanta is markedly reduced in a calcium-poor environment.[36, 37] Magnesium opposes the effect of calcium as a high extracellular magnesium concentration also reduces the number of released quanta.[36, 37, 43] The inward calcium current associated with the invasion of the nerve terminal by the action potential has a vital role in the synchronized release.[45]

Electron microscopy has revealed that the nerve terminal contains a large number of vesicles with an external diameter of about 45 nm and bound by a bilayer lipid membrane.[9, 47] These vesicles tend to congregate close to the membrane opposite the muscle end-plate and appear to form bands oriented parallel to the crests of the folds of the end-plate where the acetylcholine receptor lies.[34, 48, 49] Although they do not contain all the acetylcholine detected in or near the nerve terminal, the vesicles definitely contain a large portion of it.[50–52] Moreover, the vesicles have been found to fuse with the cell membrane when the nerve is stimulated.[49] All these findings are evidence to support the vesicular hypothesis, according to which depolarization of the nerve terminal causes the simultaneous opening of a large number of acetylcholine-containing vesicles.

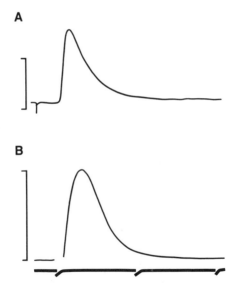

FIG 2–14.
Intracellular recordings of end-plate with nerve stimulation, **A**, and iontophoretic application of acetylcholine, **B**. The similarity of response suggests that acetylcholine is the natural transmitter. (From Krnjevic K, Miledi R: Acetylcholine in mammalian neuromuscular transmission. *Nature* 1958; 182:805–806. Used by permission.)

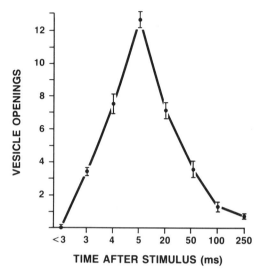

FIG 2–15.

Number of vesicle openings observed at a portion of terminal nerve membrane, as a function of time after stimulation. This number peaks much after stimulation. (From Heuse JE, Reese TS: Structural changes after transmitter release at the frog neuromuscular junction. *J Cell Biol* 1981; 88:564–580. Used by permission.)

Nonquantal Release

Chemical analysis of the released material at the neuromuscular junction suggests that no more than 2% of the acetylcholine comes from quantal release in unstimulated preparations.[19, 52] The rest probably comes from some kind of leakage from the nerve terminal and also from Schwann cells, muscles, and nonsynaptic parts of the axon, all of which contain acetylcholine.[53, 54] The role of this nonquantal release is unclear.

Vesicular Hypothesis

Evidence supports the hypothesis that an action potential invading the nerve terminal causes a calcium-mediated exocytosis of a large number of acetylcholine-containing vesicles. However, some observations are difficult to reconcile with this hypothesis. Vesicles are observed to form pits in the synaptic membrane after nerve stimulation, as would be expected if they discharged their contents into the synaptic cleft, but this process is observed a few milliseconds after stimulation (Fig 2–15).[57] This time course seems incompatible with the short duration of the synaptic delay, which is only a fraction of a millisecond. Furthermore, the incorporation of labeled acetylcholine into the nerve terminal suggests that the most recently synthesized acetylcholine is released preferentially.[58] This would be consistent with the vesicular hypothesis only if newly formed vesicles incorporated newly synthesized acetylcholine almost exclusively and displaced older vesicles as the most likely to release acetylcholine. It seems, however, that vesicles are all capable of incorporating new acetylcholine, because false transmitters, when introduced into the preparation, mix evenly with old material.[59] In addition, repetitive stimulation causes a decrease in extravesicular acetylcholine, leaving intravesicular acetylcholine contents unchanged.[60, 61]

Alternative to the Vesicular Hypothesis

The above evidence appears inconsistent with the vesicular hypothesis and has led some workers to offer alternative theories. It has been proposed[60, 61] that acetylcholine leaves the nerve terminal through channels in the membrane that open either randomly to produce MEPPs or in a concerted fashion in response to an action potential. If the extravesicular acetylcholine concentration were much greater than in the synaptic cleft, release would occur because of the concentration gradient. Vesicles could be storage sites and could be involved with calcium regulation, but the theory does not explain why they lie so close to the cell membrane and what the role of vesicle exocytosis might be. However, this nonvesicular hypothesis is also compatible with the quantal nature of acetylcholine release.

Storage and Control

There is a progressive decrease in end-plate currents with repetitive stimulation, especially in the presence of neuromuscular blocking drugs[14, 62–67] (Fig 2–16). This has given rise to the hypothesis that the pool of acetylcholine available for immediate release was in short supply.[68] However, it has been suggested that with each impulse, only 0.14% of the total acetylcholine contained in the nerve ending is released.[69] This degree of depletion is insufficient to account for the marked fade observed with d-tubocurarine.[66, 67] Thus, it has been suggested that the amount of immediately "releasable" acetylcholine is small compared with "stored" acetylcholine. High frequency stimulation would exhaust the releasable pool faster than it can be regenerated.[68] If this were true, transmitter output decrease due to high-frequency stimulation would not be affected by the presence of relaxants, and equipotent doses of different relaxants would be predicted to exhibit the same degree of fade. None of these was found to be true.[66, 67, 70]

To explain these data, the presence of a feedback loop involving acetylcholine receptors in the nerve terminal or the first node of Ranvier has been proposed. The putative role of these presynaptic receptors would be to maintain transmitter release during high-frequency stimulation. These receptors would normally be activated by acetylcholine and blocked by antagonists such as d-tubocurarine, thus causing the characteristic fade observed with nondepolarizing blockade.[64] Unfortunately, the mechanism by which these receptors exert their action is not known, and at present, their role in neuromuscular transmission should be considered a hypothesis.

ACETYLCHOLINE RECEPTOR

Recent advances in electron microscopy and histochemistry have allowed the scientific community to see what was, until only a few years ago, only a creation of the mind. Receptors are no longer fuzzy and elusive entities: they have been identified as a protein complex "sitting" across the whole thickness of the postsynaptic membrane.

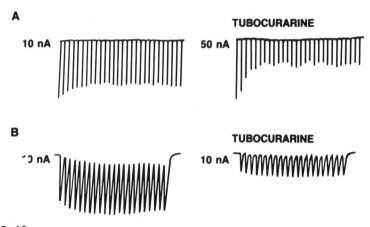

FIG 2–16.
Trains of end-plate currents produced by nerve stimulation (**A**) and with iontophoretic application (with a microelectrode) of acetylcholine (**B**) in the absence (**left**) and the presence (**right**) of d-tubocurarine. Fade of response is observed only with nerve stimulation, suggesting a presynaptic mechanism. (From Bowman WC, Marshall IG, Gibb AJ: Is there feedback control of transmitter release at the neuromuscular junction? *Semin Anesth* 1984; 3:275–283. Used by permission.)

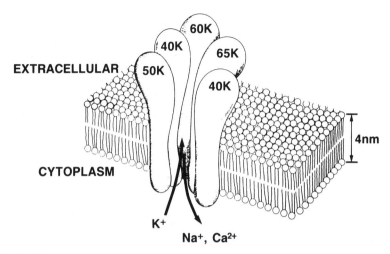

FIG 2–17.
Diagrammatic representation of the acetylcholine receptor. (From Goudsouzian NG, Standaert FG: The infant and the myoneural junction. *Anesth Analg* 1986; 65:1208–1217. Used by permission.)

Receptor Theory

The role of receptors is to act as mediators between the environment and the cell by being specific to certain agents. In the case of the nerve-muscle unit, the acetylcholine receptor is the link between a messenger (usually acetylcholine) and the effector cell (muscle). A receptor has been likened to a lock. A specific key (an agonist molecule) will fit into it and will open it (produce a response). If a slightly different key is tried, it may fit into the lock without opening it: this is analogous to antagonist molecules, which bind to the receptor without producing a response. Most biologic receptors, such as the acetylcholine receptors, consist of proteins that undergo conformational changes when bound to agonists.

Anatomy of the Acetylcholine Receptor

The acetylcholine receptor has been identified as a structure consisting of five glycoprotein subunits arranged in the form of a rosette[23, 71–73] (Fig 2–17). Two noncontiguous subunits are identical and called α. They have a molecular weight of 40,000 daltons. The other subunits (β,γ,δ) have molecular weights of 50,000, 60,000 and 65,000, respectively. Agonist binding most probably produces conformational changes such that a hole is created at the center of the rosette, allowing the passage of ions. From the size of the largest molecules that have been demonstrated to pass through, the size of the open channel is estimated to be approximately 0.65 nm in diameter.[74] The receptor itself is approximately 8.5 nm in diameter.[75] It protudes on both sides of the membrane, but more on the synaptic side.[76]

The receptors are clustered on the crests of the junctional folds, opposite the active zones of the synaptic membrane, which contain a large number of acetylcholine vesicles.[19] The receptor density in the crest area has been reported to be 5,000 to 30,000/sq μm.[56, 72, 75, 77] Each end-plate has 10^6 to 10^7 receptors.[78] This number is reduced considerably in myasthenia gravis.[87]

Effect of Agonists

The relationship between acetylcholine concentration and end-plate current is difficult to measure because of the presence of acetylcholinesterase. In addition, the presence of acetylcholine, if prolonged, causes a decreased responsiveness of the end-plate called desensitization.[78, 79, 81] Thus, dose-response curves have been established by iontophoretic application of acetylcholine, the application of a known current to a pipette with a tip in close proximity to the end-plate. Although this does not provide a very accurate estimate of the concentration at the active sites, the effect of an increase in acetylcholine can be measured[77, 78, 80] (Fig 2–18). The slope of the relationship between applied microelectrode current and end-plate current is usually between 2 and 3, indicating that more than one acetylcholine molecule is required to activate the receptor. Another possibility is that some cooperativity exists, i.e., that the binding to one molecule of acetylcholine enhances the ability of the receptor to bind to more acetylcholine molecules.[78] Recent evidence suggests that acetylcholine molecules bind to α subunits and that two α subunits must be bound to acetylcholine simultaneously for the channel to open.[72, 81, 82] This, however, does not exclude the possibility of cooperativity.

With refined electrophysiologic techniques such as noise analysis, which looks at the current fluctuations caused by the random opening and closing of channels, and the patch clamp technique, which isolates single receptors, estimates of the mean open time of channels and current passing through them could be made. In mammalian preparations at body temperature, single channel conductance is about 45 psec $(45 \times 10^{-12} \text{ ohm}^{-1})$, and is about the same for acetylcholine as for the other agonists.[72, 78] Under the same conditions, mean channel open time is about 0.3 msec for acetylcholine as an agonist, during which time some 10,000 ions are allowed to pass.[72] Conductances and open times depend on muscle type.[84] Mean open time depends on temperature and on which agonist is used. For example, the channel will stay open only a fourth as long if succinylcholine is the agonist.[72]

End-Plate Potentials

The opening of a channel allows all ions small enough to go through to move down their concentration gradient. The movement of potassium and sodium is quantitatively most important because they constitute the majority of cations intracellularly and extracellularly, respectively. At resting potential, the inward movement of sodium will be favored because sodium will also move along its electrical gradient, being attracted by the negative intracellular potential. Accumulation of intracellular sodium makes the inside of the cell less negative. If a large number of receptors opens simultaneously, the inside of the cell is depolarized sufficiently to trigger the generation of an action potential.[36] The propagation of the action potential is then quite independent of acetylcholine receptors, relying on the activation of sodium channels.

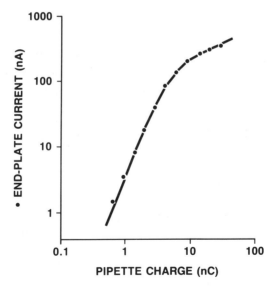

FIG 2–18.
End plate current as a function of quantity of acetylcholine (expressed as pipette charge) provided by a microelectrode near frog end-plate. (From Dreyer F, Peper K, Strez R: Determination of dose-response curves by quantitative iontophoresis at the frog neuromuscular junction. *J Physiol* 1978; 281:395–419. Used by permission.)

Termination of Effect

The acetylcholine concentration in the synaptic cleft decreases within microseconds because of diffusion of the molecule and breakdown by acetylcholinesterase.[78, 84] The decay time of an end-plate potential is much longer (0.3 msec). Thus, the duration of the effect of acetylcholine on the receptor does not depend on the decrease of agonist concentrations in the synaptic cleft but on the rate of unbinding from the receptor. Thus, rebinding is very unlikely, and channel open time is determined by the agonist used.[78]

Acetylcholinesterase is an enzyme consisting of two active binding sites. The anionic site binds to the quaternary ammonium end of the acetylcholine molecule, whereas the esteratic site has affinity for the acidic end of the molecule.[85] A cleavage of acetylcholine then occurs at the ester linkage, breaking it into its constituents, choline and acetate. The enzyme has not been localized with as much accuracy as the receptor, but it appears to be present further away from the nerve terminal than the receptor itself, such as in the junctional folds.[79, 86]

Desensitization

When the acetylcholine concentration in the synaptic cleft is not allowed to decline, the receptor becomes less responsive and is said to be "desensitized."[81, 83] The exact molecular mechanism for this phenomenon is unknown, but whatever the mechanism, it could be the basis for the blocking action of other agonists, such as succinylcholine and decamethonium. Exposure to agonists also produces depolarization, and this could also contribute to the blocking effect of these drugs.[88]

Extrajunctional Receptors

Acetylcholine receptors are not confined to the end-plate and can be found in much lower densities throughout the muscle membrane. It appears that innervation increases the stability of junctional receptors and inhibits the formation of extrajunctional receptors. The latter are destroyed after a lifetime of approximately 20 hours. They are slightly different from junctional receptors: in addition to a shorter half-life, their open time is longer. Denervation removes the essential factor in the inhibition of their synthesis, and extrajunctional receptors are found to proliferate.[100]

ANTAGONIST ACTION

Neuromuscular blocking drugs are known to compete with acetylcholine for the receptor, but they are by no means the only drugs capable of interfering with neuromuscular transmission, nor is competitive block the only mode of action of neuromuscular blockers. Some antibiotics, local anesthetics, magnesium, and inhalational agents are but a few of the agents that may produce neuromuscular block. Neuromuscular blocking drugs are also capable of producing noncompetitive block as well as decreasing transmitter output.

Receptor Blockade

Neuromuscular blocking drugs can compete with acetylcholine for the postjunctional receptors. Competitive block implies a dynamic equilibrium between agonist, antagonist, and receptor, that is, a constant movement to and from the same binding site. In a given situation, the proportion of receptors bound to the agonist depends on the affinity of the binding site for the agonist, on its affinity for the antagonist, and the concentration of agonist and antagonist. It is thought that binding of one antagonist molecule to one of the two α subunits of the receptor prevents opening of the channel because both α subunits need to be bound by acetylcholine for activation of the channel.[82]

Other Types of Receptor Interactions

Neuromuscular blocking drugs can also block the open receptor.[72, 90, 91] All nondepolarizing blockers are large molecules that can have access to the mouth of the open channel but cannot pass through, thus preventing further ionic movement. An excess of acetylcholine in the synaptic cleft would be expected to increase rather than decrease the degree of neuromuscular blockade because it increases the number of open channels. Therefore, open channel blockade is not competitive. Although some workers assign an important role to this mode of interaction between receptor and relaxant molecule, it is probably marginal as a mechanism of action of neuromuscular blocking drugs. Calculations based on the affinity of the antagonist for the receptor suggest that even after a tetanic stimulation, a very small fraction—of the order of 1%—of receptors are blocked in the open position.[65]

The receptors lie in a lipid environment, and it is reasonable to assume that any alteration in the lipid phase of the membrane might affect the performance of receptors. Lipid-soluble drugs, such as inhalational agents, might exert their effect through this mechanism. Thus, there are multiple sites, both presynaptic and postsynaptic, where these agents may cause some interference with neuromuscular transmission.[92] At the end-plate, depolarization is reduced by inhalational agents,[92-94] and the extent of this reduction correlates well with the degree of potentiation with d-tubocurarine.[95]

Desensitization (see above), that is, the decreased responsiveness of the receptor to the prolonged presence of the agonist, can be regarded as a possible mechanism for neuromuscular blockade.

Finally, drugs that reduce the acetylcholine output by the nerve terminal may produce neuromuscular blockade or potentiate it. Magnesium does this by antagonizing the essential action of calcium on the release process.[36, 37, 43] Certain antibiotics and calcium blockers may also do this.[96] At low-stimulation frequencies, it appears that neuromuscular relaxants do not affect acetylcholine output. However, there is evidence that they may do so at high frequencies.[62-67]

Margin of Safety

Only a small number of end-plate receptors needs to be activated by acetylcholine for transmission to take place, and this has been referred to as the "margin of safety" of the neuromuscular junction. An elegant demonstration of this concept has been provided by Paton and Waud[97] who estimated the proportion of receptors blocked by measuring the depolarizing effect of succinylcholine following administration of progressively greater concentrations of d-tubocurarine and measured twitch tension. In the rat diaphragm muscle, single muscle fibers were blocked when 75% to 92% of the receptors were occupied[97] (Fig 2–19). Peripheral muscles have been found to have a smaller margin of safety than the diaphragm,[98] which might be a factor in the relative resistance of the latter to muscle relaxants.

Interpretation of Fade

The progressive decrease in muscle response following high-frequency nerve stimulation is a fundamental characteristic of nondepolarizing drugs used in clinical anesthesia and is the basis of train-of-four and tetanic monitoring. The mechanism for this, however, is uncertain. It has been suggested that the releasable pool of acetylcholine is rather small and that a substantial proportion of it is released after each nerve impulse. Replenishment of the pool occurs at a rather slow rate so that acetylcholine output, although constant with low frequen-

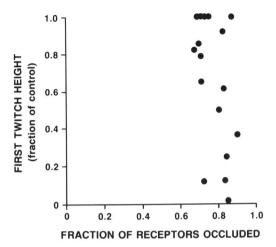

FIG 2–19.
Twitch height as a function of receptor occupancy in the rabbit tibialis anterior. (From Waud BE, Waud DR: The relation between tetanic fade and receptor occlusion in the presence of competitive neuromuscular block. *Anesthesiology* 1971; 35:456–464. Used by permission.)

cies of stimulation, cannot be maintained at higher frequencies. According to this hypothesis, muscle contraction can be sustained in the absence of neuromuscular blockers because acetylcholine output during high-frequency stimulation is still in excess of the amount needed to produce a full response. The presence of neuromuscular blocking drugs diminishes the number of postsynaptic receptors available for acetylcholine and fade becomes apparent.[68]

Experimental evidence makes this hypothesis untenable. The snake poison α-bungarotoxin, which has been shown to bind selectively and irreversibly to the postsynaptic acetylcholine receptor, does not produce train-of-four fade.[101] Moreover, the degree of fade varies markedly depending on the neuromuscular blocker used.[70] Open channel blockade has been proposed as an alternative explanation.[72] A nerve impulse would release acetylcholine and open postsynaptic channels, which would then be blocked open by the antagonist. These channels would not be available for further activation by acetylcholine until the antagonist comes out. This hypothesis explains why different drugs are different in this regard because the degree of fade depends on the drug concentration. However, it does not explain the competitive effect produced by the increase in acetylcholine concentration that is associated with the administration of anticholinesterase drugs.

Presynaptic Receptors

Fade could also be explained if one postulates the presence of a feedback loop on the nerve terminal whereby the release of acetylcholine would promote the availability of more releasable acetylcholine ready to be discharged with the next nerve impulse.[64] Agonist drugs, such as acetylcholine and succinylcholine, can produce presynaptic activity,[102–104] and this activity can be suppressed by d-tubocurarine.[103] This suppression could be accomplished through acetylcholine receptors situated at the nerve terminal membrane or further up the axon at the first node of Ranvier.[64] The mechanism of action of the suppression by these receptors is unclear.

Potentiation

Certain combinations of neuromuscular blocking drugs are synergistic, that is, the effect of a mixture of two drugs may be greater than either drug alone. For example, combinations of either pancuronium and metocurine or pancuronium and d-tubocurarine are synergistic in humans.[105] It has been suggested that such a phenomenon occurs because neuromuscular blocking drugs have different actions at various sites, presynaptic and postsynaptic, and that the mixture of two drugs with different properties at different sites might produce synergism.[105] Recently, another explanation involving only postsynaptic receptors has been proposed.[106, 107] Since neuromuscular blocking drugs can block the receptor by binding to any of the two α subunits, it is possible that they have different affinities for each subunit because each one lies in a different ionic and chemical environment. For example, pancuronium may be as much as 80 times more likely to bind to one unit rather than the other.[108] Binding of one subunit may also change the affinity of the other. In any case, the mechanism for mutual potentiation of neuromuscular drugs is not clear.

RELAXANT ANTAGONISM

In contrast to neuromuscular blocking drugs, the antagonists of neuromuscular blockade have received much less attention. The study of their effects is made even more complicated because they may have more than one site of action and the main mechanism of action might be different depending on whether or not relaxants are used concurrently.

Acetylcholinesterase Inhibition

Neuromuscular blockade antagonism is commonly accomplished with anticholinesterases. The drugs used for this purpose in clinical practice, neostigmine, edrophonium, and pyridostigmine, all bind to acetylcholinesterase and inactivate it in a reversible fashion.[85, 109] The final result is the inhibition of the enzyme, which is no longer available to break down acetylcholine. Edrophonium forms an electrostatic bond with the enzyme at the active sites, and this bond is rapidly reversible. On the other hand, both neostigmine and pyridostigmine, when attached to the enzyme, undergo hydrolysis of their ester group. An inactive, carbamylated enzyme is formed until the carbamyl group detaches. This spontaneous reaction takes place at a half-life of approximately 30 minutes.

As expected, anticholinesterases increase the decay half-time of MEPPs and EPPs.[36, 87] During stimulated release of acetylcholine, the transmitter is allowed a prolonged stay in the synaptic cleft and presumably can bind repeatedly to many receptors. This would increase the duration of the end-plate potential. In addition, since a large proportion of the acetylcholine released by the nerve is not released through stimulation, the increased concentration of acetylcholine near the receptors favors displacement of the relaxant away from them.

Other Effects

A large body of evidence has accumulated that suggests that acetylcholinesterase inhibition at the end-plate is not the sole effect of the anticholinesterase drugs. Neostigmine, pyridostigmine, and edrophonium can generate antidromic action potentials in the nerve terminal.[104, 110] These spread backward to the spinal cord and invade the other terminal branches of the same axon, producing repetitive firing. The final result is twitch potentiation, which arises because of repeated nerve terminal depolarizations.[111] Repetitive firing probably occurs because of depolarization of the nerve terminal, which is in turn caused either by a direct action of the drugs or through activation of presynaptic acetylcholine receptors. If some terminals are depolarized sufficiently to propagate an action potential, it is reasonable to assume that most, if not all, are depolarized enough to increase acetylcholine release. This might account for the increased amplitude of the end-plate potential observed in the presence of anticholinesterase drugs.[36, 87] The relative contribution of presynaptic and postsynaptic mechanisms in the reversal of nondepolarizing blockade is unknown.

Other Muscle Relaxant Antagonists

Calcium is necessary in the release process, and the addition of calcium would be expected to antagonize neuromuscular blockade. This is effective in reversing the block produced by certain antibiotics[112] (see also Chapter 11). In the presence of high calcium concentrations, the potency of d-tubocurarine and pancuronium is decreased.[113]

Drugs such as 4-aminopyridine and tetraethylammonium block potassium channels in the nerve terminal. As a result, the action potential is more prolonged, the inward calcium current is greater and more prolonged, and more acetylcholine is released.[38, 56]

CONCLUSION

In spite of important developments in electrophysiology, electron microscopy, and histochemistry, the best known receptor still appears as a source of more questions than answers. As knowledge expands, some thoughts and assumptions are being reevaluated, such as the vesicular theory, the postsynaptic site of action of relaxants, and the anticholinesterase action of reversal agents. Although all these theories may be true to a certain extent, the neuromuscular junction is probably a more complicated and sophisticated example of chemical engineering than previously assumed.

REFERENCES

1. Katz B: Nerve, Muscle and Synapse. New York, McGraw-Hill Book Co, 1966.
2. Palay SL, Chan-Palay V: General morphology of neurons and neuroglia, in Handbook of Physiology: Cellular Biology of Neurons, section 1: The Nervous System, volume 1, Part 1; ER Randel (vol ed). Bethesda, Md, American Physiological Society, 1977, pp 5–37.
3. Truex RC, Carpenter MB: Human Neuroanatomy. Baltimore, Williams & Wilkins Co, 1969.
4. Kimura J: Electrodiagnosis in Diseases of Nerve and Muscle: Principles and Practice. Philadelphia, FA Davis Co, 1983.
5. Mayer RF: Nerve conduction studies in man. Neurology 1963; 13:1021–1030.
6. Hille B: Ionic basis of resting and action potentials, in Handbook of Physiology: Cellular Biology of Neurons, section 1: The Nervous System, vol 1, pt 1; ER Randel (vol ed). Bethesda, Md, American Physiological Society, 1977, pp 99–136.

7. Buchthal F, Schmalbruch H: Motor unit of mammalian muscle. *Physiol Rev* 1980; 60:90–142.
8. Buchthal F: The general concept of the motor unit: Neuromuscular disorders. *Res Publ Assoc Res Nerv Ment Dis* 1960; 38:3–30.
9. Bowden REM, Duchen LW: The anatomy and pathology of the neuromuscular junction, in Zaimis E (ed): *Neuromuscular Junction: Handbook of Experimental Pharmacology*. Berlin, Springer-Verlag, 1976, vol 42, pp 23–97.
10. Floyd K: The physiology of striated muscle. *Br J Anaesth* 1980; 52:111–121.
11. Buller AJ: The mechanism of skeletal muscle contraction, in Scurr C, Feldman S (eds): *Scientific Foundations of Anesthesia*, ed 2. Chicago, Year Book Medical Publishers, 1982, pp 277–283.
12. Illingworth JA: Muscle biochemistry. *Br J Anaesth* 1980; 52:123–138.
13. Huxley AF: The activation of skeletal muscle and its mechanical response. *Proc R Soc Lond* 1971; 178:1–27.
14. Bowman WC: *Pharmacology of Neuromuscular Function*. Baltimore, University Park Press, 1980.
15. Morgan DL, Proske U: Vertebrate slow muscle: Its structure, pattern of innervation, and mechanical properties. *Physiol Rev* 1984; 64:103–169.
16. Buller AJ, Eccles JC, Eccles RM: Interactions between motor neurons and muscles in respect of the characteristic speeds of their responses. *J Physiol Lond* 1960; 150:417–439.
17. Keens TG, Bryan AC, Levison H, et al: Development pattern of muscle fiber types in human ventilatory muscles. *J Appl Physiol* 1978; 44:909–913.
18. Johnson MA, Polgar J, Weightman D, et al: Data on the distribution of fibre types in thirty-six human muscles: An autopsy study. *J Neurol Sci* 1973; 18:111–129.
19. Standaert FG: Release of transmitter at the neuromuscular junction. *Br J Anaesth* 1982; 54:131–145.
20. Ellisman MH, Rash JE, Staehelin A, et al: Studies of excitable membranes: II. A comparison of specializations at neuromuscular junctions and nonjunctional sarcolemmas of mammalian fast and slow twitch muscle fibers. *J Cell Biol* 1976; 68:752–774.
21. Woodbury JW: The cell membrane: Ionic and potential gradients and active transport, in Ruch TC, Patton HD, Woodbury JW, et al (eds): *Neurophysiology*, ed 2. Philadelphia, WB Saunders Co, 1965, pp 1–25.
22. Woodbury JW: Action potential: Properties of excitable membranes, in Ruch TC, Patton HD, Woodbury JW, et al (eds): *Neurophysiology*, ed 2. Philadelphia, WB Saunders Co, 1965, pp 26–72.
23. Bowman WC: The neuromuscular junction: Recent developments. *Eur J Anaesthesiol* 1985; 2:59–93.
24. Hodgkin AL, Huxley AF: A quantitative description of membrane current and its application to conduction and excitation in nerve. *J Physiol Lond* 1952; 117:500–544.

25. Kendig JJ, Trudell JR: Membrane physiology, in Scurr C, Feldman S (eds): *Scientific Foundations of Anaesthesia,* ed 3. Chicago, Year Book Medical Publishers, 1982, pp 251–259.
26. Nishizono H, Saito Y, Miyashita M: The estimation of conduction velocity in human skeletal muscle in situ with surface electrodes. *Electroencephalogr Clin Neurophysiol* 1979; 46:659–663.
27. Epstein RA, Jackson SH: Repetitive muscle depolarization from single indirect stimulation in anesthetized man. *J Appl Physiol* 1970; 28:407–410.
28. Epstein RA, Jackson SH, Wyte SR: The effects of nondepolarizing relaxants and anticholinesterases on the neuromuscular refractory period of anesthetized man. *Anesthesiology* 1969; 31:69–77.
29. Donlon JV, Savarese JJ, Ali HH: Cumulative dose-response curves for gallamine: Effect of altered resting thumb tension and mode of stimulation. *Anesth Analg* 1979; 58:377–381.
30. Mayer SE: Neurohumoral transmission and the autonomic nervous system, in Gilman AG, Goodman LS, Rall TW (eds): *The Pharmacological Basis of Therapeutics,* ed 7. New York, MacMillan Publishing Co, 1985, pp 66–99.
31. Krnjevic K, Mitchell JF: The release of acetylcholine in the isolated rat diaphragm. *J Physiol Lond* 1961; 155:246–262.
32. Vaca K, Pilar G: Mechanism controlling choline transport and acetylcholine synthesis in motor nerve terminals during electrical stimulation. *J Gen Physiol* 1979; 73:605.
33. Beach RL, Vaca K, Pilar G: Ionic and metabolic requirements for high affinity choline uptake and acetylcholine synthesis in nerve terminals at a neuromuscular junction. *J Neurochem* 1980; 34:1387–1398.
34. Standaert FG: Release of neurotransmitter at the neuromuscular junction. *Br J Anaesth* 1982; 54:131–145.
35. Fatt P, Katz B: Spontaneous subthreshold activity at motor nerve-endings. *J Physiol* 1952; 117:109–128.
36. Fatt P, Katz B: An analysis of the end-plate potential recorded with an intracellular electrode. *J Physiol* 1951; 115:320–370.
37. Del Castillo J, Katz B: Quantal components of the end-plate potential. *J Physiol* 1954; 124:560–573.
38. Katz B, Miledi R: Estimates of quantal content during 'chemical potentiation' of transmitter release. *Proc R Soc Lond* 1979; 205:369–378.
39. Hubbard JI, Wilson DF: Neuromuscular transmission in a mammalian preparation in the absence of blocking drugs and the effect of d-tubocurarine. *J Physiol* 1973; 228:307–325.
40. Ginsborg BL, Jenkinson DH: Transmission of impulses from nerve to muscle, in Zaimis E (ed): *Neuromuscular Junction: Handbook of Experimental Pharmacology.* Berlin, Springer-Verlag, 1976, pp 229–364.
41. Donati F, Beven JC, Bevan DR: Neuromuscular blocking drugs in anaesthesia. *Can Anaesth Soc J* 1984; 31:324–335.

42. Edwards RHT, Young A, Hosking GP, et al: Human skeletal muscle function: Description of tests and normal values. *Clin Sci* 1977; 52:283–290.
43. Del Castillo J, Katz B: The effect of magnesium on the activity of nerve endings. *J Physiol Lond* 1954; 124:553–559.
44. Krnjevic K, Miledi R: Acetylcholine in mammalian neuromuscular transmission. *Nature* 1958; 182:805–806.
45. Llinas RR: Calcium in synaptic transmission. *Sci Am* 1982; 247(4):56–65.
46. Martin AR: Quantal nature of synaptic transmission. *Physiol Rev* 1966; 46:51–66.
47. Hubbard JI: Microphysiology of vertebrate neuromuscular transmission. *Physiol Rev* 1973; 53:674–723.
48. Heuser JE, Reese TS: Evidence for recycling of synaptic vesicle membrane during transmitter release at the frog neuromuscular junction. *J Cell Biol* 1973; 57:315–344.
49. Heuser JE, Reese TS, Dennis MJ, et al: Synaptic vesicle exocytosis captured by quick freezing and correlated with quantal transmitter release. *J Cell Biol* 1979; 81:275–300.
50. Marchbanks RM, Israel M: The heterogeneity of bound acetylcholine and storage vesicles. *Biochem J* 1972; 129:1049–1061.
51. Miledi R, Molenaar PC, Polak RL: The effect of lanthanum ions on acetylcholine in frog muscle. *J Physiol Lond* 1980; 309:199–214.
52. Mitchell JF, Silver A: The spontaneous release of acetylcholine from the denervated hemidiaphragm of the rat. *J Physiol* 1963; 165:117–129.
53. Katz B, Miledi R: Does the motor nerve impulse evoke nonquantal transmitter release? *Proc R Soc Lond Biol* 1981; 212:131–137.
54. Katz B, Miledi R: Transmitter leakage from motor nerve endings. *Proc R Soc Lond B* 1977; 196:59–72.
55. Kuffler SW, Yoshikami D: The number of transmitter molecules in a quantum: An estimate from iontophoretic application of acetylcholine at the neuromuscular synapse. *J Physiol* 1975; 251:465–482.
56. Durant NN: The physiology of neuromuscular transmission. *Semin Anesth* 1984; 3:262–274.
57. Heuser JE, Reese TS: Structural changes after transmitter release at the frog neuromuscular junction. *J Cell Biol* 1981; 88:564–580.
58. Potter LT: Synthesis, storage and release of [^{14}C]-acetylcholine in isolated rat diaphragm muscles. *J Physiol* 1970; 206:145.
59. Whittaker VP, Luqmani YA: False transmitters in the cholinergic system: Implications for the vesicle theory of transmitter storage and release. *Gen Pharmacol* 1980; 11:7.
60. Israel M, Dunant Y, Manaranche R: The present status of the vesicular hypothesis. *Prog Neurobiol* 1979; 13:237–275.
61. Dunant Y, Israel M: The release of acetylcholine. *Sci Am* 1985; 252(4):58–66.

62. Sokoll MD, Dretchen KL, Gergis SD: d-Tubocurarine effects on nerve-terminal and neuromuscular conduction. *Anesthesiology* 1972; 36:592–597.

63. Glavinovic MI: Presynaptic action of curare. *J Physiol Lond* 1979: 290:499–506.

64. Bowman WC: Prejunctional and postjunctional cholinoceptors at the neuromuscular junction. *Anesth Analg* 1980; 59:935–943.

65. Magleby KL, Pallotta BS, Terrar DA: The effect of (+)-tubocurarine on neuromuscular transmission during repetitive stimulation in the rat, mouse, and frog. *J Physiol* 1981; 312:97–113.

66. Gibb AJ, Marshall IG: Pre- and post-junctional effects of tubocurarine and other nicotinic antagonists during repetitive stimulation in the rat. *J Physiol* 1984; 351:275–297.

67. Bowman WC, Marshall IG, Gigg AJ: Is there feedback control of transmitter release at the neuromuscular junction. *Semin Anesth* 1984; 3:275–283.

68. Ali HH, Savarese JJ: Monitoring of the neuromuscular junction. *Anesthesiology* 1976; 45:216–249.

69. Elmqvist D, Quastel DMJ: A quantitative study of end-plate potentials in isolated human muscle. *J Physiol Lond* 1965; 178:505–529.

70. Williams NE, Webb SN, Calvey TN: Differential effects of myoneural blocking drugs on neuromuscular transmission. *Br J Anaesth* 1980; 52:1111–1115.

71. Raftery MA, Hunkapiller MW, Strader CD: Acetylcholine receptor: Complex of homologous subunits. *Science* 1980; 208:1454–1457.

72. Dreyer F: Acetylcholine receptor. *Br J Anaesth* 1982; 54:115–130.

73. Goudsouzian NG, Standaert FG: The infant and the myoneural junction. *Anesth Analg* 1986; 65:1208–1217.

74. Dwyer TM, Adams DJ, Hille B: The permeability of the endplate channel to organic cations in frog muscle. *J Gen Physiol* 1980; 75:469–492.

75. Grohovaz F, Limbrick, Miledi R: Acetylcholine receptors at the rat neuromuscular junction as revealed by deep etching. *Proc R Soc Lond B* 1982; 215:147–154.

76. Ross MJ, Klymowsky MW, Agard DA: Structural studies of a membrane-bound acetylcholine receptor from *Torpedo californica*. *J Mol Biol* 1977; 116:635–659.

77. Dreyer F, Peper K, Strez R: Determination of dose-response curves by quantitative iontophoresis at the frog neuromuscular junction. *J Physiol* 1978; 281:395–419.

78. Peper K, Bradley RJ, Dreyer F: The acetylcholine receptor at the neuromuscular junction. *Physiol Rev* 1982; 62:1271–1340.

79. Adams PR: Acetylcholine receptor kinetics. *J Membr Biol* 1981; 58:161–174.

80. Dreyer F, Peper K: Density and dose-response curve of acetylcholine receptors in frog neuromuscular junction. *Nature* 1975; 253:641–643.

81. Neubig RR, Boyd ND, Cohen JB: Conformations of *Torpedo* acetylcho-

line receptor associated with ion transport and desensitization. *Biochemistry* 1982; 21:3460–3467.

82. Standaert FG: The doughnut and its hole. *Clin Anaesthesiol* 1985; 3:243–259.
83. Sakmann B, Patlak J, Neher E: Single acetylcholine-activated channels show burst-kinetics in presence of desensitizing concentrations of agonist. *Nature* 1980; 286:71–73.
84. Anderson CR, Stevens CF: Voltage clamp analysis of acetylcholine produced end-plate current fluctuations at frog neuromuscular junction. *J Physiol* 1973; 235:655–691.
85. Taylor P: Anticholinesterase agents, in Gilman AG, Goodman LS, Gilman A (eds): *The Pharmacological Basis of Therapeutics*, ed 6. New York, MacMillan Publishing Co, 1980, pp 99–119.
86. Salpeter MM: Electron microscope radio-autography as a quantitative tool in enzyme cytochemistry: I. The distribution of acetylcholinesterase at motor endplates of a vertebrate twitch muscle. *J Cell Biol* 1967; 32:379–389.
87. Cull-Candy SG, Miledi R, Trautman A: End-plate currents and acetylcholine noise at normal and myasthenic human end-plates. *J Physiol Lond* 1979; 287:247–265.
88. Zaimis E, Head S: Depolarising neuromuscular blocking drugs, in Zaimis E (ed): *Neuromuscular Junction: Handbook of Experimental Pharmacology*. Berlin, Springer-Verlag, 1976, vol 42, pp 365–419.
89. Dreyer F, Muller KD, Peper K, et al: The M. omohyoideus of the mouse as a convenient mammalian muscle preparation. *Pflugers Arch* 1976; 367:115–122.
90. Colquhoun D, Dreyer F, Sheridan RE: The actions of tubocurarine at the frog neuromuscular junction. *J Physiol* 1979; 293:247–284.
91. Lambert JJ, Durant NN, Henderson EG: Drug-induced modification of ionic conductance at the neuromuscular junction. *Annu Rev Pharmacol Toxicol* 1983; 23:505–539.
92. Kennedy RD, Galindo AD: Comparative site of action of various anaesthetic agents at the mammalian myoneural junction. *Br J Anaesth* 1975; 47:533–540.
93. Kennedy R, Galindo A: Neuromuscular transmission in a mammalian preparation during exposure to enflurane. *Anesthesiology* 1975; 42:432–442.
94. Waud BE, Waud DR: The effects of diethyl ether, enflurane, and isoflurane at the neuromuscular junction. *Anesthesiology* 1975; 42:275–280.
95. Waud BE: Decrease in dose requirement of d-tubocurarine by volatile anesthestics. *Anesthesiology* 1979; 51:298–302.
96. Marshall IG, Henderson F: Drug interactions at the neuromuscular junction. *Clin Anaesthesiol* 1985; 3:261–270.
97. Paton WDM, Waud DR: The margin of safety of neuromuscular transmission. *J Physiol* 1967; 191:59–90.

98. Waud BE, Waud DR: The margin of safety of neuromuscular transmission in the muscle of the diaphragm. *Anesthesiology* 1972; 37:417–422.

99. Waud BE, Waud DR: The relation between tetanic fade and receptor occlusion in the presence of competitive neuromuscular block. *Anesthesiology* 1971; 35:456–464.

100. Frambrough DM: Control of acetylcholine receptors in skeletal muscle. *Physiol Rev* 1979; 59:165–227.

101. Lee C, Chen D, Katz RL: Characteristics of nondepolarizing neuromuscular block: I. Post-junctional block by alpha-bungarotoxin. *Can Anaesth Soc J* 1977; 24:212–219.

102. Riker WF: Actions of acetylcholine on mammalian motor nerve terminal. *J Pharmacol Exp Ther* 1966; 152:397–416.

103. Hartman GS, Fiamengo SA, Riker WF: Succinylcholine: Mechanism of fasciculations and their prevention by d-tubocurarine or diphenylhydantoin. *Anesthesiology* 1986; 65:405–413.

104. Miyamoto MD: The actions of cholinergic drugs on motor nerve terminals. *Pharmacol Rev* 1978; 29:221–247.

105. Lebowitz PW, Ramsey FM, Savarese JJ: Potentiation of neuromuscular blockade in man produced by combinations of pancuronium and metocurine or pancuronium and d-tubocurarine. *Anesth Analg* 1980; 59:604–609.

106. Waud BE, Waud DR: Interaction among agents that block end-plate depolarization competitively. *Anesthesiology* 1985; 63:4–15.

107. Waud BE, Waud DR: Quantitative examination of the interaction of competitive neuromuscular blocking agents on the indirectly elicited twitch. *Anesthesiology* 1984; 61:420–427.

108. Sine SM, Taylor P: Relationship between reversible antagonist occupancy and the functional capacity of the acetylcholine receptor. *J Biol Chem* 1981; 256:6692–6699.

109. Pantuck EJ, Pantuck CB: Cholinesterases and anticholinesterases, in Katz RL (ed): *Muscle Relaxants: Monographs in Anesthesiology.* New York, Elsevier North-Holland, 1975, pp 143–162.

110. Riker WF: Prejunctional effects of neuromuscular blocking and facilitatory drugs, in Katz RL (ed): *Muscle Relaxants: Monographs in Anesthesiology.* New York, Elsevier North-Holland 1975, pp 59–102.

111. Hobbinger F: Pharmacology of anticholinesterase drugs, in Zaimis E (ed): *Neuromuscular Junction: Handbook of Neuromuscular Pharmacology.* Berlin, Springer-Verlag, 1976, pp 487–581.

112. Sokoll MD, Gergis SM: Antibiotics and neuromuscular function. *Anesthesiology* 1981; 55:148–159.

113. Waud BE, Waud DR: Interaction of calcium and potassium with neuromuscular blocking agents. *Br J Anaesth* 1980; 52:863–866.

3

Clinical Measurement

When muscle relaxants are used, a certain degree of paralysis is sought, without compromising recovery. Thus, the dose given will be determined on the basis of the patient's characteristics, such as weight and age, the nature of the surgery, and the duration of the procedure. However, one cannot depend on a fixed dose of drug to provide a predictable degree of relaxation for a predictable period of time. The "therapeutic window" of relaxants is narrow,[1, 2] because of the high margin of safety of the neuromuscular junction. Thus, the range of plasma concentrations over which partial neuromuscular blockade occurs is narrow[3] (Fig 3–1). Moreover, there are wide variations in the individual response to the same dose of relaxant[4, 5] (Fig 3–2). Thus, the degree of neuromuscular blockade must be assessed frequently and carefully.

CLINICAL ASSESSMENT

During anesthesia, the signs of inadequate relaxation may be spontaneous movement, triggering of the respirator, a change in the inflation pressures, paradoxical respirations, or a tight abdomen as reported by the surgeon. However, these signs are not specific for poor relaxation: they can indicate an inadequate level of anesthesia. Furthermore, the absence of these signs is not evidence of a sufficient degree of paralysis, as a rapid change in conditions, such as a sudden increase in the level of surgical stimulation, might trigger spontaneous movement.

In subjects recovering from anesthesia, the degree of residual paralysis can be assessed qualitatively by asking the patient to lift his head against force, to open his eyes, or to sustain handgrip. Tidal vol-

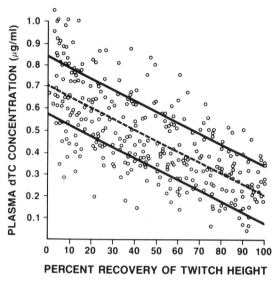

FIG 3–1.
Plasma concentration of *d*-tubocurarine (dTC) as a function of twitch height. Each dot represents an individual measurement in a patient. Merely doubling the concentration can produce a change from 0 to 100% paralysis, an indicator of the low margin of safety of the neuromuscular junction. Also, a concentration of 0.5 μ/ml can be associated with anything from almost no blockade to complete blockade. (From Matteo RS, Spector S, Horowitz PE: Relation of serum *d*-tubocurarine concentration to neuromuscular blockade in man. *Anesthesiology* 1974; 41:440–443. Used by permission.)

ume can be maintained in spite of severe weakness. Vital capacity and inspiratory force are more sensitive indicators of residual paralysis.[6, 7] The effect of depolarizing and nondepolarizing relaxants is greater on peripheral than respiratory muscles.[8–16] Thus, head lift and handgrip are more sensitive indicators of residual paralysis. However, the presence of these signs depends on patient cooperation and may be influenced by pain, narcotics, inhalational agents, poor motivation, or communication barrier. Thus, a monitoring technique specific for muscle relaxation is extremely useful in clinical anesthesia.

NERVE STIMULATION

The function of the neuromuscular junction is tested by stimulating a nerve proximal to it and measuring the response of the muscle distal to it. This allows the degree of paralysis to be assessed independently of central influences.

Physiology of Nerve Stimulation

An individual nerve axon is stimulated in an all-or-none fashion. If a sufficient current is delivered for a long enough period of time, the transmembrane potential will exceed threshold, and an action potential will be generated (see Chapter 2). If the current delivered to the axon flows in such a way as to produce hyperpolarization instead of depolarization, an action potential may be initiated at the end of the current pulse due to a rapid change in membrane potential: this is referred to as "anode-break excitation."[17] These two methods of producing an action potential have different thresholds, and it is normally easier to produce an action potential by depolarizing the membrane. This explains why a negative electrode is usually more effective in stimulating a nerve.[18, 19] If both stimulating electrodes are placed near a nerve and sufficient current is delivered, two action potentials may be generated: one near the negative and the other near the positive electrode, at the beginning and at the end of the current pulse, respectively. However, the axon is refractory to further stimulation during and shortly after an action potential. Thus, if the current pulse delivered is shorter than the refractory period (0.5 to 1 msec), only one action potential can be in-

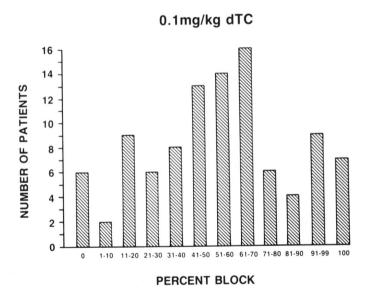

FIG 3–2.
Variability of patient response after *d*-tubocurarine (dTC), 0.1 mg/kg. (From Katz RL: Neuromuscular effects of *d*-tubocurarine, edrophonium and neostigmine in man. *Anesthesiology* 1967; 28:327–336.

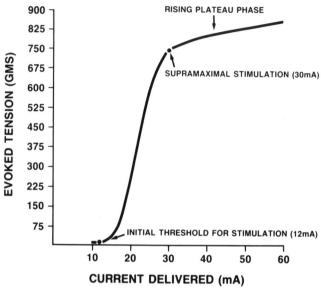

FIG 3–3.
Evoked tension of the adductor pollicis muscle as a function of current applied to the ulnar nerve. (From Kopman AF, Lawson D: Milliamperage requirements for supramaximal stimulation of the ulnar nerve with surface electrodes. *Anesthesiology* 1984; 61:83–85. Used by permission.)

itiated.[20, 21] This explains the repetitive stimulation produced by older stimulators that delivered 5-msec pulses.[22] Most modern stimulators provide pulses with a duration of 0.1 to 0.3 msec, and the problem of double stimulation is avoided.

Peripheral nerves are made up of a large number of axons. The sensitivity of each might be slightly different from the other and probably follows a normal distribution. In the absence of relaxants, the number of axons firing, and therefore the force of the muscle contraction, has a sigmoid relationship to the current delivered (Fig 3–3). Before a response is recorded, a certain minimum current must be delivered. Then an increase in stimulation current increases response markedly until a plateau is reached. This plateau corresponds to the simultaneous contraction of all muscle fibers in response to action potentials propagated down all the nerve axons. At this point, "supramaximal stimulation" is reached. This usually requires 50 to 65 mA for 0.2 msec applied to the ulnar nerve.[23] The voltage required depends on the resistance between the two electrodes, but 200 to 400 V is usually sufficient. After supramaximal stimulation is reached, the force of contraction increases slightly with increasing applied current (see Fig 3–

3). The nature of this phenomenon is unclear, but it is of little practical significance.

A supramaximal stimulus causes all nerve axons to propagate an action potential and all nerve endings to release acetylcholine. With increasing concentrations of muscle relaxants at the neuromuscular junction, a larger number of receptors are occupied. However, this will not produce any transmission failure until a large proportion of receptors is occupied. The exact proportion of receptors required for detectable block to be manifest is not exactly the same at each end-plate. As the relaxant concentration increases, no decrease in force of contraction is noticed until a certain threshold is attained. Then, the most sensitive end-plates fail to reach threshold. If relaxant concentration is increased further, more and more end-plates will fail to transmit until all end-plates are blocked, at which point no muscular activity will be detected. Thus, neuromuscular blockade is assessed by estimating the proportion of end-plates that fail to transmit.[24] The muscle response can be assessed either by measuring its electrical activity (electromyography) or its contractile force.

Types of Blockade

In the presence of nondepolarizing relaxants, repetitive stimulation is associated with fade of the evoked muscle response[24-28] (Fig 3–4).

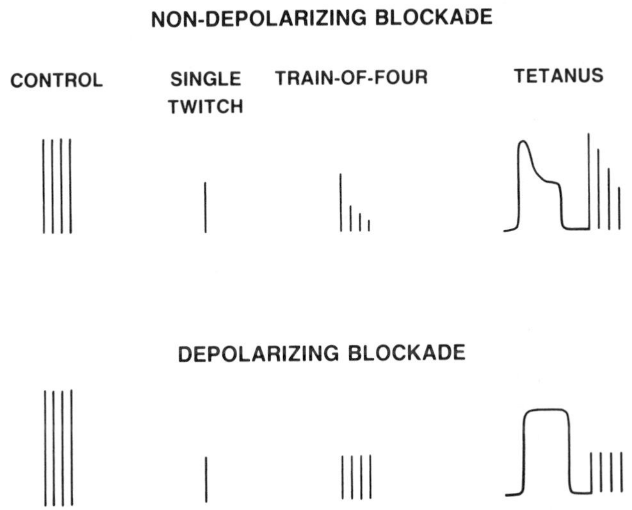

FIG 3–4.
Schematic representations of the response to single twitch, train-of-four, tetanic, and post-tetanic stimulation in the presence of nondepolarizing (*top*) and depolarizing blockers (*bottom*).

Fade is observed at stimulation frequencies greater than 0.1 Hz. In the range of 2 to 50 Hz, the degree of fade is relatively constant, and maximum depression of response usually occurs by the fourth impulse.[27, 28] The presence of fade explains why d-tubocurarine appears more potent when the frequency of stimulation is greater than 0.15 Hz.[29] This phenomenon is generally attributed to a decrease in acetylcholine release from the nerve endings with high stimulation rates.[30]

The other major feature of nondepolarizing blockade is the presence of post-tetanic facilitation[24, 25] (see Fig 3–4). Following a tetanic stimulus, the response to single stimulations is increased. The magnitude and the duration of this facilitation depend on the frequency and the duration of the tetanic stimulation. Post-tetanic facilitation is associated with an increase in both the electromyographic and mechanical responses of the muscle.[31, 32] Thus, it is due to increased acetylcholine release and/or increased sensitivity of the end-plate. It is thought that the large amount of acetylcholine released during tetanic stimulation causes competitive displacement of the relaxant from the receptor.Post-tetanic facilitation must be distinguished from post-tetanic potentiation, which occurs in certain muscles without relaxants.[33] The latter is an augmentation of twitch tension following tetanic stimulation, which is not accompanied by corresponding increases in electromyographic activity. Post-tetanic potentiation is not, like post-tetanic facilitation, a transmitter-related phenomenon but is due to an improvement in the contractile properties of muscle.[33]

Depolarizing blockade, produced by agents such as succinylcholine or decamethonium, is characterized by the lack of fade and the absence of post-tetanic facilitation (see Fig 3–4). Prolonged administration of these agents produces neuromuscular blockade characterized by tetanic fade and post-tetanic facilitation called phase II block.[32, 34] Whether the appearance of blockade, which is morphologically identical to nondepolarizing blockade, implies common mechanisms of action is an unsettled issue.

Stimulus Frequency

The simplest mode of stimulation consists in the delivery of single impulses separated by at least 10 seconds, which corresponds to the interval required to avoid the presence of fade during nondepolarizing blockade.[25, 29] However, a control, prerelaxant value is necessary to assess the degree of blockade in a quantitative manner. In addition, the presence of a full response does not guarantee full neuromuscular re-

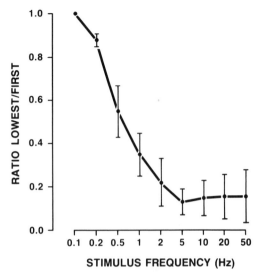

FIG 3–5.
Relationship between the ratio of the smallest electromyographic response in a train of stimulus to the first response, and stimulation frequency, in the presence of *d*- tubocurarine blockade causing 50% depression of first twitch compared with prerelaxant values. Fade is independent of frequency in the range 2 to 50 Hz. (From Lee C, Katz RL: Fade of neurally evoked compound electromyogram during neuromuscular block by *d*-tubocurarine. *Anesth Analg* 1977; 56:271–275. Used by permission.)

covery because sustained contraction depends on an appropriate response of the muscle to repetitive stimulation.[6, 35]

Tetanic fade is a more sensitive index of residual nondepolarizing blockade, especially at frequencies of 100 to 200 Hz.[36–38] However, high-frequency stimulation (100 Hz) may produce fade in the absence of neuromuscular relaxants,[39] especially in the presence of enflurane[40] or isoflurane.[41] More importantly, the application of tetanic stimulation changes the response to further stimulation for up to several minutes.[24] Thus, the use of this mode of stimulation is limited by the spurious overestimation of neuromuscular function on further testing.

The train-of-four mode of stimulation was introduced as a compromise between sensitivity and the absence of post-tetanic facilitation. Sensitivity is obtained by choosing the lowest frequency associated with significant fade.[26, 42] During *d*-tubocurarine blockade, the degree of fade is rather constant in the range 2 to 50 Hz[27] (Fig 3–5). Thus, 2 Hz appears to be an appropriate frequency, which has the advantage of being low enough so the response may be assessed visually. Since the degree of post-tetanic facilitation depends on the duration of the train of stimuli, it is important not to prolong the stimulation after the maximum fade has been attained. At 2 Hz, this occurs by the fourth impulse.[27] By applying train-of-four stimulation every 10 to 12 seconds or longer, little or no post-tetanic facilitation is observed.[26, 43]

Train-of-four stimulation is more sensitive than single twitch stimulation to small degrees of neuromuscular blockade.[28, 38, 42, 44] In addition, the degree of relaxation can be assessed without a control, prerelaxant value. The ratio of the fourth to the first response, also called train-of-four ratio (TOFR), correlates well with first twitch height[28, 42] (Fig 3–6). Usually, when TOFR exceeds 0.7, single twitch height is normal. Then, single twitch height decreases linearly with TOFR, which reaches zero when single twitch height is approximately 25% of control value. The response to the third impulse generally disappears when single twitch height is below 20%, and second response becomes zero at single twitch heights of approximately 15%. This relationship is affected by interpatient variability.[28] It also depends on which relaxant has been used: gallamine and d-tubocurarine exhibit more train-of-four fade than pancuronium[45] and atracurium more than vecuronium.[46] In addition, fade is time dependent: it is more apparent during recovery than onset.[46, 47] Despite these variations, train-of-four

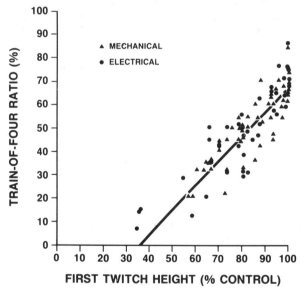

FIG 3–6.
Relationship between train-of-four ratio and first twitch height during *d*-tubocurarine blockade. (From Ali HH, Utting JE, Gray TC: Quantitative assessment of residual antidepolarizing block: Pt. I. *Br J Anaesth* 1971; 43:473–476. Used by permission.)

stimulation has emerged as the most convenient and reliable method of nondepolarizing blockade monitoring.

CLINICAL MEASUREMENT

Stimulator Characteristics

The stimulator chosen should be capable of delivering 200- to 400-V electrical impulses of 0.1- to 0.3-msec duration. Current output of at least 60 to 65 mamp should be provided over a wide range of output impedances.[23, 48] Many types of stimulators are commercially available, with a wide variety of features.[48–51] The ability to provide train-of-four stimulation at 2 Hz is an essential feature of modern stimulators. The stimulator should also be capable of delivering tetanic stimulation at 30 to 50 Hz. Higher stimulation frequencies are not necessary. Some stimulators display the current delivered to the patient. This is an advantage because a nerve responds to current, not voltage. A low current reading may indicate improper placement of the electrodes, a disconnection, and/or low stimulator battery voltage. If this information is not available, a small or absent muscle response may be misinterpreted as being the result of an excessive degree of relaxation. Needle electrodes are usually unnecessary if the stimulator can provide sufficient voltage. Silver-silver chloride electrocardiogram (ECG) electrodes, one of which must be in close proximity to the nerve to be stimulated, are usually satisfactory.[52]

Selection of Nerve for Stimulation

Theoretically, any superficial nerve supplying one or more muscles can be used for monitoring. In both research and clinical practice, the ulnar nerve is most commonly stimulated. It is accessible for stimulation either at the wrist or the elbow. The ulnar nerve supplies several hand muscles, such as the muscles of the hypothenar eminence, the interosseous muscles, and the adductor pollicis.[18] The latter adducts the thumb at the metacarpophalangeal joint. The force of this contraction can be measured with a transducer and has been considered the gold standard in research on relaxants. The muscles of the hypothenar eminence may be slightly more resistant to the action of nondepolarizing relaxants than the adductor pollicis,[32, 53] such that information obtained from this group of muscles might not be identical to that of the adductor pollicis. If stimulation is applied at the elbow, the contraction of the flexor carpi ulnaris and flexor digitorum profundus mus-

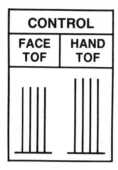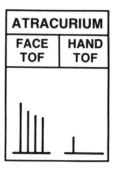

FIG 3–7.
Comparison of adductor pollicis (hand) and orbicularis oculi (face) muscles before (control) and during atracurium neuromuscular blockade. (From Caffrey RR, Warren ML, Becker KE: Neuromuscular blockade monitoring comparing the orbicularis oculi and adductor pollicis muscles. *Anesthesiology* 1986; 65:95–97. Used by permission.)

cles will also be observed. Again, the sensitivity of these muscles might be different from that of the adductor pollicis.

The facial nerve may also be accessible for most surgical procedures. Stimulating it produces a contraction of the orbicularis oculi muscle. Usually, this muscle is much more resistant to the effect of nondepolarizing relaxants than the adductor pollicis[54, 55] (Fig 3–7). Therefore, stimulating the facial nerve normally results in a marked underestimation of the intensity of neuromuscular blockade.

The median nerve can also be stimulated at the wrist, and the peroneal nerve may be accessible near the head of the fibula when access to the head and arms is difficult or impossible. However, the sensitivity of the muscles supplied by these nerves is unknown.

Theoretically, it would be advantageous to monitor respiratory muscles clinically. Stimulation of the phrenic nerve is possible and can give information on the degree of diaphragm blockade.[56, 57] Similarly, stimulation of the intercostal nerves can yield information on intercostal and abdominal muscle function.[58] However, such stimulation is technically difficult, and more importantly, it does not provide information about upper airway muscles. Thus, it seems more practical to monitor a peripheral muscle, keeping in mind the different sensitivity of respiratory muscles (Fig 3–8).

When a patient suffers from neuromuscular disease involving only part of the body, such as hemiplegia or spinal cord transection, it is important to monitor the unaffected muscle. These conditions are usually associated with relaxant resistance, and an overdose of relaxant may result from neuromuscular monitoring in affected areas.[59–61]

Evaluation of Response

Force transducers have been widely used in research to obtain quantitative results. Many versions of force transducers have been proposed for clinical use.[62–65] Most, if not all, have been designed to be used on the adductor pollicis muscle and cannot be applied to other sites. The high degree of accuracy of these devices, although useful for teaching, may be in excess of what is required in routine practice because of the differential sensitivity of other muscles in the body. Visual or tactile evaluation is adequate in most circumstances, although train-of-four fade can be grossly underevaluated.[66]

The response to nerve stimulation can also be evaluated by electromyography. This involves the measurement of the electrical activity associated with the propagation of action potentials in muscle cells that is triggered by acetylcholine-induced depolarization. The amplitude of the electromyographic (EMG) signal is directly related to the number of contracting units.[67] Since the muscle action potential travels from the neuromuscular junction to both ends of the muscle cell, the largest EMG signal is usually obtained by placing one electrode over the in-

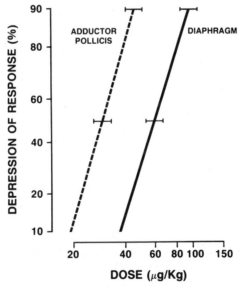

FIG 3–8.
Dose-response curves for pancuronium at the adductor pollicis and diaphragm muscles, indicating diaphragm resistance. (From Donati F, Antzaka C, Bevan DR: Potency of pancuronium at the diaphragm and the adductor pollicis in humans. *Anesthesiology* 1986; 656:1–5. Used by permission.)

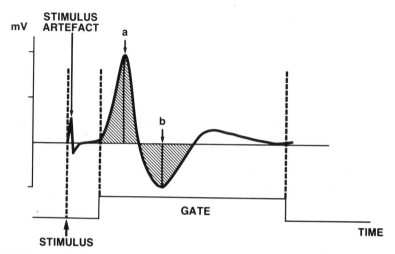

STIMULUS

FIG 3–9.
Electromyographic (EMG) signal obtained after nerve stimulation. The stimulus artifact is followed by a time delay, which corresponds to nerve conduction and synaptic delay. The EMG signal that follows is quantified either by measuring the amplitude of the first deflection *(a)* or by electronic rectification and integration, which effectively measures the area under the curve *(b)* during a 10 to 16 msec gate. (From Viby-Mogensen J: Clinical measurement of neuromuscular functions: An update. *Clin Anaesthesiol* 1985; 3:467–482. Used by permission.)

sertion of the muscle and the other near the midportion where the neuromuscular junction is most usually located. An indifferent electrode is placed nearby. The amplitude of the EMG obtained in the hypothenar or thenar eminence following ulnar nerve stimulation is usually 5 to 15 mV, and its duration is 10 to 15 msec (Fig 3–9). This is too rapid for visual observation on an oscilloscope screen, so a certain amount of electronic processing must be made. This usually involves either the measurement of the EMG amplitude,[68] or the rectification and integration of the signal.[68, 69] Electromyography has certain advantages over monitoring force: (1) it is theoretically applicable to a larger number of muscles; (2) it does not require a bulky apparatus near the muscle to be monitored; (3) it is much less sensitive than force measurement to lack of immobilization; and (4) compared with visual or tactile evaluation, it does not require access to the muscle after the system is set up. Its main disadvantages are (1) expensive equipment is needed; (2) the response is obliterated by electrocautery; (3) moving the patient or the leads can cause interference; and (4) most commercial devices do not provide the raw signal.

As expected, there is usually a very good correlation between EMG activity and force.[42, 53, 70, 71] However, several factors contribute to minor discrepancies. First, neither EMG nor force necessarily add up linearly. Second, it is generally easier to obtain force for one muscle only, whereas it is unlikely that the electrical activity picked up by skin electrodes originates in one muscle only. More important, if the electrical activity comes from a different muscle, the discrepancy may be greater because the two muscles involved may have different sensitivities. Third, the superficial part of the muscle, which lies closer to the electrodes, might contribute a disproportionately large part to the EMG signal. Finally, some drugs affect the relationship; for example, dantrolene leaves the EMG unaffected while diminishing evoked force markedly, and succinylcholine causes depolarization, repetitive firing, and possibly a direct action on muscle.[71]

APPLICATIONS

Monitoring Onset

It would be advantageous to assess the adequacy of the relaxant dose given before laryngoscopy and endotracheal intubation are attempted. Unfortunately, peripheral nerve stimulation is of limited value. The muscles of respiration are relatively more resistant than the adductor pollicis.[7–16, 56, 57] On the other hand, it appears that the onset of action of neuromuscular blockade is more rapid in the diaphragm than in the adductor pollicis, probably because of larger diaphragmatic blood perfusion.[57] It follows that if the dose is adequate, diaphragm paralysis occurs sooner than in the adductor pollicis. However, if the dose is inadequate, the diaphragm will never be blocked despite an absent adductor pollicis response. Paradoxically, the onset of apnea occurs when adductor pollicis twitch height is in the 50% to 80% range while considerable respiratory muscle power is still present[72] (Fig 3–10). The

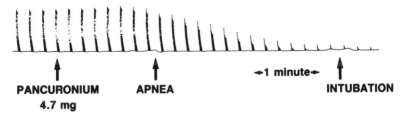

↑ **PANCURONIUM** ↑ **APNEA**　　◄—1 minute—►　↑ **INTUBATION**
4.7 mg

FIG 3–10.
Train-of-four monitoring of the twitch tension of the adductor pollicis muscle in a 78 kg patient. The patient was breathing spontaneously when pancuronium was injected. Apnea was observed when only a small depression of twitch height was seen. Manual ventilation was instituted. The intubating conditions 2.5 minutes later were poor, in spite of 90% adductor pollicis blockade.

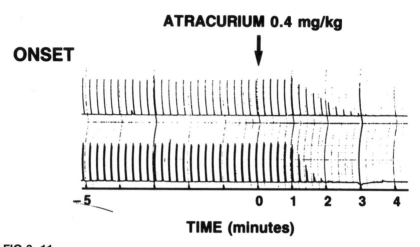

FIG 3–11.
Onset of neuromuscular blockade in a patient given atracurium. Both adductor pollicis muscles were monitored simultaneously with either single twitch *(top)* or train-of-four *(bottom)*
stimulation. Onset time as measured with train-of-four stimulation is markedly reduced. (From
Curran MJ, Donati F, Bevan DR: Onset and recovery of atracurium and suxamethonium-
induced neuromuscular blockade with simultaneous train-of-four and single twitch stimulation.
Br J Anaesth 1987; 59:989–994. Used by permission.)

reason for this is unclear, but apnea cannot be relied on as a sign of
good intubating conditions.[72] Finally, the type of stimulation itself may
modify time of onset of action markedly: measured onset times for
atracurium and succinylcholine were found to be markedly reduced
by the application of train-of-four stimulation when compared with
single twitch[73] (Fig 3–11). It follows that it is impossible to define a
degree of peripheral twitch depression that corresponds invariably with
good intubating conditions.

Monitoring Surgical Relaxation

The degree of neuromuscular blockade required during a surgical
procedure depends on many factors, such as the patient's musculature,
the type of surgery, and the amount of inhalational anesthetics given.
The major problem associated with the administration of large doses
of relaxants once the airway has been secured is the lack of reversibility
of intense neuromuscular blockade.[74, 75] The effectiveness of reversal
agents is markedly impaired if they are administered when first twitch
height is less than 10% of control. On the other hand, surgical conditions are very often not satisfactory when first twitch height is greater
than 25%. Fortunately, train-of-four monitoring is very easy in this

range of blockade because the fourth twitch usually disappears when first twitch height is approximately 25%. At 10% first twitch height, usually only one twitch is visible. Thus, a useful indicator of the degree of relaxation is to count the number of twitches following train-of-four stimulation.[28] This type of stimulation should not be repeated more often than every 10 to 12 seconds to allow the neuromuscular junction to recover completely between trains.

When the response to train-of-four stimulation is visible, it is not necessary to use tetanic stimulation, which causes post-tetanic facilitation and may render the neuromuscular junction spuriously more responsive to further testing. However, the presence of post-tetanic facilitation may be useful in certain circumstances. When no response is seen after train-of-four stimulation, a 50-Hz, 5-second train may produce sufficient facilitation to make the neuromuscular junction responsive to further stimulation. The post-tetanic count technique involves the application of tetanic stimulation, followed by 1-Hz stimulation: the number of twitches observed is inversely related to the degree of blockade[76, 77] (Fig 3–12). The usefulness of this technique,

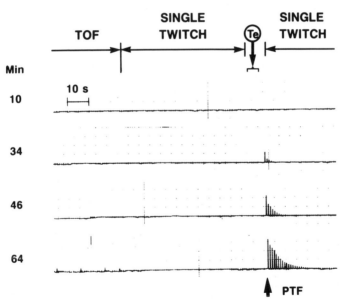

FIG 3–12.
Post-tetanic count with pancuronium blockade, after injection of 0.1 mg/kg of the drug. With spontaneous recovery, the number of visible single twitches elicited after tetanic stimulation increases, although no response is seen to either train-of-four *(TOF),* single twitch, or tetanic stimulation. (From Viby-Mogensen J: Clinical assessment of neuromuscular transmission. *Br J Anaesth* 1982; 54:209–223. Used by permission.)

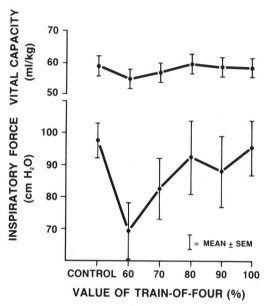

FIG 3–13.
Vital capacity and inspiratory force in awake volunteers given *d*-tubocurarine as a function of train-of-four ratio. (From Ali HH, Wilson RS, Savarese JJ, et al: The effect of tubocurarine on indirectly elicited train-of-four muscle response and respiratory measurements in humans. *Br J Anaesth* 1975; 47:570–574. Used by permission.)

however, is limited because (1) it is applicable to situations of intense block, when no more relaxant is required and reversal is not possible; and (2) the response to subsequent testing is modified.

Monitoring Recovery

Before a reversal agent is administered, the response to train-of-four stimulation of an unconditioned neuromuscular junction should be one visible twitch, and preferably more. No tetanic stimulation should have been applied during the previous 5 to 10 minutes. The response of the adductor pollicis muscle is preferred to that of other muscles because of its relative sensitivity to relaxants. Thus, full recovery of neuromuscular function in this muscle is strongly indicative of recovery in the more resistant respiratory muscles.

An adductor pollicis train-of-four ratio of 0.7 or greater was found to correspond to the ability to lift the head[78] and adequate respiratory parameters such as inspiratory force and vital capacity[6] (Fig 3–13). However, this relationship is not necessarily true in all clinical situations. Thus, it is essential to assess the patient's ability to breathe, cough, and maintain a patent airway. Furthermore, it appears that experienced clinicians cannot detect reliably train-of-four fade with either tactile or visual evaluation, even if train-of-four ratio is as low as 0.3[66] (Fig 3–14). Such an overevaluation of train-of-four response makes clinical assessment mandatory.

CONCLUSION

Neuromuscular monitoring should be considered an integral part of anesthetic practice. It is noninvasive, inexpensive, and can make the management of surgical relaxation much more rational and individualized. However, such a technique is an aid, not a substitute, for sound clinical observation and judgment. Muscle relaxants can be lethal, largely because of their effects on the respiratory system. For this reason, mechanical ventilation should be continued or instituted until there is sufficient clinical evidence for the full return of neuromuscular function.

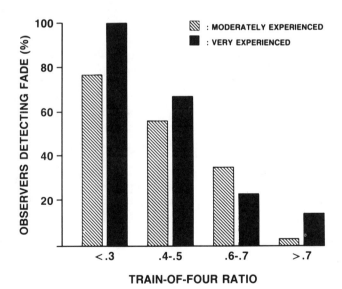

FIG 3–14.
Number of observers detecting fade by visual or tactile evaluation vs. train-of-four fade ratio, as measured by a force transducer. A substantial number of observers could not detect fade when train-of-four ratio was 0.7 or less. (Data from Viby-Mogensen J, Jensen NH, Engbaek J, et al: Tactile and visual evaluation of the response to train-of-four stimulation. *Anesthesiology* 1985; 63:440–443.)

REFERENCES

1. Paton WDM, Waud DR: The margin of safety of neuromuscular transmission. *J Physiol* 1967; 191:59–90.
2. Waud BE, Waud DR: The margin of safety of neuromuscular transmission in the muscle of the diaphragm. *Anesthesiology* 1972; 37:417–422.
3. Matteo RS, Spector S, Horowitz PE: Relation of serum d-tubocurarine concentration to neuromuscular blockade in man. *Anesthesiology* 1974; 41:440–443.
4. Katz RL: Neuromuscular effects of d-tubocurarine, edrophonium and neostigmine in man. *Anesthesiology* 1967; 28:327–336.
5. Katz RL, Stirt J, Murray AL, et al: Neuromuscular effects of atracurium in man. *Anesth Analg* 1982; 61:730–734.
6. Ali HH, Wilson RS, Savarese JJ, et al: The effect of tubocurarine on indirectly elicited train-of-four muscle response and respiratory measurements in humans. *Br J Anaesth* 1975; 47:570–574.
7. Rosenbaum SH, Askanazi J, Hyman AI, et al: Breathing patterns during curare-induced muscle weakness. *Anesth Analg* 1983; 62:809–814.
8. Johansen SH, Jorgensen M, Molbech S: Effect of tubocurarine on respiratory and nonrespiratory muscle power in man. *J Appl Physiol* 1964; 19:990–994.
9. Gal TJ, Smith TC: Partial paralysis with d-tubocurarine and the ventilatory response to CO_2: An example of respiratory sparing? *Anesthesiology* 1976; 45:22–28.
10. Wymore ML, Eisele JH: Differential effects of d-tubocurarine on inspiratory muscles and two respiratory muscle groups in anesthetized man. *Anesthesiology* 1978; 48:360–362.
11. De Troyer A, Bastenier J, Delhez L: Function of respiratory muscles during partial curarization in humans. *J Appl Physiol* 1980; 49:1049–1056.
12. Gal TJ, Goldberg SK: Diaphragmatic function in healthy subjects during partial curarization. *J Appl Physiol* 1980; 48:921–926.
13. Foldes FF, Monte AP, Brunn HM, et al: Studies with muscle relaxants in unanesthetized subjects. *Anesthesiology* 1961; 22:230–236.
14. Jorgensen M, Molbech S, Johansen SH: Effect of decamethonium on head lift, hand grip, and respiratory muscle power in man. *J Appl Physiol* 1966; 21:509–512.
15. Gal Tj, Goldberg SK: Relationship between respiratory muscle strength and vital capacity during partial curarization in awake subjects. *Anesthesiology* 1981; 54:141–147.
16. Williams JP, Bourke DL: Effects of succinylcholine on respiratory and nonrespiratory muscle strength in humans. *Anesthesiology* 1985; 63:299–303.
17. Aidley DJ: *The Physiology of Excitable Cells.* Cambridge, Cambridge University Press, 1971.
18. Rosenberg H, Greenhow DE: Peripheral nerve stimulator performance:

The influence of output polarity and electrode placement. *Can Anaesth Soc J* 1978; 25:424–426.

19. Berger JJ, Gravenstein JS, Munson ES: Electrode polarity and peripheral nerve stimulation. *Anesthesiology* 1982; 56:402–404.

20. Epstein RA, Jackson SH, Wyte SR: The effects of nondepolarizing relaxants and anticholinesterases on the neuromuscular refractory period of anesthetized man. *Anesthesiology* 1969; 31:69–77.

21. Epstein RA, Jackson SH: Repetitive muscle depolarization from single direct stimulation in anesthetized man. *J Appl Physiol* 1970; 28:407–410.

22. Epstein RA, Wyte SR, Jackson SH, et al: The electromechanical response to stimulation by the block-aid monitor. *Anesthesiology* 1969; 30:43–47.

23. Kopman AF, Lawson D: Milliamperage requirements for supramaximal stimulation of the ulnar nerve with surface electrodes. *Anesthesiology* 1984; 61:83–85.

24. Ali HH, Savarese JJ: Monitoring of neuromuscular function. *Anesthesiology* 1976; 45:216–249.

25. Gissen AJ, Katz RL: Twitch, tetanus and posttetanic potentiation as indices of nerve-muscle block in man. *Anesthesiology* 1969; 30:481–487.

26. Ali HH, Utting JE, Gray C: Stimulus frequency in the detection of neuromuscular block in humans. *Br J Anaesth* 1970; 42:967–978.

27. Lee C, Katz RL: Fade of neurally evoked compound electromyogram during neuromuscular block by d-tubocurarine. *Anesth Analg* 1977; 56:271–275.

28. Lee C: Train-of-four quantitation of competitive neuromuscular block. *Anesth Analg* 1975; 54:649–653.

29. Ali HH, Savarese JJ: Stimulus frequency and dose-response curve to d-tubocurarine in man. *Anesthesiology* 1980; 52:36–39.

30. Bowman WC, Marshall IG, Gibb AJ: Is there feedback control of transmitter release at the neuromuscular junction? *Semin Anesth* 1984; 4:275–283.

31. Epstein RA, Epstein RM: The electromyogram and the mechanical response of indirectly stimulated muscle in anesthetized man following curarization. *Anesthesiology* 1973; 38:212–223.

32. Katz RL: Electromyographic and mechanical effects of suxamethonium and tubocurarine on twitch, tetanic and posttetanic responses. *Br J Anaesth* 1973; 45:849–859.

33. Bowman WC: *Pharmacology of Neuromuscular Function.* Baltimore, University Park Press, 1980.

34. Lee C: Train-of-four fade and edrophonium antagonism of neuromuscular block by succinylcholine in man. *Anesth Analg* 1976; 55:663–667.

35. Ali HH, Savarese JJ, Lebowitz PW, et al: Twitch, tetanus and train-of-four as indices of recovery from nondepolarizing neuromuscular blockade. *Anesthesiology* 1981; 54:294–297.

36. Waud BE, Waud DR: The relation between tetanic fade and receptor oc-

clusion in the presence of competitive neuromuscular block. *Anesthesiology* 1971; 35:456–464.

37. Kopman AF, Epstein RH, Flashburg MH: Use of 100-Hertz tetanus as an index of recovery from pancuronium-induced nondepolarizing neuromuscular blockade. *Anesth Analg* 1982; 61:439–441.

38. d'Hollander AA, Duvaldestin P, Delcroix C, et al: Evolution of single twitch and train-of-four responses and of tetanic fade in relation to plasma concentrations of fazadinium in man. *Anesth Analg* 1982; 61:225–230.

39. Stanec A, Heyduk J, Stanec G, et al: Tetanic fade and post-tetanic tension in the absence of neuromuscular blocking agents in anesthetized man. *Anesth Analg* 1978; 57:102–107.

40. Fogdall RP, Miller RD: Neuromuscular effects of enflurane, alone and combined with d-tubocurarine, pancuronium, and succinylcholine, in man. *Anesthesiology* 1975; 42:173–178.

41. Miller RD, Eger EI II, Way WL, et al: Comparative neuromuscular effects of Forane and halothane alone and in combination with d-tubocurarine in man. *Anesthesiology* 1971; 35:38–42.

42. Ali HH, Utting JE, Gray TC: Quantitative assessment of residual antidepolarizing block: I. *Br J Anaesth* 1971; 43:473–476.

43. Lee C, Katz RL: Neuromuscular pharmacology: A clinical update and commentary. *Br J Anaesth* 1980; 52:173–188.

44. Waud BE, Waud DR: The relation between the response to "train-of-four" stimulation and receptor occlusion during competitive neuromuscular block. *Anesthesiology* 1972; 37:413–416.

45. Williams NE, Webb SN, Calvey TN: Differential effects of myoneural blocking drugs on neuromuscular transmission. *Br J Anaesth* 1980; 52:1111–1115.

46. Pearce AC, Casson WR, Jones M: Factors affecting train-of-four fade. *Br J Anaesth* 1985; 57:602–606.

47. Robbins R, Donati F, Bevan DR, et al: Differential effects of myoneural blocking drugs on neuromuscular transmission in infants. *Br J Anaesth* 1984; 56:1095–1099.

48. Mylrea KC, Hameroff SR, Calkins JM, et al: Evaluation of peripheral nerve stimulators and relationship to possible errors in assessing neuromuscular blockade. *Anesthesiology* 1984; 60:464–466.

49. Viby-Mogensen J, Hansen PH, Jorgensen BC, et al: A new nerve stimulator (Myotest). *Br J Anaesth* 1980; 52:547–550.

50. Drummond GB, Wright ADJ: A new multifunction nerve stimulator. *Anaesthesia* 1982; 37:842–846.

51. Viby-Mogensen J: Clinical measurement of neuromuscular function: An update. *Clin Anaesthesiol* 1985; 3:467–482.

52. Kopman AF: A safe surface electrode for peripheral nerve stimulation. *Anesthesiology* 1976; 44:343–345.

53. Kopman AF: The relationship between evoked electromyographic and

mechanical responses following atracurium in humans. *Anesthesiology* 1985; 63:208–211.

54. Stiffel P, Hameroff SR, Blitt CD, et al: Variability in assessment of neuromuscular blockade. *Anesthesiology* 1980; 52:436–437.

55. Caffrey RR, Warren ML, Becker KE: Neuromuscular blockade monitoring comparing the orbicularis oculi and adductor pollicis muscles. *Anesthesiology* 1986; 65:95–97.

56. Donati F, Antzaka C, Bevan DR: Potency of pancuronium at the diaphragm and the adductor pollicis in humans. *Anesthesiology* 1986; 65:1–5.

57. Chauvin M, Lebreault C, Duvaldestin P: The neuromuscular blocking effect of vecuronium on human diaphragm. *Anesth Analg* 1987; 66:117–122.

58. Wright ADG, Drummond GB: A technique for comparison of two muscle sites during neuromuscular block. *Br J Anaesth* 1983; 55:1164P.

59. Moorthy SS, Hilgenberg JC: Resistance to non-depolarizing muscle relaxants in paretic upper extremities of patients with residual hemiplegia. *Anesth Analg* 1980; 59:624–627.

60. Graham DH: Monitoring neuromuscular block may be unreliable in patients with upper motor-neuron lesions. *Anesthesiology* 1980; 52:74–75.

61. Shayevitz JR, Matteo RS: Decreased sensitivity to metocurine in patients with upper motoneuron disease. *Anesth Analg* 1985; 64:767–772.

62. Nemazie AS, Kitz RJ: A quantitative technique for the evaluation of peripheral neuromuscular blockade in man. *Anesthesiology* 1967; 28:215–217.

63. Walts LF, Lebowitz M, Dillon JB: A means of recording force of thumb adduction. *Anesthesiology* 1968; 29:1054–1055.

64. Karis JP, Burton LW, Karis JH: A quantitative neuromuscular blockade monitor. *Anesth Analg* 1980; 59:308–310.

65. Stanec A, Stanec G: The adductor pollicis monitor: Apparatus and method for the quantitative measurement of the isometric contraction of the adductor pollicis muscle. *Anesth Analg* 1983; 62:602–605.

66. Viby-Mogensen J, Jensen NH, Engbaek J, et al: Tactile and visual evaluation of the response to train-of-four stimulation. *Anesthesiology* 1985; 63:440–443.

67. Lam HS, Morgan DL, Lampard DG: Derivation of reliable electromyograms and their relation to tension in mammalian skeletal muscles during synchronous stimulation. *Electroencephalogr Clin Neurophysiol* 1979; 46:72–80.

68. Pugh ND, Kay B, Healy TEJ: Electromyography in anaesthesia: A comparison between two methods. *Anaesthesia* 1984; 39:574–577.

69. Lam HS, Cass NM, Ng KC: Electromyographic monitoring of neuromuscular block. *Br J Anaesth* 1981; 53:1351–1357.

70. Shanks CA, Jarvis JE: Electromyographic and mechanical twitch responses following suxamethonium administration. *Anaesth Intensive Care* 1980; 8:341–344.

71. Donati F, Bevan DR: Muscle electromechanical correlations during succinylcholine infusion. *Anesth Analg* 1984; 63:891–894.

72. Bencini A, Newton DEF: Rate of onset of good intubating conditions, respiratory depression and hand muscle paralysis after vecuronium. *Br J Anaesth* 1984; 56:959–965.

73. Curran MJ, Donati F, Bevan DR: Onset and recovery of atracurium and suxamethonium-induced neuromuscular blockade with simultaneous train-of-four and single twitch stimulation. *Br J Anaesth* 1987; 59:989–994.

74. Katz RL: Clinical neuromuscular pharmacology of pancuronium. *Anesthesiology* 1971; 34:550–556.

75. Rupp SM, McChristian JW, Miller RD, et al: Neostigmine and edrophonium antagonism of varying intensity neuromuscular blockade induced by atracurium, pancuronium, or vecuronium. *Anesthesiology* 1986; 64:711–717.

76. Viby-Mogensen J, Howardy-Hansen P, Chraemmer-Jorgensen B, et al: Posttetanic count (PTC): A new method of evaluating an intense nondepolarizing neuromuscular blockade. *Anesthesiology* 1981; 55:458–461.

77. Viby-Mogensen J: Clinical assessment of neuromuscular transmission. *Br J Anaesth* 1982; 54:209–223.

78. Ali HH, Utting JE, Gray TE: Quantitative assessment of residual antidepolarizing block: II. *Br J Anaesth* 1971; 43:478–485.

4

Pharmacodynamic Principles

Drugs produce a dose-dependent effect that is usually mediated through an interaction between the drug molecule and a receptor. Muscle relaxants, which are effective at the neuromuscular junction, are no exception. Thus, it is important to characterize the relationship between drug concentration in the vicinity of the receptor and receptor occupancy. Unfortunately, neither of these two variables is easy to measure, especially in anesthetized humans, so indirect estimates must be made.

It is almost impossible to measure the concentration of a relaxant drug at the neuromuscular junction. However, it is reasonable to assume, under certain conditions, that the concentration near the receptor is in dynamic equilibrium with the medium perfusing it. This medium is a bath containing a known concentration of drug during in vitro experiments, or blood in the case of patients. Thus, provided that there is no significant net movement of drug to or away from the neuromuscular junction, plasma concentrations of a relaxant drug may be taken as a reasonable estimate of the concentration at the effector site. In the absence of a reliable assay, it may be assumed that for a relatively homogeneous group of patients, the maximum concentration at the effector site is related directly to the dose given. Therefore, the dose given is often substituted for the concentration at the effector site in the description of pharmacokinetic properties of the drug.

In most if not all circumstances, it is not possible to measure receptor occupancy. In the case of the acetylcholine receptor in skeletal muscle, it is easier to measure the effect of receptor occupancy, i.e., the degree of depolarization produced either by the administration of a known quantity of agonist or by nerve stimulation. However, these experiments can be performed only in vitro. In the clinical setting, the effect measured is the consequence of depolarization, which is either the contractile force or the electromyographic activity associated with muscle activity. This measurement is directly related, but in a nonlinear fashion, to the degree of membrane depolarization because it is the macroscopic result of multiple all-or-none phenomena occurring at each end-plate.

Strictly speaking, pharmacodynamics are restricted to drug-receptor interactions and deal with the relationship between receptor occupancy and drug concentration. However, it is both more practical and more meaningful to express drug concentration at the effector site in terms of dose, and receptor occupancy in terms of neuromuscular block produced. This process generates dose-response relationships, at the core of which lies the interaction between the drug molecule and the receptor.

AGONIST-RECEPTOR INTERACTIONS

Interactions Involving One Molecule

An agonist can be defined as an agent that, when bound to a receptor, produces an effect. Acetylcholine and succinylcholine are agonists at the neuromuscular junction because the doughnut-shaped receptor opens in response to them, causing a change in membrane potential. The simplest interaction between a drug and a receptor occurs when only one agonist molecule binds to the receptor and when the affinity of the drug for the receptor is independent of the drug concentration or the number of receptors bound. In this circumstance, the following reversible reaction takes place:

$$D + R \rightleftharpoons DR, \qquad (4.1)$$

where D represents a drug molecule, R a receptor, and DR, a drug-receptor complex. In this context, the drug-receptor relationship is described by

$$[D][R] = K_d[DR], \qquad (4.2)$$

where [D] denotes the concentration of the drug; [R], the concentration of free receptors; [DR], the concentration of receptors bound to the drug; and K_d the dissociation constant.[1-5] Knowing that the number of free receptors,

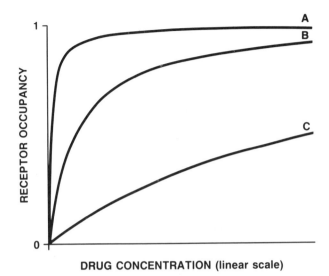

FIG 4–1.
Receptor occupancy vs. dose, according to the Clarke model, for three drugs *(A,B,C)* whose potencies vary by a factor of 10.

$$[R] = R_t - [DR], \tag{4.3}$$

where R_t represents the total number of receptors, equation 4.2 can be rearranged to yield

$$\frac{[DR]}{R_t} = \frac{[D]}{[D] + K_d} \tag{4.4}$$

where $[DR]/R_t$ represents the fraction of receptors occupied by the drug. The dissociation constant has the units of concentration and represents the concentration of drug at which 50% of the receptors are occupied.[2–4]

If the fraction of occupied receptors is plotted against concentration of drug, a curve tending asymptotically toward 1 is obtained (Fig 4–1). This representation is not very useful, especially if several drugs whose potency may vary manyfold are compared. Thus it is more common to plot the fraction of receptors occupied vs. the logarithm of the dose, in which case a sigmoid relationship is obtained. Between 20% and 80% receptor occupancy, the curve is reasonably linear. If several drugs with different potencies are compared, the curves are parallel and can be shown on the same graph (Fig 4–2).

Both sides of equation 4.2 can be divided by the number of free receptors [R]:

$$[D] = K_d[DR]/[R]$$

Dividing again by K_d,

$$[DR]/[R] = [D]/K_d$$

Taking the logarithm on both sides, one gets

$$\log([DR]/[R]) = \log([D]/K_d)$$

which is equivalent to

$$\log([DR]/[R]) = \log[D] - \log K_d \qquad (4.5)$$

which indicates that the logarithm of ratio of drug-bound receptors to free receptors is linearly related to the logarithm of the dose. This straight line can be represented graphically and is referred to as a Hill plot[6] (Fig 4–3). Calculating the logarithm of the ratio of free to bound receptors is also referred to as taking its "logit" transformation.[4] The logit scale runs from minus infinity to plus infinity.

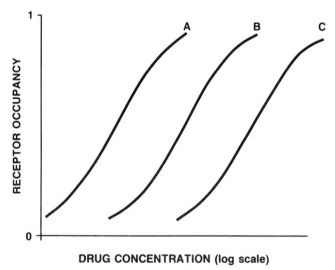

FIG 4–2.
Receptor occupancy vs. dose, on log scale, for the same drugs as Figure 4–1.

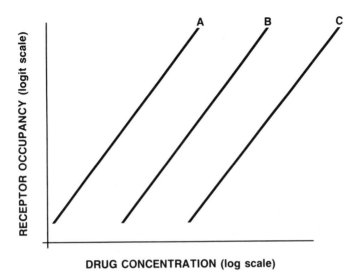

FIG 4–3.
Ratio of occupied to unoccupied receptors, on a logit scale, vs. dose, on log scale (Hill plot), for the same drugs as in Figure 4–1.

The above model predicts that 50% receptor occupancy will occur at a drug concentration K_d. If this concentration is doubled, two thirds of the receptors will be occupied. At four times K_d, 80% of the receptors are bound with the drug, and at 10 times K_d, 91% receptor occupancy is attained.

Probit (or probability) scales are also used in dose-response studies. They are based on the probability that a receptor will be occupied at a given dose, and the scale is arranged in such a way as to give equal weight to each standard deviation unit. For example, the difference between the mean (50%) and one standard deviation above the mean (84%) has a value of one on the probit scale, and the difference between one standard deviation above the mean (84%) and two standard deviations above the mean (97.5%) also has a value of one. This transformation effectively "stretches" the scale in the vicinity of 0% and 100%. In practice, there is little difference between the results expressed by their logit or probit transformations.[4]

Interactions Involving Two Molecules

When two agonist molecules bind to the same receptor, the reaction is

$$2 D + R \rightleftharpoons D_2R \qquad (4.6)$$

where D_2R represents a drug-receptor complex containing two drug molecules. In this case, equations 4.2 and 4.5 are modified slightly to become

$$[D]^2[R] = K_d[D_2R] \tag{4.7}$$

and

$$\log\{[D_2R]/(R_t - [D_2R])\} = 2 \log [D] - \log (K_d) \tag{4.8}$$

where $[D_2R]$ is the number of receptors occupied by two molecules of agonist, and $R_t - [D_2R]$ represents the number of receptors occupied by fewer than two molecules.[4] In other words, the logarithm of the ratio of the number of receptors occupied by two molecules of agonist to the number of receptors occupied by fewer than two molecules of agonist is proportional to the logarithm of the drug concentration, and the slope of this relationship is 2 (Fig 4–4). In this case, 50% receptor occupancy corresponds to a concentration equal to the square root of K_d. Doubling the drug concentration will produce an 80% receptor occupancy, and doubling it again will cause the proportion of receptors bound to two molecules of agonist to increase to 94%. Thus, receptor occupancy changes much more rapidly to an increase of agonist concentration in the case of two than one molecule binding to one receptor. Equation 4.7 can be generalized to any number (n) of agonist molecules, the slope, also called the Hill coefficient, being equal to n.

The simple model described above predicts that the Hill coefficient can only be an integer and its slope numerically equal to the number of agonist molecules binding to one receptor. However, if some cooperativity exists, that is, if binding increases the tendency for more binding, the Hill coefficient increases and may take a noninteger value.[2, 7]

Acetylcholine Dose-Response Curves

Receptor occupancy is difficult to measure, and it is more practical to measure an effect that is directly proportional to receptor occupancy. The current across the membrane with voltage being kept artificially constant (voltage clamp experiments) is probably directly proportional to the number of open channels and, therefore, to the number of drug-receptor complexes. Such an experiment has been conducted in a number of preparations[8, 9] (Fig 4–5). The slope of the Hill plot is between 1.5 and 2.9.[7] Because of the experimental error involved in these experiments, the results can be regarded as supporting the hypothesis

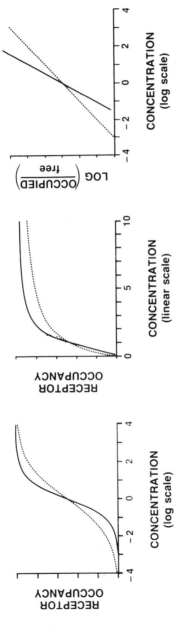

FIG 4–4.
Receptor occupancy vs. log dose *(left)*, receptor occupancy vs. dose (linear scale) *(middle)*, and Hill plot *(right)* in case of two agonist molecules for each receptor. The case for one molecule interaction is shown as dashed lines.

that two acetylcholine molecules must bind to the receptor for the channel to open.

However, the Hill coefficient was found to vary slightly with changing conditions such as pH and temperature,[7] and these findings are compatible with the presence of some cooperativity or with a different affinity of the two receptor subunits binding to acetylcholine.

EFFECTS OF ANTAGONISTS

Antagonists bind to the receptor but do not produce any effect and thus prevent agonist action. If the interaction of both antagonist and agonist is competitive, the inhibiting effect of the antagonist can be overridden by increasing the dose of the agonist. The net effect is a shift of the receptor occupancy-concentration relationship to the right (Fig 4–6). However, if the interaction between antagonist and receptor

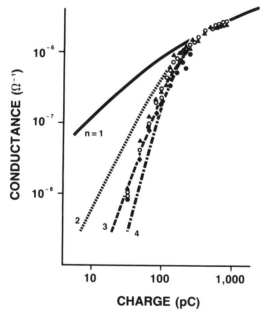

FIG 4–5.
Acetylcholine dose-response curve at the frog neuromuscular junction. These results were obtained by applying an acetylcholine-filled microelectrode close to the neuromuscular junction, applying a varying current for a short time (pipette charge), and measuring the peak current across the membrane. Experimental data are consistent with a Hill coefficient of 3. (From Dreyer F, Peper K: Density and dose-response curve of acetylcholine receptors in frog neuromuscular junction. *Nature* 1975; 253:641–643. Used by permission.)

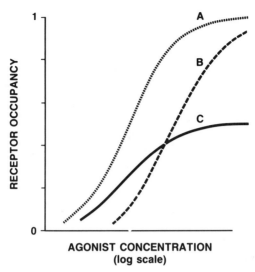

FIG 4–6.
Receptor occupancy by agonist vs. concentration in the absence of antagonist *(A)* and in the presence of a competitive *(B)* and noncompetitive antagonist *(C)*.

is of the noncompetitive type, the presence of antagonist limits the number of receptors available to bind with the agonist (see Fig 4–6). Most of the interactions between nondepolarizing muscle relaxants and acetylcholine at the neuromuscular junction are thought to be competitive.[10, 11]

During competitive interaction, the antagonist drug binds to the receptor in much the same way as the agonist:

$$A + R \rightleftharpoons AR \tag{4.9}$$

where A represents the antagonist. The dissociation constant for the antagonist is defined as

$$K_a = [A][R]/[AR] \tag{4.10}$$

When both agonist and antagonist are present, it can be shown that the fraction of receptors occupied by the agonist is[4]

$$[DR]/R_t = [D]/\{[D] + K_d(1 + [A]/K_a)\} \tag{4.11}$$

In other words, the presence of a concentration [A] of antagonist causes an increase of the apparent dissociation constant of the agonist by a factor $(1 + [A]/K_a)$. Thus, the dose-response of the agonist is shifted to the right, depending on the concentration of the antagonist [A] and its affinity for the receptor (see Fig 4–6).

Usually, the effects of antagonists are expressed as a shift in the concentration-response curve of the agonist produced by a certain concentration of antagonist. In the case of the neuromuscular junction, this approach is not practical: it is usually more convenient to vary the antagonist (relaxant) concentration rather than the agonist (acetylcholine) concentration. The proportion of receptors $[AR]/[R_t]$ occupied by the antagonist when a concentration [D] of agonist is present is expressed by an equation which has the same form as equation 4.11:

$$[AR]/[R_t] = [A]/\{[A] + K_a(1 + [D]/K_d)\} \qquad (4.12)$$

If the effect of the agonist is proportional to receptor occupancy, $[AR]/[R_t]$ represents inhibition of effect. At low agonist concentrations, the dose of antagonist that produces 50% inhibition is close to the antagonist dissociation constant K_a.[4]

NERVE STIMULATION

So far, it has been assumed that the measured effect was directly proportional to receptor occupancy. This assumption is not valid in the clinical setting where either force of contraction or electromyographic activity is measured. At the cellular level, the degree of depolarization, which depends directly on the number of open channels, results in either a full contraction or a subthreshold depolarization. A muscle contains a large number of such cells, and the force of contraction that results from supramaximal nerve stimulation depends directly on the number of units in which depolarization exceeds threshold.[12]

It follows that depression of twitch height in a muscle depends on the variability between its end-plates and not on a graded response at the cellular level. Consequently, if one assumes the sensitivity of end-plates to be normally distributed, the probit (or probability scale) is the most suitable in the description of dose-response relationships. However, probit and logit transformations yield very similar results, and either may be used in practice.[4, 13]

The arcsine transformation of the response is sometimes used in the construction of dose-response curves.[13–15] As with probit and logit transformations, it expands the scale at both extremes (close to 0% and 100%). However, it assigns a finite value to 0% and 100% points, which neither probit nor logit transformations do.[13, 16] Thus, dose-response relationships established with the use of arcsine transformations yield results comparable to logit or probit transformations unless there are values outside the range of 5% to 95%. In fact, if all points are in the range of 20% to 80%, the relationship between response and the logarithm of the dose is sufficiently linear to preclude the need for any mathematical transformation (see Fig 4–2).

The dependence of response on end-plate variability has another consequence: the numerical value of the slope of concentration-response or dose-response curves is not necessarily equal to the number of receptor sites occupied by the antagonist molecule. It also depends on the range of receptor occupancy values over which neuromuscular block occurs (Fig 4–7). Animal experiments suggest that this range is rather narrow. Using receptor-occlusion techniques, the transition from 0% to 100% single twitch depression has been estimated to occur when receptor occupancy changes from approximately 75% to 92%.[17–19] This explains why concentration-response or dose-response curves for relaxants are steep.

If only one molecule of relaxant can bind to the acetylcholine receptor, one can show from equation 4.5 that a change from 75% to 92% occupancy occurs with a 3.3-fold increase in relaxant concentration.

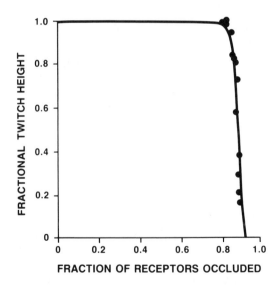

FIG 4–7.
Twitch height vs. fraction of receptors occupied in cat tibialis anterior muscle.[20] Receptor occupancy by antagonist and neuromuscular blockade vs. antagonist concentration. The range of concentrations over which neuromuscular blockade occurs is much narrower than that over which receptor occupancy occurs because no effect results from receptor occupancy less than 75%.

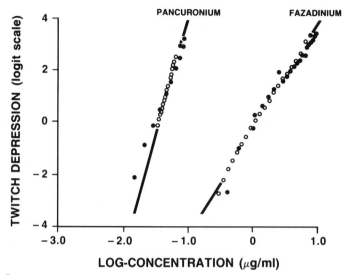

FIG 4–8.
Concentration-response curves for pancuronium and fazadinium. The logit transformation of twitch height depression is shown against the logarithm of the concentration. The slopes are not parallel. (From Hull CJ, English MJM, Sibbald A: Fazadinium and pancuronium: A pharmacodynamic study. *Br J Anaesth* 1980; 52:1209–1221. Used by permission.)

Thus, if this is the range of detectable neuromuscular blockade, a change from 0% to 100% paralysis can be effected by increasing relaxant concentration by a factor of 3.3.[20] However, if the relaxant molecule can bind with equal affinity to any of the two subunits that have the capability to accept the acetylcholine molecule, a 75% receptor occupancy will occur if only 50% of each of the subunits is bound, and 92% occupancy of the receptor will be the result of a 71% occupancy of the subunits. Thus, a 2.5-fold increase in relaxant concentration may result in a change from no paralysis to total paralysis. There is evidence that relaxants may not have the same affinity for each of the two subunits in the acetylcholine receptor.[21, 22] This might explain, at least in part, the differences in slope between the dose-response curves of different relaxants[2] (Fig 4–8).

   The above considerations suggest that the dissociation constant K_a of a relaxant drug cannot be determined from the relationship between twitch depression and dose, even if steady state conditions are met.[2] Strictly speaking, K_a is defined as the concentration at which 50% of receptors are occupied, using a one molecule per receptor model. Therefore, K_a is not the concentration corresponding to 50% twitch depression because this occurs at 80% to 85% receptor occupancy. However, the concentration of relaxant corresponding to 50% depression of twitch height, also called EC50 (for effective concentration for 50% block) is a very useful parameter in the comparison of different drug potencies. Since surgical relaxation requires deep blockade, the EC90 and EC95 are also useful.

OTHER TYPES OF RECEPTORS AND INTERACTIONS

Receptors

The previous discussion was based on the assumption that only one type of receptor exists at the neuromuscular junction. This is difficult to reconcile with all the experimental evidence.[23, 24] It appears that presynaptic receptors are responsible for the control of acetylcholine output from the nerve terminal.[25] Theoretically, these receptors could function in the same way as postsynaptic receptors, but their sensitivity to relaxants might be greater.[26] Presynaptic receptors are thought to be responsible for train-of-four and tetanic fade that is observed following repetitive stimulation in the presence of nondepolarizing relaxants. This, however, does not rule out the influence of presynaptic action on dose-response relationships for single twitch height.

Types of Interactions

When an agent interacts with the receptor in a competitive manner, it is assumed that the reaction between drug and receptor is reversible, that the drug may be displaced by a large concentration of either agonist or antagonist, and that unbinding leaves both drug and receptor unchanged. These conditions are probably not true under all circumstances at the neuromuscular junction. A noncompetitive type of block may occur when a drug blocks open channels.[5, 26, 27] This reaction cannot be reversed by an antagonist, and the rate of binding is proportional to the number of open channels, i.e., it is a use-dependent reaction. Also, the receptor might be changed after binding to an agonist, and a desensitized state might exist for some time after dissociation of the molecule with the receptor. Finally, some molecules may alter the relationship between agonist and receptor indirectly by changing the ionic or lipid environment of the receptor.[26] These types of interactions are more difficult to describe mathematically than the usual competitive interaction. The relative role of noncompetitive interactions at the neuromuscular junction is unknown. However, the excellent correlation between experimental data and theory based on competitive interactions suggests that the role of noncompetitive channel blockade is minor.

Transient Effects

Dose-response relationships describe the interaction of a drug with a receptor at equilibrium. Such a state is not reached until there are as many drug-receptor complexes unbinding as there are drug molecules binding with free receptors. Thus, the time to reach equilibrium depends on the rate of drug association with and dissociation from the receptor. If a step increase in agonist or antagonist concentration occurs in the vicinity of the neuromuscular junction, the equilibrium is reached exponentially at a rate that depends on the association constant, the drug concentration, and the dissociation constant.[2] If the drug concentration decreases to zero in an instantaneous fashion, the proportion of receptors occupied will decrease exponentially at a rate that depends exclusively on the dissociation constant.[2] It appears that the offset halftimes at the receptor level for d-tubocurarine are no greater than a few seconds,[2, 28, 29] and the onset halftimes might even be shorter.[29] In the rat hemidiaphragm preparation, recovery from either pancuronium or succinylcholine neuromuscular blockade occurred at similar rates (1 to 2 minutes), which were dependent on drug washout.[30] These results indicate strongly that the termination of relaxant action is not dependent on its rate of dissociation from the receptor. Similarly, the rate of association to the receptor does not appear to be the limiting factor in the onset time of relaxant drugs.

Access to the Neuromuscular Junction

The drug concentration at the acetylcholine receptor of the neuromuscular junction does not normally change abruptly, except in the case of acetylcholine release from the nerve terminal. Following the injection of a drug, many factors determine the time delay until stable concentrations are achieved near the receptor. These factors are (1) blood flow to the neuromuscular junction, which affects the rate of delivery of the drug to the effector site; (2) the rate of diffusion from the intravascular compartment to the vicinity of the receptor; and (3) the extent of specific and nonspecific binding in muscle tissue, which represents the amount of drug required to saturate the target tissues.[31]

If a concentration of drug C_a is delivered to an organ, the change in tissue concentrations of drug is described[32] by

$$\frac{dC_t}{dt} = (C_a - C_t)F/\lambda \qquad (4.12)$$

where C_a and C_t are arterial and tissue drug concentrations, respectively, λ is the partition coefficient of the drug, and F is the perfusion of the tissue. The expression dC_t/dt represents the change in tissue concentration with time. This equation is analogous to that used for inhalational agents. It assumes that the drug concentration in the organ is in equilibrium with venous blood draining it. If the arterial concentration of drug is held constant, and if the partition coefficient does not change with drug concentration, the solution for this differential equation would be

$$C_t = C_a(1 - e^{-(F/\lambda)t}) \qquad (4.13)$$

The concentration of drug in tissue reaches arterial concentration asymptotically, with a time constant of λ/F. In other words, an equilibrium will be reached more rapidly if either organ perfusion is large or the partition coefficient is small. The partition coefficient of relaxants in muscle tissue is relatively small. These drugs are ionized and do not have access to the intracellular compartment. Thus, in the absence of protein binding, the muscle-to-plasma partition coefficient would be determined by the size of the extracellular fluid volume compared with total muscle volume, in the range 0.2 to 0.4.[33, 34]

The muscle-to-plasma partition coefficient is increased if extensive binding occurs in muscle tissue and decreased if significant binding occurs in plasma. The amount of plasma protein binding for relaxants is not extensive,[80] and no large error is likely to be made by assuming that all relaxant is free in the plasma.

Binding of relaxant occurs at the neuromuscular junction, and some nonspecific binding may also occur at other sites in muscle tissue. When radiolabeled d-tubocurarine is injected into an animal, most of the radioactivity is later found in a narrow band of muscle that coincides with the anatomical location of the neuromuscular junction, suggesting that little binding takes place in nonjunctional areas.[35] However, the concentration of receptors at the junction is so great that at 50% receptor occupancy, it has been estimated that only 1 out of 300 d-tubocurarine molecules is free.[29] The free drug fraction is expected to be even smaller in the case of more potent drugs such as pancuronium and vecuronium. However, the size of the synaptic cleft is negligible compared with the volume of distribution of the drug in the body, so that at equilibrium only a small portion of the total dose of relaxant is actually bound to acetylcholine receptors at the neuromuscular junction. If one assumes no binding to either plasma or tissue, the partition coefficient of relaxant drugs, which are ionized molecules and do not penetrate cells, is about 0.3, that is, the ratio of extracellular water to total body water. For a muscle blood flow at rest of 5 ml/100 gm of tissue per minute, the halftime for drug access to the neuromuscular junction can be calculated to be approximately 4 minutes. This corresponds to calculations obtained from experimental data with d-tubocurarine (4.7 to 7.9 minutes),[33, 36] pancuronium (3.3 minutes),[37] vecuronium (3.7 minutes),[38, 39] and atracurium (6.9 minutes).[40]

ONSET AND OFFSET OF NEUROMUSCULAR BLOCKADE

Diffusion to and From the Neuromuscular Junction

At the molecular level, the rates of association with and dissociation from the receptor are extremely rapid. However, this assumes that drug molecules have ready access to the synaptic cleft. It has been estimated that d-tubocurarine can diffuse in and out of the cleft in 1 msec.[41] However, more time must be required to diffuse from the intravascular space into the cleft. In addition, the neuromuscular junction has a very high concentration of receptors, most of which must be bound to relaxant molecules for neuromuscular blockade to be detected. Because of this "sink" effect of the neuromuscular junction, no blockade can be detected until a large number of relaxant molecules have gained access to the active site. Considering that for each free relaxant molecule in the synaptic cleft, a few hundred or thousand molecules are bound, it is conceivable that equilibrium might not be reached for as long as a few seconds.[2, 29] This time delay is likely to be more important for potent drugs because of the small number of molecules available to bind to the same number of receptors. This might explain why the time from injection until the first sign of neuromuscular blockade increases with drug potency (fazadinium<d-tubocurarine<pancuronium).[42] Also, the artery-to-muscle latency times observed by Minsaas and Stovner[43] were directly related to potency (pancuronium: 32 seconds; d-tubocurarine: 21 seconds, and fazadinium: 9 seconds). Nevertheless, the time delays involved are small compared with the time to maximum neuromuscular blockade for nondepolarizing relaxants.

It has been suggested that the time to onset of neuromuscular blockade might be related to molecular weight.[44] One would expect that diffusion of small molecules from the intravascular space to the synaptic cleft would be faster. However, this effect, which modifies an effect that is small already, is expected to have little influence on overall onset time.

Role of Blood Flow

Whereas diffusion is complete within a few seconds, the relaxant drug caried via the bloodstream takes a few minutes to equilibrate with the muscle tissue (see above). Therefore, blood flow appears to be a determinant factor in the onset time of relaxants. The onset of action of gallamine was found to be delayed markedly by a decrease in blood flow to the muscle tested (Fig 4–9).[45] Similarly, the time from injection to maximum succinylcholine blockade correlated strongly with arm-to-arm circulation time (Fig 4–10).[46] However, the duration of action of the long-acting relaxant gallamine was unrelated to muscle blood flow,[45] indicating that recovery is governed mainly by the rate of decrease of plasma concentrations of relaxant.

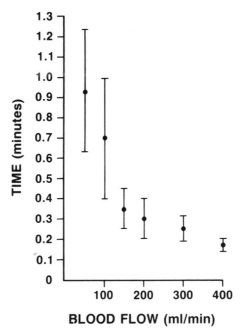

FIG 4–9.
Dependence of onset time on muscle blood flow after injection of gallamine (From Goat VA, Yeung ML, Blakeney C, et al: The effect of blood flow upon the activity of gallamine triethiodide. *Br J Anaesth* 1976; 48:69. Used by permission.)

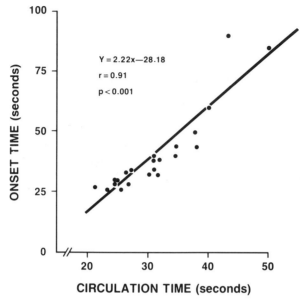

FIG 4–10.
Relationship between succinycholine onset time and circulation time in surgical patients
(From Harrison GA, Junius F: The effect of circulation time on the neuromuscular action of
suxamethonium. *Anaesth Intensive Care* 1972; 1:33–40. Used by permission.)

Dose

During onset of neuromuscular blockade, the time required to
achieve a submaximal degree of receptor occupancy depends mainly
on the number of relaxant molecules delivered to the neuromuscular
junction. By increasing the dose given, the number of molecules delivered also increases, neuromuscular blockade occurs faster, and maximum receptor occupancy is more intense. However, the time required
to reach maximum receptor occupancy is unaltered by increasing the
dose because the administration of a high dose does not change the
rate of the processes (blood flow, diffusion) that control the onset time.
It follows that, for doses producing less than 100% blockade, the time
to maximum effect is independent of the dose. However, time to minimum blockade is reduced considerably if the dose given produces total
paralysis (Fig 4–11)[47] because the receptor occupancy corresponding
to 100% blockade will be reached before maximal receptor occupancy
is attained.

Recovery

Theoretically, the rate of dissociation of the relaxant from the receptor, the diffusion of the drug away from the neuromuscular junction, and the perfusion of the neuromuscular junction have some influence on recovery. However, the rate of recovery is usually limited by the presence of a very small concentration gradient of relaxant between neuromuscular junction and plasma, the latter being determined by the relatively slow elimination of the drug.[31] Theoretically, the role of plasma concentration on the termination of action of relaxant drugs can be eliminated by the "isolated arm technique." This involves the intravenous administration of a small dose of relaxant in an arm isolated from the rest of the circulation by a cuff inflated above arterial pressure.[48] The recovery index, i.e., the time from 25% to 75% recovery of twitch height, was found to be 9 to 15 minutes for most of the relaxants tested.[48, 49] For pancuronium, the mean recovery index was 23 minutes after a bolus injection, compared with only 10 minutes with the isolated arm.[49] As expected, the plasma concentrations were considerably less in the latter case. It follows that, at least in the case of long acting drugs, the rate of decrease of plasma concentrations is the major determinant of the duration of action of relaxants. Therefore, it is not surprising to find that blood flow has very little effect on recovery from gallamine[45] or pancuronium[50] blockade.

There has been some dispute regarding the role of blood flow in

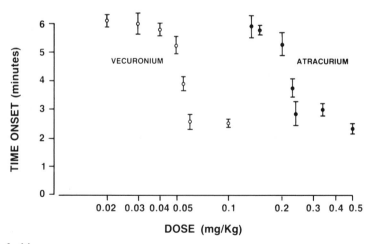

FIG 4–11.
Relationship between onset time and dose of atracurium and vecuronium (From Healy TEJ, Pugh ND, Kay B, et al: Atracurium and vecuronium: Effect of dose on time of onset. *Br J Anaesth* 1986; 58:620–624. Used by permission.)

the interpretation of isolated arm experiments. The theoretical calculations suggest that blood flow alone could produce recovery indices ranging from 4[51] to 9[52] minutes. The discrepancy hinges on the estimates of plasma concentrations after tourniquet release, the drug concentrations corresponding to 25% and 75% twitch height, and the estimate of muscle time constant. Nevertheless, in the absence of more reliable data, one could conclude that blood flow plays a major role in the termination of action in the isolated arm experiment, and no other factor could be identified.

If the elimination of the drug is very rapid, as is the case for succinylcholine, plasma concentrations of the drug fall so rapidly that the time from injection to maximum receptor occupancy is shortened, compared with longer-acting relaxants. Thus, its onset of action is shortened. Because of its rapid breakdown in plasma, which can take place near the neuromuscular junction, termination of effect of succinylcholine does not depend on washout of the drug from muscle. Thus recovery rate is more rapid (time from 10% to 90% recovery of 2 to 4 minutes[53, 54]) than for nondepolarizing relaxants during the isolated arm experiments. In patients with abnormal pseudocholinesterase who eliminate the drug slowly, both onset and recovery times are prolonged.[55]

PLASMA CONCENTRATIONS

It is normally impossible to measure the concentration of drug at the neuromuscular junction. However, plasma concentrations can be measured more easily. Therefore, one can obtain the relationship between concentration and effect only when there is no concentration gradient between the neuromuscular junction and plasma. This occurs when (1) maximum blockade is reached after administration of a bolus dose or (2) during a constant infusion, when neuromuscular blockade is stable. In the latter case, there is constant equilibrium between plasma and effector site, and in the first case, maximum blockade occurs when no net transfer of drug occurs between plasma and neuromuscular junction, that is, when the concentration of drug is equal at both sites. During recovery, the plasma concentrations are close to the concentrations at the effector site provided that the elimination of the drug is long compared with the rate of washout at the neuromuscular junction. Even in the case of long-acting relaxants such as pancuronium, the plasma concentrations are smaller, at an identical degree of blockade, than those prevailing during a constant infusion.[49] The discrepancy is probably even greater in the case of faster acting relaxants. For vecuronium, concentrations corresponding to 50% block were determined either with a constant infusion,[38] or after administration of a bolus dose but correcting for the rate of washout from the neuromuscular junction.[39, 56, 57]

Within the limitations of the assay, it is then possible to measure the plasma concentration at equilibrium, corresponding to a given degree of block. A concentration yielding 50%, 90%, and 95% blockade can be determined (these are called $C_{pss}50$, $C_{pss}90$, and $C_{pss}95$, respectively, and are referred to as plasma concentrations at steady state). Theoretically, potency ratios between relaxants can be obtained from comparisons of $C_{pss}50$ values. However, the assays based on different techniques performed in different laboratories yield results that may not be comparable. For example, the $C_{pss}50$ of atracurium evaluated by Ward and Wright[58] is 0.29 μg/ml, much lower than that reported by Weatherley and co-workers[40] (0.652 μg/ml).

DOSE-RESPONSE RELATIONSHIPS

Measuring plasma concentrations is cumbersome, often difficult, and expensive. However, in every patient, there is a direct relationship between plasma concentration and dose given, and dose is measured much more easily. This relationship is determined by the volume into which a dose is distributed, which can be obtained by pharmacokinetic analysis. Provided that a relatively homogeneous population is chosen, whose individuals have approximately the same relationship between dose and concentration, dose can be taken as a measure of concentration, and the relationship between effect and dose can be established. This is the most common way of investigating the potency of muscle relaxants in clinical practice, and such a relationship has been measured for most available relaxants (Fig 4–12). Using appropriate logit or probit transformations of twitch height (see section on nerve stimulation), effective doses expected to produce 50%, 90%, and 95% blockade can be evaluated (ED50, ED90, ED95).[80]

The standard method to obtain dose-response curves is to administer a certain number (3 to 6) of predetermined doses randomly to a group of patients, each patient receiving a single dose. This method has two drawbacks: the treatment of 0% and 100% twitch depression is difficult on probit or logit scales,[16] and a large number of patients is required. These problems are largely avoided if a "cumulative" method is used. This consists in the administration of incremental doses of the relaxant when neuromuscular blockade is stable until 100% paralysis is attained[59] (Fig 4–13). The accuracy of the method depends on two

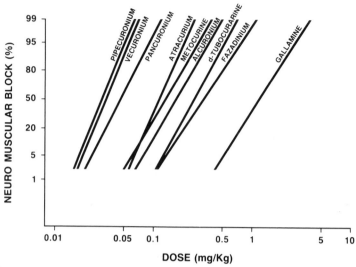

FIG 4–12.

Dose-response curves for the nondepolarizing agents. The potency of relaxants depends on many factors, such as the background anesthetic, the population studied, and the geographic site of the study. Therefore, this graph should be taken as a rough guide only. (From Bevan DR: Neuromuscular blocking drugs. *Can Anaesth Soc J* 1983; 30:556–561. Used by permission.)

GALLAMINE
CUMULATIVE DOSE RESPONSE STUDY

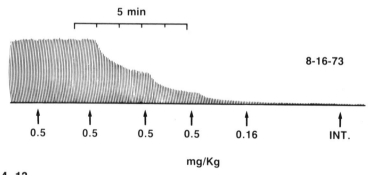

FIG 4–13.

Administration of cumulative doses of gallamine. (From Donlon JV, Savarese JJ, Ali HH, et al: Human dose-response curves for neuromuscular blocking drugs: A comparison of two methods of construction and analysis. *Anesthesiology* 1980; 53:161–166. Used by permission.)

major assumptions: the effect of relaxants is concentration-dependent only, as a given dose given in increments will yield the same result as if all the drug had been given in a single bolus, and little elimination occurs during the period of administration. For long-acting relaxants, the cumulative technique has been shown to yield results very similar to the single-dose technique[60] (Fig 4–14). Shorter-acting drugs, such as vecuronium and atracurium, tend to have lower apparent potencies with the cumulative technique as compared with the single-bolus method.[14, 15, 61]

FACTORS AFFECTING DOSE-RESPONSE RELATIONSHIPS

The sensitivity of otherwise comparable individuals to the same dose of muscle relaxant may vary markedly. For example, a dose of 0.1 mg/kg of d-tubocurarine or atracurium may produce as little as 0% or as much as 100% neuromuscular blockade.[62, 63] This wide interindividual variability is due in part to the dispersion of kinetic parameters and to the varying sensitivity of the acetylcholine receptor at the neuromuscular junction. It is also the consequence of the narrow spectrum of concentrations over which detectable neuromuscular blockade occurs.[65]

Age can also modify the pharmacodynamics of relaxants. For example, neonates have a lower $C_{pss}50$ for d-tubocurarine[64] and vecuronium[39] than adults. However, the volume of distribution of these relaxants, which corresponds to the extracellular water volume, is larger on a milliliter-per-kilogram basis in neonates.[39, 64] The net effect is that neonates require approximately the same milligram per kilogram dose as older individuals. In the elderly, the concentration or dose of pancuronium required for a given degree of neuromuscular blockade was not significantly different from that in younger adults.[66]

Many drugs affect the response to nondepolarizing relaxants. The previous administration of an intubating dose of succinylcholine shifts the dose-response curve to the left, i.e., the nondepolarizing relaxants are more potent.[67–69] The administration of mixtures of relaxants, such as pancuronium and d-tubocurarine, or pancuronium and metocurine, results in more profound neuromuscular blockade than each individual drug given alone.[70] The inhalational agents enflurane, isoflurane, and halothane also potentiate the effect of d-tubocurarine,[71, 72] pancuronium,[71, 72] vecuronium,[73] and atracurium[74, 75] in a dose-dependent manner. Although the exact mechanism for these interactions is unknown, it appears that all these agents do not modify the distribution of the relaxants but affect their interactions with the receptors at the neuromuscular junction.[76–78]

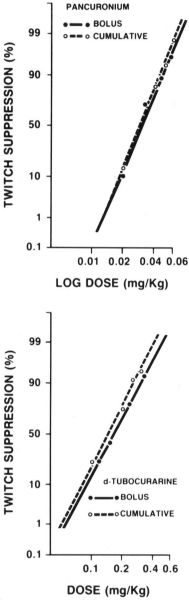

FIG 4–14.

Comparison of pancuronium and d-tubocurarine dose-response curves obtained by the single-bolus *(solid lines)* and cumulative *(dashed lines)* method. (From Donlon JV, Savarese JJ, Ali HH, et al: Human dose-response curves for neuromuscular blocking drugs: A comparison of two methods of construction and analysis. *Anesthesiology* 1980; 53:161–166. Used by permission.)

REFERENCES

1. Clark AJ: *The Mode of Action of Drugs on Cells*. London, Edward Arnold, 1923.
2. Hull CJ: Pharmacodynamics of non-depolarizing neuromuscular blocking agents. *Br J Anaesth* 1982; 54:169–182.
3. Wood AJJ: Drug receptor interactions, in Wood M, Wood AJJ (eds): *Drugs and Anesthesia: Pharmacology for Anesthesiologists*. Baltimore, Williams & Wilkins Co, 1982, pp 77–96.
4. Norman J: Drug receptor reaction, in Prys-Roberts C, Hug CC (eds): *Pharmacokinetics of Anaesthesia*. Oxford, Blackwell Scientific Publications, 1984, pp 25–37.
5. Rang HP: Drugs and ionic channels: Mechanisms and implications. *Postgrad Med J* 1981; 57(suppl 1):89–97.
6. Hill AV: The possible effect of aggregation of the molecules of haemoglobin on its dissociation curves. *J Physiol Lond* 1910; 40:190.
7. Peper K, Bradley RJ, Dreyer F: The acetylcholine receptor at the neuromuscular junction. *Physiol Rev* 1982; 62:1271–1340.
8. Dreyer F, Peper K, Sterz R: Determination of dose-response curves by quantitative ionophoresis at the frog neuromuscular junction. *J Physiol Lond* 1978; 281:395–419.
9. Dionne VE, Steinbach JH, Stevens CF: An analysis of the dose-response relationship at voltage clamped frog neuromuscular junctions. *J Physiol Lond* 1978; 281:421–444.
10. Durant NN: The physiology of neuromuscular transmission. *Semin Anesth* 1984; 3:262–274.
11. Magleby KL, Pallotta BS, Terrar DA: The effect of (+)-tubocurarine on neuromuscular transmission during repetitive stimulation in the rat, mouse, and frog. *J Physiol* 1981; 312:97–113.
12. Ali HH, Savares JJ: Monitoring of the neuromuscular junction. *Anesthesiology* 1976; 45:216–249.
13. Armitage P: *Statistical Methods in Medical Research*. Oxford, Blackwell Scientific Publications, 1971.
14. Gibson FM, Mirakhur RK, Lavery GG, et al: Potency of atracurium: A comparison of single dose and cumulative dose techniques. *Anesthesiology* 1985; 62:657–659.
15. Gibson FM, Mirakhur RK, Clark RSJ, et al: Comparison of cumulative and single bolus dose techniques for determining the potency of vecuronium. *Br J Anaesth* 1985; 57:1060–1062.
16. Litchfield JT, Wilcoxon F: A simplified method of evaluating dose-effect experiments. *J Pharmacol Exp Ther* 1949; 96:99–113.
17. Paton WDM, Waud DR: The margin of safety of neuromuscular transmission. *J Physiol* 1967; 191:59–90.
18. Waud BE, Waud DR: The margin of safety of neuromuscular transmission in the muscle of the diaphragm. *Anesthesiology* 1972; 37:417–422.

19. Waud BE, Waud DR: The relation between tetanic fade and receptor occlusion in the presence of competitive neuromuscular block. *Anesthesiology* 1971; 35:456–464.

20. Waud BE: Neuromuscular blocking agents, in Gallagher TJ (ed): *Advances in Anesthesia*. Chicago, Year Book Medical Publishers, 1984, pp 337–382.

21. Weiland G, Taylor P: Ligand specificity and state transitions in the cholinergic receptor: Behavior of agonists and antagonists. *Mol Pharmacol* 1979; 15:197–212.

22. Sine SM, Taylor P: Relationship between reversible antagonist occupancy and the functional capacity of the acetylcholine receptor. *J Biol Chem* 1981; 256:6692–6699.

23. Bowman WC: Prejunctional and postjunctional cholinoceptors at the neuromuscular junction. *Anesth Analg* 1980; 59:935–943.

24. Bowman WC, Marshall IG, Gibb AJ: Is there feedback control of transmitter release at the neuromuscular junction? *Semin Anesth* 1984; 4:275–283.

25. Sokoll MD, Dretchen KL, Gergis S, et al: *d*-Tubocurarine effects on nerve-terminal and neuromuscular conduction. *Anesthesiology* 1972; 36:592–597.

26. Dreyer F: Acetylcholine receptor. *Br J Anaesth* 1982; 54:115–130.

27. Trautmann A: Curare can open and block ionic channels associated with cholinergic receptors. *Nature* 1982; 298:272–275.

28. Waud DR: The rate of action of competitive neuromuscular blocking agents. *J Pharmacol Exp Ther* 1967; 158:99–114.

29. Armstrong DL, Lester HA: The kinetics of d-tubocurarine action and restricted diffusion within the synaptic cleft. *J Physiol* 1979; 294:365–386.

30. Bartkowski RR: Recovery of neuromuscular function in the perfused rat diaphragm after succinylcholine and pancuronium blockade. *Anesthesiology* 1983; 58:409–413.

31. Hennis PJ, Stanski DR: Pharmacokinetic and pharmacodynamic factors that govern the clinical use of muscle relaxants. *Semin Anesth* 1985; 4:21–30.

32. Eger EI II: *Anesthetic Uptake and Action*. Baltimore, Williams & Wilkins, 1975.

33. Stanski DR, Ham J, Miller RD, et al: Pharmacokinetics and pharmacodynamics of *d*-tubocurarine during nitrous oxide-narcotic and halothane anesthesia in man. *Anesthesiology* 1979; 51:235–241.

34. Cohen EN, Corbascio A, Fleischli G: The distribution and fate of d-tubocurarine. *J Pharmacol Exp Ther* 1965; 147:120–129.

35. Waser PG: Molecular basis of curare action, in Katz RL (ed): *Muscle Relaxants*. New York, Elsevier North-Holland, Inc, 1975, pp 102–123.

36. Stanski DR, Ham J, Miller RD, et al: Time-dependent increase in sensitivity to *d*-tubocurarine during enflurane anesthesia in man. *Anesthesiology* 1980; 52:483–487.

37. Hull CJ, English MJM, Sibbald A: Fazadinium and pancuronium: A pharmacodynamic study. *Br J Anaesth* 1980; 52:1209–1221.
38. Van der Veen F, Bencini A: Pharmacokinetics and pharmacodynamics of ORG NC 45 in man. *Br J Anaesth* 1980; 52:37S–41S.
39. Fisher DM, Castagnoli K, Miller RD: Vecuronium kinetics and dynamics in anesthetized infants and children. *Clin Pharmacol Ther* 1985; 37:402–406.
40. Weatherley BC, Williams SG, Neill EAM: Pharmacokinetics, pharmacodynamics and dose-response relationships of atracurium administered i.v. *Br J Anaesth* 1983; 551(suppl 1): 39S–45S.
41. Eccles JC, Jaeger JC: The relationship between the mode of operation and the dimension of the junctional regions at synapses and motor end-organs. *Proc R Soc Lond B* 1958; 148:38.
42. Blackburn CL, Morgan M: Comparison of speed of onset of fazadinium, tubocurarine and suxamethonium. *Br J Anaesth* 1978; 50:361–364.
43. Minsaas B, Stovner J: Artery-to-muscle onset time for neuromuscular blocking drugs. *Br J Anaesth* 1980; 52:403–407.
44. Ramzan IM: Molecular weight of cation as a determinant of speed of onset of neuromuscular blockade. *Anesthesiology* 1982; 57:247–248.
45. Goat VA, Yeung ML, Blakeney C, et al: The effect of blood flow upon the activity of gallamine triethiodide. *Br J Anaesth* 1976; 48:69–73.
46. Harrison GA, Junius F: The effect of circulation time on the neuromuscular action of suxamethonium. *Anaesth Intensive Care* 1972; 1:33–40.
47. Healy TEJ, Pugh ND, Kay B, et al: Atracurium and vecuronium: Effect of dose on time of onset. *Br J Anaesth* 1986; 58:620–624.
48. Feldman SA, Tyrrell MF: A new theory of the termination of action of the muscle relaxants. *Proc R Soc Med* 1970; 63:692–695.
49. Agoston S, Feldman SA, Miller RD: Plasma concentrations of pancuronium and neuromuscular blockade after injection into the isolated arm, bolus injection, and continuous infusion. *Anesthesiology* 1979; 51:119–122.
50. Heneghan CPH, Findley IL, Gillbe CE, et al: Muscle blood flow and rate of recovery from pancuronium neuromuscular blockade in dogs. *Br J Anaesth* 1978; 50:1105–1108.
51. Kopman AF: More on pharmacokinetics and dynamics of muscle relaxants, letter. *Anesthesiology* 1980; 52:454–455.
52. Stanski DR, Sheiner LB: More on the pharmacokinetics and dynamics of muscle relaxants, reply. *Anesthesiology* 1980; 52:456–457.
53. Walts LF, Dillon JB: Clinical studies with succinylcholine chloride. *Anesthesiology* 1967; 28:372–376.
54. Katz RL, Ryan JF: The neuromuscular effects of suxamethonium in man. *Br J Anaesth* 1969; 41:381–390.
55. Cass NM, Doolan LA, Gutteridge GA: Repeated administration of suxamethonium in a patient with atypical cholinesterase. *Anaesth Intensive Care* 1982; 10:25–28.

56. Cronnelly R, Fisher DM, Miller RD, et al: Pharmacokinetics and pharmacodynamics of vecuronium (ORG NC45) and pancuronium in anesthetized patients. *Anesthesiology* 1983; 58:405–408.
57. Sohn YJ, Bencini AF, Scaf AHJ, et al: Comparative pharmacokinetics and dynamics of vecuronium and pancuronium in anesthetized patients. *Anesth Analg* 1986; 65:233–239.
58. Ward S, Wright D: Combined pharmacokinetic and pharmacodynamic study of a single bolus dose of atracurium. *Br J Anaesth* 1983; 55:35S–38S.
59. Donlon JV, Ali HH, Savarese JJ: A new approach to the study of four nondepolarizing relaxants in man. *Anesth Analg* 1974; 53:934–939.
60. Donlon JV, Savarese JJ, Ali HH, et al: Human dose-response curves for neuromuscular blocking drugs: A comparison of two methods of construction and analysis. *Anesthesiology* 1980; 53:161–166.
61. Fisher DM, Fahey MR, Cronnelly R, et al: Potency determination for vecuronium (ORG NC45): Comparison of cumulative and single-dose techniques. *Anesthesiology* 1982; 57:309–310.
62. Katz RL: Neuromuscular effects of d-tubocurarine, edrophonium and neostigmine in man. *Anesthesiology* 1967; 28:327–336.
63. Katz RL, Stirt J, Murray AL, et al: Neuromuscular effects of atracurium in man. *Anesth Analg* 1982; 61:730–734.
64. Fisher DM, O'Keeffe C, Stanski DR, et al: Pharmacokinetics and pharmacodynamics of d-tubocurarine in infants, children, and adults. *Anesthesiology* 1982; 57:203–208.
65. Matteo RS, Spector S, Horowitz PE: Relation of serum d-tubocurarine concentration to neuromuscular blockade in man. *Anesthesiology* 1974; 41:440–443.
66. Duvaldestin P, Saada J, Berger JL, et al: Pharmacokinetics, pharmacodynamics, and dose-response relationships of pancuronium in control and elderly subjects. *Anesthesiology* 1982; 56:36–40.
67. Katz RL: Modification of the action of pancuronium by succinylcholine and halothane. *Anesthesiology* 1971; 35:602–606.
68. Krieg N, Hendrickx HHL, Crul JF: Influence of suxamethonium on the potency of ORG NC 45 in anesthetized patients. *Br J Anaesth* 1981; 53:259–262.
69. Stirt JA, Katz RL, Murray AL, et al: Modification of atracurium blockade by halothane and by suxamethonium. *Br J Anaesth* 1983; 55:71S–75S.
70. Lebowitz PW, Ramsey FM, Savarese JJ, et al: Potentiation of neuromuscular blockade in man produced by combinations of pancuronium and metocurine or pancuronium and d-tubocurarine. *Anesth Analg* 1980; 59:604–609.
71. Miller RD, Way WL, Dolan WM, et al: The dependence of pancuronium- and d-tubocurarine-induced neuromuscular blockades on alveolar concentrations of halothane and Forane. *Anesthesiology* 1972; 37:573–581.
72. Fogdall RP, Miller RD: Neuromuscular effects of enflurane, alone and combined with d-tubocurarine, pancuronium, and succinylcholine in man. *Anesthesiology* 1975; 42:173–178.

73. Rupp SM, Miller RD, Gencarelli PJ: Vecuronium-induced neuromuscular blockade during enflurane, isoflurane, and halothane anesthesia in humans. *Anesthesiology* 1984; 60:102–105.

74. Rupp SM, McChristian JW, Miller RD: Neuromuscular effects of atracurium during halothane-nitrous oxide and enflurane-nitrous oxide anesthesia in humans. *Anesthesiology* 1985; 63:16–19.

75. Brandom BW, Cook DR, Woelfel SK, et al: Atracurium infusion requirements in children during halothane, isoflurane, and narcotic anesthesia. *Anesth Analg* 1985; 64:471–476.

76. Kennedy R, Galindo A: Neuromuscular transmission in a mammalian preparation during exposure to enflurane. *Anesthesiology* 1975; 42:432–442.

77. Waud BE, Waud DR: The effects of diethyl ether, enflurane, and isoflurane at the neuromuscular junction. *Anesthesiology* 1975; 42:275–280.

78. Waud BE: Decrease in dose requirement of d-tubocurarine by volatile anesthetics. *Anesthesiology* 1979; 51:298–302.

79. Dreyer F, Peper K: Density and dose-response curve of acetylcholine receptors in frog neuromuscular junction. *Nature* 1975; 253:641–643.

80. Shanks CA: Pharmacokinetics of the nondepolarizing neuromuscular relaxants applied to the calculation of bolus and infusion dosage regimens. *Anesthesiology* 1986; 64:72–86.

5

Pharmacokinetic Principles

Muscle relaxants gain access to the body via the intravenous route. Then, the drug is distributed, redistributed, and eliminated in ways that are usually not dependent on its pharmacologic action but that vary according to the patient's characteristics. In other words, the study of pharmacokinetics is concerned with how the body handles a drug, instead of how the drug affects the body.

A description of pharmacokinetics, which entails a simplification of the intricate processes that take place in a living organism, is not possible without the help of models. A simplified representation is needed to make the mathematical formulation of the problem more manageable. However, the model can be no better than the assumptions on which it is based. Thus, all models have some limitations. In this context, it is obvious that no model will be satisfactory in all circumstances. It is more important to determine which pharmacokinetic model is best suited for the solution of a given problem rather than find the "true" pharmacokinetic parameters for a given drug.

Pharmacokinetic parameters are determined from the mathematical analysis of serial plasma samples obtained over time. Therefore, the accuracy of the determined parameters depends directly on the sensitivity and specificity of the assay and the frequency of blood sampling. Biologic variability adds another factor: the accuracy of mean parameters determined from a given population depends directly on the number of subjects involved and the degree of variability between individuals. The usefulness of a pharmacokinetic model can be assessed on the basis of its ability to predict the degree and time course of drug action.

Thus, models should not be considered as real, physical entities, but as mental "as if" representations that may not have much physical meaning.

COMPARTMENTAL ANALYSIS

One-Compartment Model

The simplest way to consider the time course of drug action in the body is to assume that the drug is distributed evenly and instantaneously into a given volume and is eliminated at a rate proportional to drug concentration (Fig 5–1). The size of the compartment is the volume of distribution (V), and the initial concentration (C_o) is[1] (Fig 5–2)

$$C_o = D/V \qquad (5.1)$$

where D is the dose given. If the rate of elimination is proportional to the concentration, then the relationship of concentration (C) vs. time (t) is described by an exponential process:

$$C = (C_o)(e^{-kt}) \qquad (5.2)$$

where k is the rate constant and t represents time. The half-life $(t_{1/2})$ is defined as the time necessary for the concentration to decrease by half:[2]

$$t_{1/2} = \ln(2)/k = 0.693/k \qquad (5.3)$$

where ln(2) is the natural logarithm (base e logarithm) of 2. Clearance

FIG 5–1.
One-compartment pharmacokinetic model. The drug is injected into a compartment of volume V and is eliminated at a rate K.

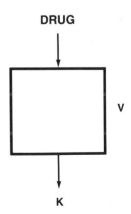

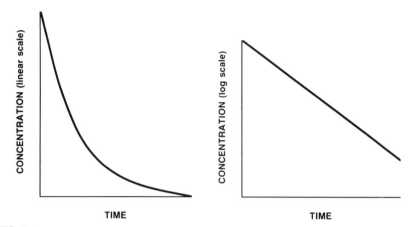

FIG 5–2.
Drug concentrations vs. time with the one-compartment model plotted on a linear scale *(left)* and on a logarithmic scale *(right)*. The elimination is an exponential process. (From Stanski DR, Watkins WD: *Drug Disposition in Anesthesia*. New York, Grune & Stratton, 1982, p 7. Used by permission.)

(Cl) is defined as the volume of plasma that is cleared of drug per unit time:[4]

$$Cl = Vk = V(0.693)/t_{1/2} \qquad (5.4)$$

Despite its simplicity, the one-compartment model provides a certain number of useful concepts. Of these, half-life is perhaps the most important clinically because it is a reflection of the duration of action of the drug, as long as effect follows plasma concentrations. The volume of the compartment determines the relationship between dose and initial concentration. Finally, clearance can provide information on the importance of the various organs of elimination in the excretion or metabolism of the drug.[3]

Two-Compartment Model

The one-compartment model is usually not adequate to describe the variations, with time, of plasma concentrations of nondepolarizing relaxants and their antagonists. The biphasic character of these concentrations (Fig 5–3) is accounted for much more accurately by a two-compartment model that involves a central and a peripheral compartment (Fig 5–4). The drug is injected into and eliminated from the central compartment. It may also diffuse into and from the peripheral compartment, depending on the direction of the concentration gradient. The rate of elimination is assumed to be proportional to the concentration in the central compartment, and the rates of diffusion between the compartments are also linearly related to the concentration gradient. The relationship between concentration and time is described by a

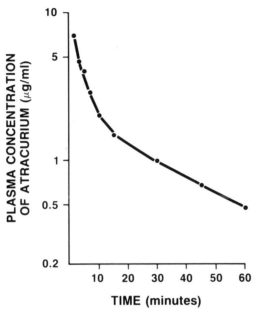

FIG 5–3.
Plasma concentrations of atracurium (log scale) plotted against time in one patient. The one-compartment model, which predicts a straight line in this case (Fig 5–4), is obviously not satisfactory. A two compartment model accounts for the data much more closely. (From Stiller RL, Brandom BW, Cook DR: Determination of atracurium in plasma by high performance liquid chromatography. *Anesth Analg* 1985; 64:58–62. Used by permission.)

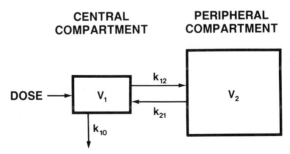

FIG 5–4.
Two compartment pharmacokinetic model. (Modified from Stanski DR, Watkins WD: *Drug Disposition in Anesthesia*. New York, Grune & Stratton, 1982, p 13.)

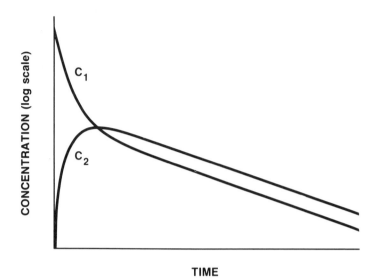

TIME

FIG 5–5.
Drug concentrations in the central (C_1) and peripheral (C_2) compartments as predicted by a two-compartment model. (From Hull CJ: General principles of pharmacokinetics, in Prys-Roberts C, Hug CC (eds): *Pharmacokinetics of Anaesthesia*. Oxford, England, Blackwell Scientific Publications, 1984, p 15. Used by permission.)

biexponential process (Fig 5–5). For the central compartment, after the injection of a single dose,[2, 4]

$$C_1 = A\ e^{-\alpha t} + B\ e^{-\beta t} \qquad (5.5)$$

and for the peripheral compartment,

$$C_2 = Q\ e^{-\alpha t} - Q\ e^{-\beta t} \qquad (5.6)$$

where A, B, and Q are constants that depend on the dose given, α is the distribution rate constant, and β is the elimination rate constant. Notice that the parameters of the model, namely the volumes of the central (V_1) and peripheral compartments (V_2), and the rate constants k_{10}, k_{12}, and k_{21} do not appear directly in equations 5.5 and 5.6. In fact, the rate constants α and β are a function of the k constants and the volumes V_1 and V_2. Thus α and β are termed hybrid rate constants.[2, 4]

Four parameters are required to characterize a two-compartment model. The volume of the central compartment (V_1), the distribution volume (V_d), the distribution half-life ($t_{1/2\alpha}$), and elimination half-life ($t_{1/2\beta}$) are used most commonly. The half-lives are related to the rate constants used in equations 5.5 and 5.6 in the following way:

$$t_{1/2\alpha} = \ln(2)/\alpha = 0.693/\alpha \qquad (5.7)$$

and

$$t_{1/2\beta} = \ln(2)/\beta = 0.693/\beta \qquad (5.8)$$

The volume of distribution is the sum of the central and peripheral volumes:

$$V_d = V_1 + V_2 \qquad (5.9)$$

At time zero, the concentration of drug (C_0) in the central compartment depends on central volume and dose (D):[3]

$$C_0 = D/V_1 \qquad (5.10)$$

Thus, an estimate of central compartment volume can be made by extrapolating the plasma concentration curve back to time zero. The volume of distribution can be estimated according to various methods.[4, 6] The most accurate of these is to measure the drug concentration at steady state when the concentrations in both central and peripheral compartments are equal. This condition is obtained by a continuous infusion of drug to compensate exactly losses by elimination, and the value obtained for the volume of distribution is referred to as V_{dss}, or "volume of distribution at steady state." It is mathematically equal to the sum of the individual compartment volumes. Another estimate of V_d (V_d^β) can be made by extrapolating the distribution phase of the central compartment concentration profile back to time zero, neglecting the distribution phase. Such a calculation, although simpler to perform, leads to an overestimate of the volume of distribution.[4, 6] This is because the concentration in the peripheral compartment is always higher than that in the central compartment during the elimination phase, whereas the calculation assumes a uniform concentration throughout. The discrepancy depends directly on the elimination rate of the drug, and volumes of distribution estimated by this method are notoriously inaccurate for short-acting drugs. A third way of estimating distribution volume is by computing the area under the plasma concentration vs. time curve ($V_{d\ area}$). This calculation is based on the definition of clearance (equation 5.4), and it assumes a homogeneous distribution of drug at all times. In fact, $V_{d\ area}$ may be closer to V_{dss} than V_d^β because the larger drug concentrations in the peripheral compartment when compared with the central compartment are at least partially compensated for by lesser concentrations during the distribution phase.

Three-Compartment Model

The three-compartment model involves a central compartment into which drug is injected and from which it is eliminated, plus two peripheral compartments (a shallow one and a deep one), which may exchange drug only with the central compartment (Fig 5–6). The relationship between plasma concentration and time is expressed with three exponentials:

$$C_1 = P\,e^{-\pi t} + A\,e^{-\alpha t} + B\,e^{-\beta t} \tag{5.11}$$

where π and α are the rapid and slow distribution rate constants, respectively, and β the elimination rate constant. These constants are inversely related to the rapid distribution, slow distribution, and elimination half-lives ($t_{1/2\pi}$, $t_{1/2\alpha}$, $t_{1/2\beta}$), respectively (Fig 5–7). The constants P, A, and B are dose-related. The principles underlying the estimation of volume of distribution discussed above also apply to the three-compartment model.

PHARMACOKINETICS OF RELAXANTS AND THEIR ANTAGONISTS

Measurement of Plasma Samples

The study of pharmacokinetics is based on the analysis of drug concentrations in plasma. Thus, a reliable, accurate, quantitative method must be developed for each relaxant studied. Radioimmunoassays[7] have been developed for d-tubocurarine[8–16] and modified for meto-

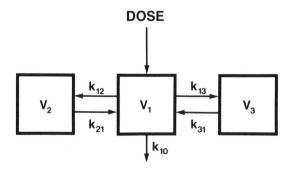

FIG 5–6.
Three-compartment pharmacokinetic model. (From Hull CJ: General principles of pharmacokinetics, in Prys-Roberts C, Hug CC (eds): *Pharmacokinetics of Anaesthesia.* Oxford, England, Blackwell Scientific Publications, 1984, p 20. Used by permission.)

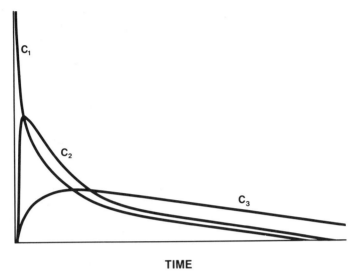

TIME

FIG 5–7.
Predicted plasma concentrations (log scale) vs. time for each of the three compartments in Figure 5–6. (From Hull CJ: General principles of pharmacokinetics, in Prys-Robert C, Hug CC (eds): *Pharmacokinetics of Anaesthesia*. Oxford, England, Blackwell Scientific Publications, 1984, p 20. Used by permission.)

curine.[16–19] Fluorimetric techniques[20] have been applied to the study of pancuronium,[21–29] vecuronium,[29, 30] fazadinium,[31–33] gallamine,[34–36] and d-tubocurarine.[37] High performance liquid chromatography is used commonly to measure atracurium concentrations,[5, 38–40, 62] but the technique has also been applied to vecuronium.[41–43] Mass spectrometry has been proposed as an alternate method for pancuronium and vecuronium.[44–45] Plasma concentration of reversal agents are usually assayed by chromatographic methods.[46–51] A summary of these analytic techniques is presented elsewhere.[52] Most of these are cumbersome and time-consuming, and this explains the relatively small number of patients in published pharmacokinetic studies.

The number and frequency of blood samples required for a certain experiment depends on the type of information sought. If an analysis of differences in elimination half-life is desired between two groups of patients, the period over which samples are obtained must be several times that of the anticipated half-life,[53] whereas frequent sampling during the distribution phase will be of little value. For example, the estimate of d-tubocurarine elimination half-life was found by Fisher et al.[13] to vary from 174 minutes in the neonatal age group to 89 minutes in the adult population. Matteo et al.[15] obtained, for the same age groups, 311 and 164 minutes, respectively. The sampling period was 4 hours in the first study and 24 hours in the second. Another example refers to the suggestion that the elimination half-life of d-tubocurarine was not increased as much as that of pancuronium in renal failure.[54] This was based on pharmacokinetic data that were obtained over 3 hours in the case of d-tubocurarine[55] and over 5 hours for pancuronium.[21] The error involved in the calculation of the elimination half-lives, which were estimated to be 2.2 and 8.1 hours, respectively, is probably too great to draw any conclusions. However, these large discrepancies in the various estimates of elimination half-life have little influence on the predictions of duration of the neuromuscular blockade and plasma concentrations during the first hour or two (Fig 5–8).

The other assumption made in the pharmacokinetic modeling is that instantaneous mixing occurs at all times in all compartments, including the central compartment, from which samples are taken. This

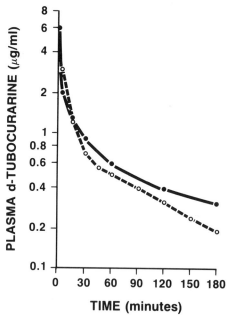

FIG 5–8.
Plasma concentrations after injection of *d*-tubocurarine, 0.3 mg/kg, as predicted by two models. The *dashed line* has an elimination half-life of 1.4 hours and the *solid line* 5.8 hours. Both predict similar times to 50% twitch height. (Adapted from Miller RD, Matteo RS, Benet LZ, et al: The pharmacokinetics of *d*-tubocurarine in man with and without renal failure. *J Pharmacol Exp Ther* 1977; 202:1–7 and Meijer DKF, Weitering JG, Vermeer GA, et al: Comparative pharmacokinetics of *d*-tubocurarine and metocurine in man. *Anesthesiology* 1979; 51:402–407.)

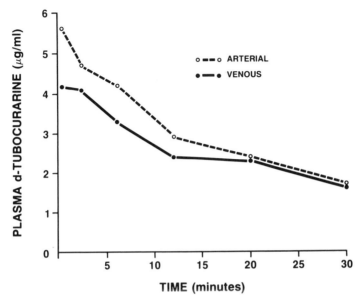

FIG 5–9.
Arterial and peripheral venous concentrations after injection of *d*-tubocurarine, 0.22 mg/kg.

assumption is probably adequate when there are small changes in plasma concentrations, such as during the elimination phase of most relaxants, when a pseudoequilibrium exists. However, after the injection of a bolus dose, the arterial concentrations of d-tubocurarine were found to exceed the peripheral venous concentrations for at least 15 minutes[56] (Fig 5–9). This occurs because the rapid uptake of the drug by tissues may introduce marked differences between arterial and venous concentrations and between venous concentrations sampled at different sites in the body. For this reason, it is probably preferable to take arterial samples. Central venous samples, although mixed, are expected to yield lower concentrations than arterial samples. Another approach is to infuse the drug over 5 to 10 minutes, which decreases arteriovenous differences, and take peripheral venous blood. The importance of these methodological differences has not been studied, but it is expected that only kinetic parameters pertaining to the rapid distribution phase of the drug would be affected.

Comparison of Results

Comparisons of pharmacokinetic data obtained with different assays, different frequency and number of samples, and different compartmental models should be made with extreme caution. A thorough analysis of the factors that may modify the estimates of the various parameters is necessary to interpret pharmacokinetic data correctly.

The calculation of central and distribution volumes is a function of the accurate determination of both dose and concentration. Of these, concentration is most difficult to measure accurately, and a systematic error could lead to gross errors in the determination of central or distribution volumes. Most nondepolarizing muscle relaxants have a volume of distribution in the range 0.2 to 0.3 L/kg (Table 5–1), which is approximately equal to the extracellular fluid volume in humans. This observation is consistent with the physical properties of relaxants, which are ionized molecules that do not penetrate cell membranes well. Exceptions to this rule include tubocurarine and metocurine, which have a volume of distribution that exceeds extracellular fluid volume. This might be due to extensive drug binding to connective tissue and ground substances composed of mucopolysaccharides.[1] If plasma sampling is continued for 96 hours, the volume of distribution of d-tubocurarine is very high (3.36 L/kg).[11] On the other hand, atracurium has a volume of distribution that is lower than that of extracellular volume. This may be the result of the assumptions made in the two compartmental model. All drug is assumed to be eliminated via the central compartment, and this may not be the case for atracurium, which undergoes spontaneous degradation through the Hofmann reaction. It can be shown that a model that does not allow for elimination of the drug in the peripheral compartment can account for the time course of the plasma concentrations. However, the calculated volume of distribution would be spuriously low, compared with a model that allows peripheral elimination of the drug (Fig 5–10).[58]

The estimation of the elimination half-life is not affected by systematic errors in the analysis of plasma concentrations. For instance, if all measured values are 50% larger than true values, the calculated volume of distribution would be altered markedly, but the half-lives would remain unchanged. However, other factors affect the estimate of elimination half-life, such as the accuracy of low concentration values, the model chosen, and the timing of blood samples. Essentially, elimination half-life is determined from the slope of the terminal portion of the log plasma concentration curve. It follows that an error of, say, 10 ng/ml will be more important on the smallest than the largest values. Also, accuracy increases if either the number of samples or the duration of sampling or both are increased. Finally, estimates of half-lives are model-dependent: Using the same data, elimination half-lives are longer if a model using a larger number of compartments is used. For example,

TABLE 5–1.
Volume of Distribution of Nondepolarizing Relaxants in Normal Adults

DRUG	VOLUME OF DISTRIBUTION, L/KG	REFERENCE
d-Tubocurarine	0.387	Meijer et al.[57]
	0.96	Martyn et al.[14]
	0.29	Stanski et al.[10]
	0.292	Ham et al.[12]
	0.472	Brotheton and Matteo[18]
	0.65	Ramzan et al.[37]
	0.375	Matteo et al.[15]
	0.470	Matteo et al.[16]
	0.425	Matteo et al.[17]
	0.42	Matteo el al.[11]
	0.3	Fisher et al.[13]
Metocurine	0.422	Miller et al.[55]
	0.446	Matteo et al.[17]
	0.513	Matteo et al.[16]
Pancuronium	0.148	McLeod et al.[21]
	0.338	Somogyi et al.[23]
	0.275	Duvaldestin et al.[28]
	0.339	Somogyi et al.[22]
	0.130	Hull et al.[32]
	0.480	Sohn et al.[29]
	0.261	Somogyi et al.[88]
	0.284	Westra et al.[89]
Gallamine	0.210	Ramzan et al.[34]
	0.207	Ramzan et al.[35]
	0.291	Shanks et al.[36]
Fazadinium	0.287	Duvaldestin et al.[33]
	0.234	Duvaldestin et al.[31]
	0.187	Hull et al.[32]
Alcuronium	0.400	Walker et al.[74]
Atracurium	0.157	Ward et al.[39]
	0.159	Ward and Neill[40]
	0.182	Fahey et al.[62]
Vecuronium	0.246	Lebreault et al.[30]
	0.179	Van der Veen and Bencini[43]
	0.194	Fahey et al.[42]
	0.270	Cronnelly et al.[44]
	0.246	Sohn et al.[29]
	0.247	Lebreault et al.[60]
	0.510	Bencini et al.[95]

Matteo and co-workers[11] found, using data from the same individuals, that the terminal half-life of *d*-tubocurarine was 166 minutes with a three-model compartment and as high as 40 hours with a four-compartment model.[11] Table 5–2 lists the mean elimination half-lives obtained for nondepolarizing relaxants, the number of compartments in the model, and the period of sampling.

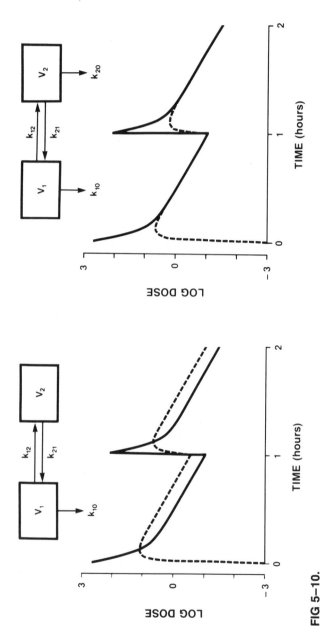

FIG 5–10.
Central (*solid lines*) and peripheral (*dashed lines*) compartment atracurium concentrations based on atracurium pharmaco-kinetic data. Type A model (*left*) involves elimination from the central compartment only. In type B model (*right*), elimination can also take place from the peripheral compartment. Both models give absolutely indistinguishable plasma concentration profiles. However, the volume of distribution is greater for type B (0.23 L/kg vs. 0.13 L/kg for type A). (From Hull CJ: A model for atracurium?, editorial. *Br J Anaesth* 1983; 55:95–96. Used by permission.)

Because of these methodological limitations, it appears futile to attach much importance to the differences reported for the long-acting nondepolarizing relaxants. Pancuronium, gallamine, d-tubocurarine, metocurine, and alcuronium all have similar elimination half-lives and similar volumes of distribution. They also have similar clearances, in the 1 to 2–ml/kg/minute range.[61] These clearance values are approximately equal to the glomerular filtration rate in normal patients, and renal excretion is a major route of drug disposition for all these relaxants. It follows that relaxants with shorter duration of action cannot depend on the kidney for their excretion. Vecuronium has a clearance of 3 to 5 ml/kg/minute[28–30, 42, 44, 45] and must depend more on the liver for its excretion. Indeed, its clearance is reduced in patients with cirrhosis[30] and cholestasis.[60] The clearance of atracurium is in the range of 5 to 7 ml/kg/minute,[39, 40, 62] a consequence of its metabolism by plasma esterases and its spontaneous degradation through the Hofmann elimination.[63, 64] Although organ elimination remains a possibility,[65] the elimination half-life of atracurium is not altered significantly by renal[62] or hepatic[40] failure.

Reversal Agents

Although less attention has been directed to the pharmacokinetics of the reversal agents, the data suggest little difference between edrophonium, pyridostigmine, and neostigmine. All three drugs have larger volumes of distribution (0.5 to 1.2 L/kg) and larger clearances (8 to 10 ml/kg/minute) than the long-acting nondepolarizing relaxants.[48–51, 66–70] They are characterized by a very important and rapid distribution phase, which implies that the plasma concentrations obtained immediately after injection of the drug are much greater than those during the elimination phase (Fig 5–11). It follows that the estimates of elimination half-lives are consistently lower in studies involving a short sampling period. For example, the elimination half-life of neostigmine was found to be 15 to 30 minutes in patients whose plasma was sampled for 60 minutes,[67] and 67 to 80 minutes in studies involving a 240-minute sampling period.[48–50] Similarly, the elimination half-life of edrophonium has been evaluated to be 33 minutes[68] and 114 minutes[69] for 60- and 240-minute sampling periods, respectively. For pyridostigmine, values of 46[51] and 112[70] minutes have been reported for identical sampling periods, indicating that other factors, such as the assay technique or the method of drug administration (bolus vs. 2-minute infusion) might affect the results.

TABLE 5–2.
Elimination Half-Lives Obtained for Nondepolarizing Relaxants in Normal Adults

DRUG	ELIMINATION HALF-LIFE, MIN	COMPARTMENT, NO.	SAMPLING TIME, MIN	REFERENCE
d-Tubocurarine	107	2	?	Stanski et al.[10]
	103	2	?	Stanski et al.[59]
	76	2	240	Ham et al.[12]
	372	2	1,440	Martyn et al.[14]
	89	2	240	Fisher et al.[13]
	164	3	1,440	Matteo et al.[15]
	173	3	1,440	Matteo et al.[17]
	190	3	2,880	Matteo et al.[16]
	347	3	720	Meijer et al.[57]
	166	3	360	Matteo et al.[11]
	2400	4	5,760	Matteo et al.[11]
Metocurine	360	3	360	Brotherton and Matteo[18]
	345	3	2,880	Matteo et al.[16]
	216	3	720	Meijer et al.[57]
Pancuronium	100	2	120	Hull et al.[32]
	107	2	1,440	Duvaldestin et al.[28]
	132	2	480	Somogyi et al.[23]
	86	2	300	McLeod et al.[21]
	133	2	360	Somogyi et al.[88]
	141	2	480	Westra et al.[89]
	140	3	480	Cronnelly et al.[44]
	190	3	300	Sohn et al.[29]
Gallamine	135	2	600	Ramzan et al.[35]
	247	3	720	Shanks et al.[36]
Fazadinium	42	2	120	Hull et al.[32]
	76	2	300	Duvaldestin et al.[31]
	82	2	360	Duvaldestin et al.[33]

Drug				Reference
Alcuronium	200	2	720	Cronnelly et al.[70]
Atracurium	21	2	180	Ward and Neill[40]
	20	2	120	Ward and Neill[39]
	21	2	240	Fahey et al.[62]
Vecuronium	31	2	?	Van der Veen and Bencini[43]
	80	2	240	Fahey et al.[42]
	58	2	210	Lebreault et al.[30]
	58	2	210	Lebreault et al.[60]
	34	2	100	Bencini et al.[95]
	71	3	1,440	Cronnelly et al.[44]
	71	3	240	Fisher et al.[45]
	116	3	300	Miller et al.[29]
	117	3	300	Bencini et al.[95]

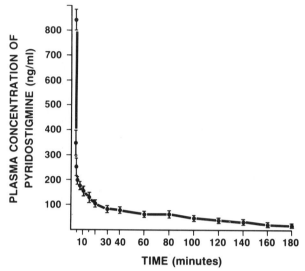

FIG 5–11.
Plasma concentration of pyridostigmine vs. time after bolus injection of 0.21 mg/kg. A marked decrease occurs during the distribution phase. (From Williams NE, Calvey TN, Chan K, et al: Plasma concentration of pyridostigmine during the antagonism of neuromuscular block. *Br J Anaesth* 1983; 55:27–31. Used by permission.)

RELATIONSHIP OF CONCENTRATION TO EFFECT

The final purpose of pharmacokinetics is to make useful predictions about the action of drugs. As long as the neuromuscular blocking effect of relaxants is related to plasma concentration, knowledge of kinetic parameters is extremely useful. This assumption is often valid during the recovery phase of relaxant action but falls short of expectations during onset.

Prediction of Recovery Times

During spontaneous recovery from neuromuscular blockade induced by long-acting nondepolarizing relaxants, a strong correlation exists between neuromuscular blockade and plasma concentration.[8, 71, 72] This occurs because the factor controlling the termination of action of relaxants is their rate of elimination, and the concentration gradient between active site and plasma is small.[27] It follows that return of neuromuscular function will occur when the plasma concentration falls below a certain threshold. After administration of a bolus dose of relaxant, the duration of action of relaxants depends on the time interval between injection and return to this critical concentration. This, in turn, depends on the dose given (Fig 5–12) and the rate of distribution and/or elimination of the drug.[75]

In the case of a one-compartment model, the rate of drug elimination is constant with time. It follows that once plasma concentrations fall below the critical level at which neuromuscular transmission is detected, recovery proceeds at the same rate, irrespective of the dose given. The same applies to the case of two- or three-compartment models, provided that recovery occurs after the distribution phase is complete. For most relaxants administered in the usual doses, detectable spontaneous recovery occurs during the elimination phase. Thus, for most nondepolarizing relaxants, the recovery index, defined as the time from 25% to 75% recovery of first twitch height, is a direct function of elimination half-life (Table 5–3). However, vecuronium does not appear to follow this pattern. Although there is considerable scatter in the various estimates of its elimination half-life (30 to 120 minutes) (see Table 5–2), the recovery index after usual doses of vecuronium is comparable to that of atracurium, with a half-life of only 20 minutes. This discrepancy is probably due to the relatively important distribution process associated with the administration of vecuronium. In the clinically useful range, recovery from vecuronium neuromuscular blockade occurs because of redistribution rather than elimination (Fig 5–13). It follows that the administration of very large doses of the drug is more likely to be associated with recoveries beyond the distribution phase and to exhibit larger recovery indices.[76] The administration of 0.28 mg/kg was found to be associated with a much greater recovery index (38 minutes) than administration of 0.1 mg/kg (8 minutes).[77] This is in contrast to atracurium recovery indices, which were found to be constant for initial doses ranging from 0.2 to 0.6 mg/kg.[78]

Prediction of Onset: The Concept of Biophase

With the two-compartment model, the drug concentration in the central compartment is greatest at time zero. Thus, if one assumes the neuromuscular junction to be in the central compartment, neuromuscular blockade would be expected to be immediate. On the other hand, if the pharmacologic site of action of relaxants were located in the peripheral compartment, maximum blockade would occur at the end of the distribution phase, a time much longer than onset times measured clinically. Thus, the time course of neuromuscular effect can be accounted for only if another compartment, called "biophase" or "effect" compartment, is added[9, 72] (Fig 5–14).

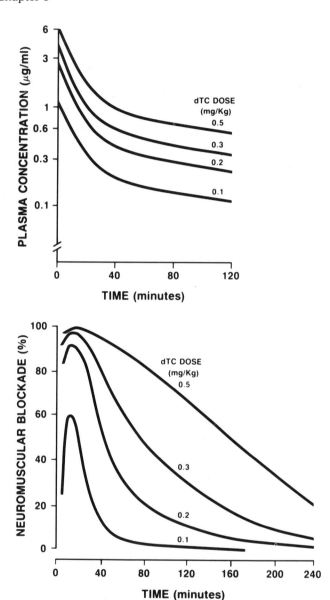

FIG 5–12.
Computer generated plasma concentration profiles *(top)* for various doses of *d*-tubocurarine
(dTC) and corresponding neuromuscular blockade *(bottom),* as a function of time. Small
doses have a rapid recovery rate, which corresponds to the distribution of the drug. At higher
doses, a slower recovery is observed because it coincides with the elimination phase (From
Hennis PJ, Stanski DR: Pharmacokinetic and pharmacodynamic factors that govern the
clinical use of muscle relaxants. *Semin Anesth* 1985. Used by permission.)

TABLE 5–3.
Comparison of Elimination Half-Lives and Recovery Index (Time From 25% to 75% Twitch Height Recovery in Normal Adults)

DRUG AND DOSE	ELIMINATION HALF-LIFE, MIN	RECOVERY INDEX, MIN	REFERENCES
d-Tubocurarine, 0.3 mg/kg	76–372	49	Matteo et al.[17]
Pancuronium, 0.04–0.1 mg/kg	86–190	24–47	Fahey et al.[77]; Katz[79]; Noeldge et al.[80]; Engbaek et al.[81]
Metocurine 0.3 mg/kg	216–360	47	Matteo et al.[17]
Atracurium, 0.2–0.6 mg/kg	20–21	11	Basta et al.[78]
Succinylcholine, 0.5–4 mg/kg	4	2	Cook et al.[73]
Vecuronium, 0.03–15 mg/kg	31–116	8–15	Fahey et al.[77]; Noeldge et al.[80]; Engbaek et al.[81]

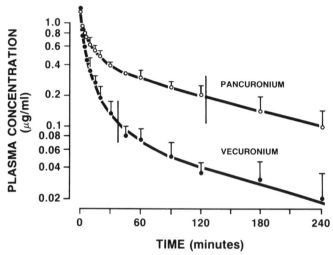

FIG 5–13.
Plasma concentrations of vecuronium and pancuronium after injection of a bolus dose of 0.1 mg/kg. Vertical bars indicate the time to return of 50% single twitch height. This occurs during the distribution phase for vecuronium and during the elimination phase for pancuronium. This might explain why spontaneous recovery is more rapid for vecuronium, in spite of an elimination half-life comparable with that of pancuronium. (From Sohn YJ, Bencini AF, Scaf AHJ, et al: Comparative pharmacokinetics and dynamics of vecuronium and pancuronium in anesthetized patients. *Anesth Analg* 1986; 65:233–239. Used by permission.)

The size of this compartment is assumed to be infinitely small, so that the quantity of drug in it is negligible. Thus, the concentrations in the other compartments are unchanged by the addition of this new compartment. In addition, the concentration of drug in the biophase compartment is directly related to effect at all times (Fig 5–15), so that the biophase concentration at a certain degree of blockade during onset is equal to that at the same degree of blockade during recovery. The addition of a biophase compartment involves the addition of another parameter, k_{13}, the biophase rate constant, which determines the rate of access to the biophase.

The biophase rate constant relating adductor pollicis blockade with pharmacokinetics is remarkably relaxant-independent. The biophase half-time, which is inversely related to the biophase rate constant, is one of the parameters that determines the time to onset of neuromuscular blockade.[75] Its value has been found to be in same range (3 to 7 minutes) for d-tubocurarine,[9, 10, 12, 13] vecuronium,[43, 45] pancuronium,[32, 72] fazadinium,[32] alcuronium,[74] and atracurium.[82] This seems to indicate that the factors that govern the onset of action of muscle relaxants are quantitatively similar for all drugs used. These are the perfusion of the neuromuscular junction, the rate of diffusion from the intravascular space into the synaptic cleft, the rate of association with the receptor, and the extent of nonspecific binding.[75] It follows that

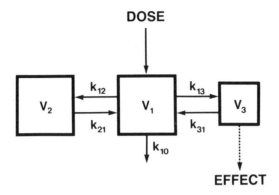

FIG 5–14.
Two-compartment model with biophase. The size of the biophase compartment (V_3) is infinitely small, and the concentration of relaxant in it is directly related to effect. (From Hull CJ, English MJM, Sibbald A: Fazadinium and pancuronium: A pharmacodynamic study. *Br J Anaesth* 1980; 52:1209–1221. Used by permission.)

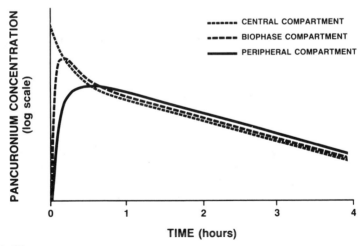

FIG 5–15.
Calculated pancuronium concentrations in the central, peripheral, and biophase compartments. During the recovery phase, biophase concentrations are very close to plasma concentrations. However, the discrepancies are large during onset. (From Hull CJ, English MJM, Sibbald A: Fazadinium and pancuronium: A pharmacodynamic study. *Br J Anaesth* 1980; 52:1209–1221. Used by permission.)

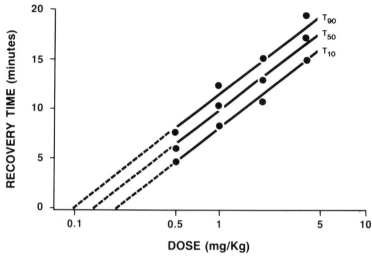

FiG 5–16.

Recovery time to 10%, 50%, and 90% twitch height vs. succinylcholine dose, on a logarithmic scale. Doubling the dose increases duration by one half-life. (From Stanski DR, Watkins DW: *Drug Disposition in Anesthesia.* New York, Grune & Stratton, 1982. Used by permission.)

equipotent doses of nondepolarizing relaxants yield comparable onset times of neuromuscular blockade. Thus, time to maximum blockade can only be reduced if the dose is increased.[75] The administration of a large dose can be accomplished safely if the drug is free from side effects and if its elimination or redistribution is rapid enough to avoid prolonged blockade.

Deriving Pharmacokinetics From Pharmacodynamics

The relationship between kinetics and dynamics can be taken one step further. When dealing with a one-compartment model, it is predicted that doubling the initial dose will shift the concentration curve to the right by one half-life[1, 73] In other words, spontaneous recovery of neuromuscular function will be delayed by one half-life. This concept has been applied to the kinetics of succinylcholine, a drug which is difficult to measure in plasma because of the rapid hydrolysis of the molecule by plasma cholinesterase. Such an analysis yields estimates of half-lives ranging from 2 minutes in children to 4 minutes in adults[73] (see Fig 5–16). For atracurium, the elimination half-life has been calculated to be 16.5 minutes from pharmacodynamic data,[83] a figure comparable with that obtained from pharmacokinetic data.

Cumulation

Once neuromuscular blockade recovers spontaneously, small doses of relaxant are usually administered to keep relaxation at a certain level. Generally, the duration of effect of the first additional dose is shorter than that of identical doses administered later. This phenomenon has been called "cumulation" and has a pharmacokinetic basis[76, 84, 85] (Fig 5–17). Linear analysis predicts that the concentrations produced by two or more doses of the same drug is the sum of the concentrations of each dose if given alone. Detailed calculations yield the following predictions: (1) cumulation occurs when the first additional dose is administered during the distribution phase, and (2) the degree of cumulation depends on the relative importance of the distribution phase[85] (see Fig 5–17). Therefore, cumulation is unlikely to occur when spontaneous recovery occurs after the distribution phase, i.e., when a large initial dose has been given. This is the case of atracurium, which has a very rapid distribution half-life (2 minutes).[86] Long-acting relaxants such as *d*-tubocurarine and pancuronium show some degree of cumulation[77, 80, 84] because the distribution phase is usually not complete after the first dose. Vecuronium is reported as exhibiting little cumulation, although distribution still takes place during spontaneous recovery from a 0.075- to 0.1-mg/kg dose.[76, 86, 87] The reason why only little cumulation was noted is unclear, but it might be related to the rather short observation time period in the studies that investigated the problem.

PHARMACOKINETIC ALTERATIONS

The mean values reported for pharmacokinetic parameters do not apply to all patients. Any condition that is associated with alterations in the volume of distribution or with interference with the function of the organs of elimination is likely to cause profound disturbances in the kinetics of muscle relaxants.

Age

The volume of extracellular fluid as a proportion of total body weight decreases markedly during the first few years of life. This decrease is matched by a similar decrease in volume of distribution of relaxants, at least for *d*-tubocurarine[13, 15] and vecuronium.[45] The infant's clearance of *d*-tubocurarine is similar,[13] or perhaps decreased,[15] com-

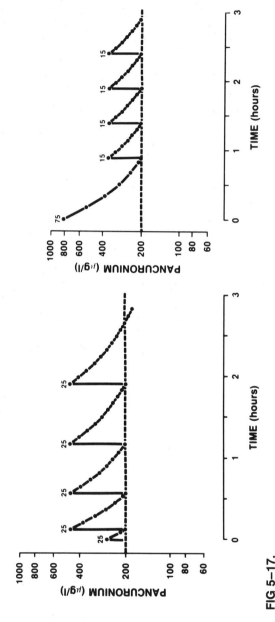

FIG 5–17.

Computed pancuronium plasma concentrations with a bolus dose followed by incremental doses when concentrations fall below 200 µg/L. The numbers indicate the size of each dose in micrograms per kilogram. Cumulation is observed *(left)* when additional doses are given during the distribution phase of the initial dose. If a large initial dose is given *(right)* additional doses will be expected to have the same duration of action (From Norman J: Pharmacokinetics of non-depolarizing muscle relaxant. *Clin Anaesthesiol* 1985; 3:273–282. Used by permission.)

pared with that of adults. This normal or lower than normal clearance associated with a larger volume of distribution provides the infant with a longer elimination half-life. This does not necessarily imply a prolonged duration of action at all doses because the presence of a large volume of distribution accentuates the effect of the distribution phase.[15] Young infants have been found to be sensitive to *d*-tubocurarine[13] and vecuronium,[45] but the increased *d*-tubocurarine sensitivity has not been confirmed in another study.[15] Data on other relaxants are lacking.

In the elderly, glomerular filtration rate[90] and liver blood flow decrease. As a result, the elimination half-life and duration of action of most relaxants is expected to increase. A notable exception is atracurium, which depends largely on spontaneous degradation and ester hydrolysis for the termination of its effect. The atracurium requirement to maintain stable blockade and the recovery index were similar in young and older adults.[91] In contrast, the vecuronium infusion required for stable blockade decreased with time in individuals aged 60 years and over, and the recovery index was markedly greater (45 minutes) than in patients younger than 40 years of age (16 minutes).[92] The elimination half-life of pancuronium[28] (Fig 5–18), *d*-tubocurarine,[17] and

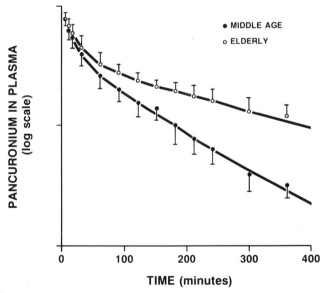

FIG 5–18.
Plasma pancuronium concentrations in middle-aged (25 to 60 years old) and elderly (>75 years old) patients. (From Duvaldestin P, Saada J, Berger LJ, et al: Pharmacokinetics, pharmacodynamics, and dose-response relationships of pancuronium on control and elderly subjects. *Anesthesiology* 1982; 56:36–40. Used by permission.)

metocurine[17] is prolonged, and clearance is decreased in the elderly. No pharmacodynamic differences have been identified in the geriatric population.[17, 28] Thus, muscle relaxation in the geriatric patient is normally achieved with the usual loading dose, followed by maintenance doses given at longer intervals than in younger individuals.

Renal Failure

The elimination half-life of all nondepolarizing relaxants, except atracurium,[62] has been found to be increased to a varying degree in renal failure. This increase is large in the case of gallamine,[93] which depends almost exclusively on the kidney for its elimination, intermediate for d-tubocurarine[55] and pancuronium,[21, 23] which also rely on metabolism and biliary excretion, and small for vecuronium,[42] which depends more on liver function for its excretion. The volume of distribution of most nondeplarizing relaxants is increased slightly in renal failure, indicating the tendency in these patients for volume overload. The reversal agents neostigmine,[48] pyridostigmine,[70] and edrophonium[69] all have prolonged elimination half-lives in patients with absent renal function. The decreases in the clearances exceed by far the glomerular filtration rate, suggesting that these drugs are secreted by the kidney.

Hepatic Disease and Biliary Obstruction

The muscle relaxants that depend on liver function for their elimination or metabolism tend to have longer elimination half-lives in patients with liver disease. Volume overload also tends to increase the volume of distribution.[94] The elimination half-lives of fazadinium,[33] pancuronium,[88, 89] and vecuronium[30, 60] were found to be increased in these patients. However, no significant alteration in the elimination half-life of atracurium[40] has been detected.

Patient Variability

The data presented above reflect the mean values obtained from a limited number of patients who are assumed to be representative of the general population. These numbers are associated with a rather large dispersion, which implies that the pharmacokinetic parameters may vary markedly from one patient to the next. Unfortunately, it is impossible to determine a priori these parameters in any given patient. Thus, the clinician should keep in mind that the response of a given patient might deviate considerably from the norm. Pharmacokinetics can help in the prediction of the range of responses to expect from a given dose. However, proper dosing tailored to suit the patient's needs requires neuromuscular monitoring.

REFERENCES

1. Stanski DR, Watkins DW: *Drug Disposition in Anesthesia.* New York, Grune & Stratton, 1982.
2. Hug CC: Pharmacokinetics of drugs administered intravenously. *Anesth Analg* 1980; 57:704–723.
3. Wood AJJ: Drug disposition and pharmacokinetics, in Wood M, Wood AJJ (eds): *Drugs and Anesthesia: Pharmacology for Anesthesiologists.* Baltimore, Williams & Wilkins Co, 1982.
4. Hull CJ: Pharmacokinetics and pharmacodynamics. *Br J Anaesth* 1979; 51:579–594.
5. Stiller RL, Brandom BW, Cook DR: Determination of atracurium in plasma by high-performance liquid chromatography. *Anesth Analg* 1985; 64:58–62.
6. Hull CJ: General principles of pharmacokinetics, in Prys-Roberts C, Hug CC (eds): *Pharmacokinetics of Anaesthesia.* Oxford, England, Blackwell Scientific Publications, 1984, pp 1–24.
7. Horowitz PE, Spector S: Determination of serum d-tubocurarine concentration by radioimmunoassay. *J Pharmacol Exp Ther* 1973; 185:94–100.
8. Matteo RS, Spector S, Horowitz PE: Relation of serum d-tubocurarine concentration to neuromuscular blockade in man. *Anesthesiology* 1974; 41:440–443.
9. Sheiner LB, Stanski DR, Vozek S, et al: Simultaneous modelling of pharmacokinetics and dynamics: Application to d-tubocurarine. *Clin Pharmacol Ther* 1979; 25:358–371.
10. Stanski DR, Ham J, Miller RD, et al: Pharmacokinetics and pharmacodynamics of d-tubocurarine during nitrous oxide-narcotic and halothane anesthesia in man. *Anesthesiology* 1979; 51:235–341.
11. Matteo RS, Nishitateno K, Pua EK, et al: Pharmacokinetics of d-tubocurarine in man: Effect of an osmotic diuretic on urinary excretion. *Anesthesiology* 1980; 52:335–338.
12. Ham J, Stanski DR, Newfield P, et al: Pharmacokinetics and dynamics of d-dubocurarine during hypothermia in humans. *Anesthesiology* 1981; 55:631–635.
13. Fisher DM, O'Keefe C, Stanski DR, et al: Pharmacokinetics and pharmacodynamics of d-tubocurarine in infants, children, and adults. *Anesthesiology* 1982; 57:203–208.
14. Martyn JAJ, Matteo RS, Greenblatt DJ, et al: Pharmacokinetics of d-tubocurarine in patients with thermal injury. *Anesth Analg* 1982; 61:241–246.

15. Matteo RS, Lieberman IG, Salanitre E, et al: Distribution, elimination, and action of d-tubocurarine in neonates, infants and children. *Anesth Analg* 1984; 63:799–804.

16. Matteo RS, Brotherton WP, Nishitateno K, et al: Pharmacodynamics and pharmacokinetics of metocurine in humans: Comparison to d-tubocurarine. *Anesthesiology* 1982; 57:183–190.

17. Matteo RS, Backus WW, McDaniel DD, et al: Pharmacokinetics and pharmacodynamics of d-tubocurarine and metocurine in the elderly. *Anesth Analg* 1985; 64:23–29.

18. Brotherton WP, Matteo RS: Pharmacokinetics and pharmacodynamics of metocurine in humans with and without renal failure. *Anesthesiology* 1981; 55:273–276.

19. Martyn JAJ, Goudsouzian NG, Matteo RS, et al: Metocurine requirements and plasma concentrations in burned paediatric patients. *Br J Anaesth* 1983; 55:263–268.

20. Kersten UW, Meijer DKF, Agoston S: Fluorimetric and chromatographic determination of pancuronium bromide and its metabolites in biological materials. *Clin Chim Acta* 1973; 44:59–66.

21. McLeod K, Watson MJ, Rawlins MD: Pharmacokinetics of pancuronium in patients with normal and impaired renal function. *Br J Anaesth* 1976; 48:341–345.

22. Somogyi AA, Shanks CA, Triggs EJ: Clinical pharmacokinetics of pancuronium bromide. *Eur J Clin Pharmacol* 1976; 10:367–372.

23. Somogyi AA, Shanks CA, Triggs EJ: The effect of renal failure on the disposition and neuromuscular blocking action of pancuronium bromide. *Eur J Clin Pharmacol* 1977; 12:23–29.

24. Hull CJ, Van Beem HBH, McLeod K, et al: A pharmacokinetic model for pancuronium. *Br J Anaesth* 1978; 50:1113–1122.

25. Miller RD, Agoston S, Booij LHDJ, et al: The comparative potency and pharmacokinetics of pancuronium and its metabolites in anesthetized man. *J Pharmacol Exp Ther* 1978; 207:539–543.

26. Shanks CA, Somogyi AA, Triggs EJ: Dose-response and plasma concentration-response relationships of pancuronium in man. *Anesthesiology* 1979; 51:111–118.

27. Agoston S, Feldman SA, Miller RD: Plasma concentrations of pancuronium and neuromuscular blockade after injection into the isolated arm, bolus injection, and continuous infusion. *Anesthesiology* 1979; 51:119–122.

28. Duvaldestin P, Saada J, Berger JL, et al: Pharmacokinetics, pharmacodynamics, and dose-response relationships of pancuronium in control and elderly subjects. *Anesthesiology* 1982; 56:36–40.

29. Sohn YJ, Bencini AF, Scaf AHJ, et al: Comparative pharmacokinetics and dynamics of vecuronium and pancuronium in anesthetized patients. *Anesth Analg* 1986; 65:233–239.

30. Lebreault C, Berger JL, d'Hollander AA, et al: Pharmacokinetics and pharmacodynamics of vecuronium (ORG NC 45) in patients with cirrhosis. *Anesthesiology* 1985; 62:601–605.

31. Duvaldestin P, Henzel D, Demetriou M, et al: Pharmacokinetics of fazadinium in man. *Br J Anaesth* 1978; 50:773–777.
32. Hull CJ, English MJM, Sibbald A: Fazadinium and pancuronium: A pharmacodynamic study. *Br J Anaesth* 1980; 52:1209–1221.
33. Duvaldestin P, Saada J, Henzel D, et al: Fazadinium pharmacokinetics in patients with liver disease. *Br J Anaesth* 1980; 52:789–794.
34. Ramzan MI, Triggs EJ, Shanks CA: Pharmacokinetic studies in man with gallamine triethiodide: I. Single and multiple clinical doses. *Eur J Clin Pharmacol* 1980; 17:135–143.
35. Ramzan IM, Shanks CA, Triggs EJ: Pharmacokinetics and pharmacodynamics of gallamine triethiodide in patients with total biliary obstruction. *Anesth Analg* 1981; 60:289–296.
36. Shanks CA, Funk DI, Avram MJ, et al: Gallamine administered by combined bolus and infusion. *Anesth Analg* 1982; 61:847–852.
37. Ramzan MI, Shanks CA, Triggs EJ: Pharmacokinetics of tubocurarine administered by combined i.v. bolus and infusion. *Br J Anaesth* 1980; 52:893–899.
38. Neill EAM, Jones CR: Determination of atracurium besylate in human plasma. *J Chromatogr* 1983; 274:409–412.
39. Ward S, Neill EAM, Weatherley BC, et al: Pharmacokinetics of atracurium besylate in healthy patients (after a single i.v. bolus dose). *Br J Anaesth* 1983; 55:113–118.
40. Ward S, Neill EAM: Pharmacokinetics of atracurium in acute hepatic failure (with acute renal failure). *Br J Anaesth* 1983; 55:1169–1172.
41. Paanakker JE, Van de Laar GLM: Determination of Org NC 45 (a myoneural blocking agent) in human plasma using high-performance normal-phase liquid chromatography. *J Chromatogr* 1980; 183:459–466.
42. Fahey MR, Morris RB, Miller RD, et al: Pharmacokinetics of ORG NC 45 (Norcuron) in patients with and without renal failure. *Br J Anaesth* 1981; 53:1049–1053.
43. Van der Veen F, Bencini A: Pharmacokinetics and pharmacodynamics of ORG NC 45 in man. *Br J Anaesth* 1980; 52:37S–41S.
44. Cronnelly R, Fisher DM, Miller RD, et al: Pharmacokinetics and pharmacodynamics of vecuronium (ORG NC 45) and pancuronium in anesthetized humans. *Anesthesiology* 1983; 58:405–408.
45. Fisher DM, Castagnoli K, Miller RD: Vecuronium kinetics and dynamics in anesthetized infants and children. *Clin Pharmacol Ther* 1985; 37:402–406.
46. Chan K, Williams NE, Baty JD, et al: A quantitative gas-liquid chromatographic method for the determination of neostigmine and pyridostigmine in human plasma. *J Chromatogr* 1976; 120:349–358.
47. De Ruyter MGM, Cronnelly R, Castagnoli N: Reversed-phase, ion-pair chromatography of quaternary ammonium compounds: Determination of pyridostigmine, neostigmine and edrophonium in biological fluids. *J Chromatogr* 1980; 183:193–201.

48. Cronnelly R, Stanski DR, Miller RD, et al: Renal function and the pharmacokinetics of neostigmine in anesthetized man. *Anesthesiology* 1979; 51:222–226.

49. Morris RB, Cronnelly R, Miller RD, et al: Pharmacokinetics of edrophonium and neostigmine when antagonizing d-tubocurarine neuromuscular blockade in man. *Anesthesiology* 1981; 54:399–402.

50. Fisher DM, Cronnelly R, Miller RD, et al: The neuromuscular pharmacology of neostigmine in infants and children. *Anesthesiology* 1983; 59:220–225.

51. Williams NE, Calvey TN, Chan K, et al: Plasma concentration of pyridostigmine during the antagonism of neuromuscular block. *Br J Anaesth* 1983; 55:27–31.

52. Sear JW, Trafford DJH, Makin HLJ: General methods of measuring drug concentrations in plasma, urine and other tissues, in Prys-Roberts C, Hug CC (eds): *Pharmacokinetics of Anaesthesia.* Oxford, England, Blackwell Scientific Publications, 1984, pp 38–63.

53. Morgan DJ, Blackman GL, Paull JD, et al: Pitfalls in deriving pharmacokinetic variables, letter. *Anesthesiology* 1982; 56:237–239.

54. Miller RD: Pharmacokinetics of muscle relaxants and their antagonists, in Prys-Roberts C, Hug CC (eds): *Pharmacokinetics of Anaesthesia.* Oxford, England, Blackwell Scientific Publications, 1984, pp 246–269.

55. Miller RD, Matteo RS, Benet LZ, et al: The pharmacokinetics of d-tubocurarine in man with and without renal failure. *J Pharmacol Exp Ther* 1977; 202:1–7.

56. Cohen EN, Paulson WJ, Elert B: Studies of d-tubocurarine with measurements of concentration in human blood. *Anesthesiology* 1957; 18:300–309.

57. Meijer DKF, Weitering JG, Vermeer GA, et al: Comparative pharmacokinetics of d-tubocurarine and metocurine in man. *Anesthesiology* 1979; 51:402–407.

58. Hull CJ: A model for atracurium?, editorial. *Br J Anaesth* 1983; 55:95–96.

59. Stanski DR, Ham J, Miller RD, et al: Time-dependent increase in sensitivity to d-tubocurarine during enflurane anesthesia in man. *Anesthesiology* 1980; 52:483–487.

60. Lebreault C, Duvaldestin P, Henzel D, et al: Pharmacokinetics and pharmacodynamics of vecuronium in patients with cholestasis. *Br J Anaesth* 1986; 58:983–987.

61. Shanks CA: Pharmacokinetics of the nondepolarizing neuromuscular relaxants applied to calculation of bolus and infusion dosage regimens. *Anesthesiology* 1986; 64:72–86.

62. Fahey MR, Rupp SM, Fisher DM, et al: The pharmacokinetics and pharmacodynamics of atracurium in patients with and without renal failure. *Anesthesiology* 1984; 61:699–702.

63. Merrett MA, Thompson CW, Webb FW: In vivo degradation of atracurium in human plasma. *Br J Anaesth* 1983; 55:61–66.

64. Stiller RL, Cook RD, Chakravorti S: In vitro degradation of atracurium in human plasma. *Br J Anaesth* 1985; 57:1085–1088.

65. Fisher DM, Canfell PC, Fahey MR, et al: Elimination of atracurium in humans: Contribution of Hofmann elimination and ester hydrolysis versus organ-based elimination. *Anesthesiology* 1986; 65:6–12.

66. Cronnelly R: Kinetics of anticholinesterases. *Clin Anesthesiol* 1985; 3:315–328.

67. Williams NE, Calvey TN, Chan K: Clearance of neostigmine from the circulation during the antagonism of neuromuscular block. *Br J Anaesth* 1978; 50:1065–1067.

68. Calvey TN, Williams NE, Muir KT, et al: Plasma concentration of edrophonium in man. *Clin Pharmacol Ther* 1976; 19:813–820.

69. Morris RB, Cronnelly R, Miller RD, et al: Pharmacokinetics of edrophonium in anephric and renal transplant patients. *Br J Anaesth* 1981; 53:1311–1314.

70. Cronnelly R, Stanski DR, Miller RD, et al: Pyridostigmine kinetics with and without renal function. *Clin Pharmacol Ther* 1980; 28:78–81.

71. Agoston S, Crul JF, Kersten UW, et al: Relationship of the serum concentration of pancuronium to its neuromuscular activity in man. *Anesthesiology* 1977; 47:509–512.

72. Hull CJ, Van Beem HBH, McLeod K, et al: A pharmacokinetic model for pancuronium. *Br J Anaesth* 1978; 50:1113–1122.

73. Cook DR, Wingard LB, Taylor FH: Pharmacokinetics of succinylcholine in infants, children and adults. *Clin Pharmacol Ther* 1976; 20:493–498.

74. Walker JS, Shanks CA, Brown KF: Alcuronium kinetics and plasma concentration-effect relationship. *Clin Pharmacol Ther* 1983; 33:510–516.

75. Hennis PJ, Stanski DR: Pharmacokinetic and pharmacodynamic factors that govern the clinical use of muscle relaxants. *Semin Anesth* 1985; 4:21–30.

76. Fisher DM, Rosen JI: A pharmacokinetic explanation for increasing recovery time following larger or repeated doses of nondepolarizing muscle relaxants. *Anesthesiology* 1986; 65:286–291.

77. Fahey MR, Morris RB, Miller RD, et al: Clinical pharmacology of ORG NC45 (Norcuron): A new nondepolarizing muscle relaxant. *Anesthesiology* 1981; 55:6–11.

78. Basta SJ, Ali HH, Savarese JJ, et al: Clinical pharmacology of atracurium besylate (BW 33A): A new non-depolarizing muscle relaxant. *Anesth Analg* 1982; 61:723–729.

79. Katz RL: Clinical neuromuscular pharmacology of pancuronium. *Anesthesiology* 1971; 34:550–556.

80. Noeldge G, Hinsken H, Buzello W: Comparison between the continuous infusion of vecuronium and the intermittent administration of pancuronium and vecuronium. *Br J Anaesth* 1984; 56:473–477.

81. Engbaek J, Ording H, Viby-Mogensen J: Neuromuscular blocking effects of vecuronium and pancuronium during halothane anaesthesia. *Br J Anaesth* 1983; 55:497–500.

82. Weatherly BC, Williams SG, Neill EAM: Pharmacokinetics, pharmacodynamics and dose-response relationships of atracurium administered i.v. *Br J Anaesth* 1983; 55:39S–45S.

83. Donati F, Bevan DR: The pharmacodynamic half-life of atracurium. *Can Anaesth Soc J* 1985: 32:S56–S57.

84. Gibaldi M, Levy G, Hayton W: Kinetics of the elimination and neuromuscular blocking effect of d-tubocurarine in man. *Anesthesiology* 1972; 36:213–218.

85. Norman J: Pharmacokinetics of non-depolarizing muscle relaxants. *Clin Anaesthesiol* 1985; 3:273–282.

86. Ali HH, Savarese JJ, Basta SJ, et al: Evaluation of cumulative properties of three non-depolarizing neuromuscular blocking drugs BW A444U, atracurium and vecuronium. *Br J Anaesth* 1983; 55:107S–111S.

87. Bevan DR, Donati F, Gyasi H, et al: Vecuronium in renal failure. *Can Anaesth Soc J* 1984; 31:491–495.

88. Somogyi AA, Shanks CA, Triggs EJ: Disposition kinetics of pancuronium bromide in patients with total biliary obstruction. *Br J Anaesth* 1977; 49:1103–1108.

89. Westra P, Vermeer GA, de Lange AR, et al: Hepatic and renal disposition of pancuronium and gallamine in patients with extrahepatic cholestasis. *Br J Anaesth* 1981; 51:331–338.

90. Ritschel WA: Pharmacokinetic approach to drug dosing in the aged. *J Am Geriatr Soc* 1976; 24:344–354.

91. d'Hollander AA, Luyckx C, Barvais L, et al: Clinical evaluation of atracurium besylate requirement for a stable muscle relaxation during surgery: Lack of age-related effects. *Anesthesiology* 1983; 59:237–240.

92. d'Hollander A, Massaux F, Nevelsteen M, et al: Age-dependent dose-response relationship of ORG NC45 in anaesthetized patients. *Br J Anaesth* 1982; 54:653–657.

93. Ramzan MI, Shanks CA, Triggs EJ: Gallamine disposition in surgical patients with chronic renal failure. *Br J Clin Pharmacol* 1981; 12:141–147.

94. Duvaldestin P, Lebreault C, Chauvin M: Pharmacokinetics of muscle relaxants in patients with liver disease. *Clin Anaesthesiol* 1985; 3:293–306.

95. Bencini AF, Scaf AHJ, Sohn YJ: Disposition and urinary excretion of vecuronium bromide in anesthetized patients with normal renal function or renal failure. *Anesth Analg* 1986; 65:245–251.

6

Nondepolarizing Relaxants

In the last 45 years, nearly 50 nondepolarizing relaxants have been introduced into clinical practice. Discussion in this chapter will be limited to those in current use in North America and Europe: alcuronium, atracurium, fazadinium, gallamine, metocurine, pancuronium, d-tubocurarine, and vecuronium. Inevitably, investigation of the newer agents, atracurium and vecuronium, has been more extensive and systematic than for the older drugs. Indeed, some details of the latter only became available when they were compared with the former. Despite this, there remain gaps in our knowledge, particularly of alcuronium, fazadinium, and metocurine, and as a result, myths of their supposed pattern of action remain and influence clinical opinion.

ALCURONIUM

Alcuronium (Fig 6–1), a semisynthetic nondepolarizing neuromuscular blocking drug (NMBD), was introduced in 1961.[1] It is a bis-quaternary ammonium compound derived from the naturally occurring curare alkaloid, C-toxiferine-I. It was developed as an alternative to d-tubocurarine and is thought by many to have a shorter duration of action than either pancuronium or d-tubocurarine.

Metabolism and Excretion

Alcuronium is probably not metabolized and, as a water-soluble, ionized compound, is excreted unchanged in the urine. Alcuronium is

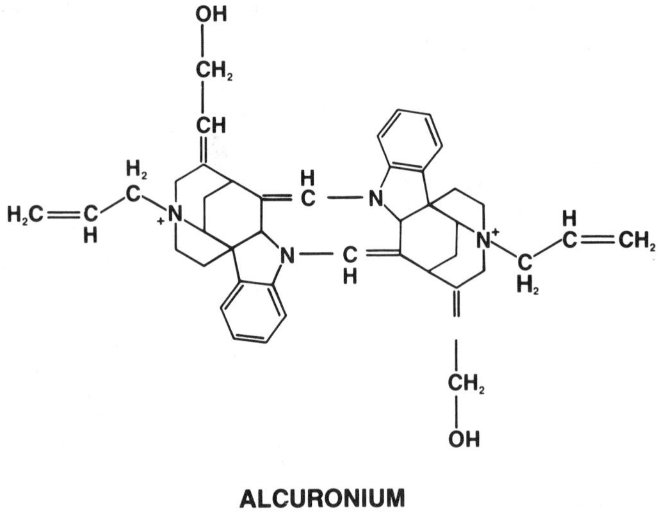

ALCURONIUM

FIG 6–1.
Structure of alcuronium.

TABLE 6–1.
Pharmacokinetic Median Values (Range) or ±SD for Alcuronium From Several Studies*

	DISTRIBUTION VOLUME (V_{dss}), (L/KG)	PLASMA CLEARANCE (C_p), (ML/KG/MIN)	ELIMINATION HALF-LIFE ($t_{1/2\,\beta}$), (MIN)	REFERENCE
Normal	0.32 (0.27–0.4)	1.3 (1.3–1.4)	200 (198–207)	Raaflaub and Frey[3], Buzello and Agoston,[4] Walker et al.,[5,6]
Elderly	0.32 ± 0.08	0.53 ± 0.24	439 ± 171	Stephens et al.[7]

*Adapted from Shanks CA: Pharmacokinetics of the nondepolarizing neuromuscular relaxants applied to calculation of bolus and infusion dose regimens. *Anesthesiology* 1986; 64:72–86.

about 40% protein bound,[2] and this is mainly to albumin.

Pharmacokinetics

Plasma concentrations of alcuronium may be measured using high-performance liquid chromatography (HPLC) method.[2] Median values, obtained from data in several studies,[3–7] are shown in Table 6–1 and are very similar to those for pancuronium and d-tubocurarine.[8]

Neuromuscular Blockade

Potency

Alcuronium is about 1.5 times as potent as d-tubocurarine. In conscious volunteers, grip strength was reduced by 50% following administration of a cumulative dose of 42 μg/kg compared with 55 μg/kg for d-tubocurarine.[9] Cumulative dose-response curves using ulnar nerve stimulation at 0.1 Hz produced an ED50 of about 70 μg/kg and an ED95 of about 145 μg/kg (Fig 6–2).[10] Dose-response curves obtained during a continuous infusion with ulnar nerve stimulation at 0.1 Hz gave an ED50 of 161 μg/kg and an ED95 of 286 μg/kg. In the same study, electromyographic (EMG) response gave a lower ED50, 135 μg/kg, than the twitch tension.[11] Thus, as for other relaxants, the derived potency is influenced by the method of measurement.

Alcuronium is potentiated by volatile anesthetic agents. At concentrations of 1 minimal alveolar concentration (MAC), the ED50 was reduced from 106 μg/kg during nitrous oxide (N_2O)-narcotic anesthesia to 90.5 μg/kg with halothane, 92.6 μg/kg with enflurane, and 80.5 μg/kg with isoflurane anesthesia.[12]

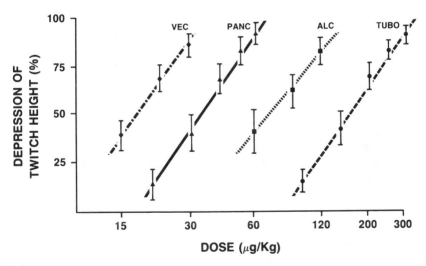

FIG 6–2.
Dose-response curves for vecuronium, pancuronium, alcuronium, and d-tubocurarine. (From Krieg N, Crul JF, Booij LHDJ: Relative potency of vecuronium, pancuronium, alcuronium and tubocurarine in anesthetized man. *Br J Anaesth* 1980; 52:783–787. Used by permission.)

Onset and Duration of Block

When approximately equipotent doses were used, the onset of maximum block (5.9 ± 0.4 minutes), time to 90% recovery (62.5 ± 7.5 minutes), and 25% to 75% recovery index (29.0 ± 2.3 minutes), obtained using ulnar nerve stimulation at 0.1 Hz and during N_2O-narcotic anesthesia, were similar to those obtained with pancuronium[10] and similar to three times as potent doses of atracurium.[13, 14] This confirms that the rate of recovery and restoration of respiration is no quicker with alcuronium than pancuronium.[15]

Cardiovascular Actions

Hughes and Chapple[16] investigated the simultaneous effects of several NMBDs on muscle relaxation and autonomic mechanisms. Parasympathetic effects were investigated by stimulating the celiac end of the cut vagus nerve. Sympathetic mechanisms were studied by stimulation of the preganglionic sympathetic nerve and recording contractions of the nictitating membrane. Atropinic effects were assessed by inducing bradycardia with methacholine. The paralysis from alcuronium was associated with vagal blockade due to an atropinic effect, but effects were minimal on sympathetic mechanisms (Fig 6–3).

In man, the vagolytic effect results in a slight, 9% to 10%, increase in heart rate after a dose of 0.15 mg/kg.[17] Alcuronium seems to affect blood pressure very little,[17, 18] although it has been blamed for a hypotensive effect[19–21] in the ill patient; this may be a result of a weak ganglionic blocking action.

The vagal blocking actions of alcuronium make its use more appropriate in the prevention of the bradycardia during strabismus surgery—oculocardiac reflex—than d-tubocurarine, pancuronium, or vecuronium.[22]

Alcuronium does not release histamine, although anaphylaxis has been reported following its use.[23]

Age

The plasma clearance is decreased, and the terminal half-life of alcuronium is prolonged in the elderly[7] (see Table 6–1). These changes resemble those of pancuronium and are probably a result of the age-related decrease in glomerular filtration rate. Although pharmacodynamic data are not available, prolonged duration of action of alcuronium is expected in the aged.

ALCURONIUM

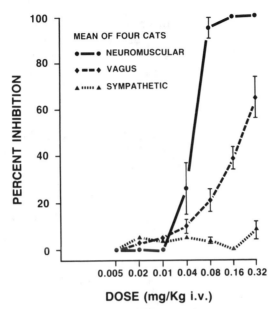

FIG 6–3.
Autonomic mechanisms of alcuronium in the cat. (From Hughes R, Chapple DJ: Effects of non-depolarizing neuromuscular blocking agents on peripheral autonomic mechanisms in cats. *Br J Anaesth* 1976; 48:59–68. Used by permission.)

Intraocular Pressure

In common with other nondepolarizing NMBDs, intraocular pressure (IOP) is reduced after alcuronium. Following injection of thiopental and alcuronium, 0.25 to 0.3 mg/kg, IOP decreased from control values of 15.3 ± 2.3 mm Hg to 8.9 ± 2.5 mm Hg, which increased after intubation to 12.6 ± 3.1 mm Hg.[24]

Modes of Administration

The onset of action of alcuronium is too slow for it to be recommended for intubation although it may be accelerated with a priming dose. When a total dose of 0.2 mg/kg was used with various priming doses of 20, 35, or 50 μg/kg given 2 minutes earlier, intubating conditions following the second dose improved, the larger the priming dose. It was calculated that intubation would be best with a dose of

106 µg/kg.[25] When principal doses of 0.15, 0.2, or 0.3 mg/kg were preceded 4 minutes earlier by priming doses of 0.04, 0.08, or 0.12 mg/kg,
priming accelerated the onset of neuromuscular blockade but only to
a limited degree.[26] Thus the place of priming remains controversial,
particularly as the initial dose may produce considerable weakness and
respiratory paralysis and increases the risk of aspiration.

More commonly, alcuronium is used as a bolus of 0.2 to 0.3 mg/kg
after intubation has been facilitated with succinylcholine. Muscle relaxation may be maintained with repeated doses one quarter of the
initial dose.

It has been demonstrated that a stable block can be achieved with
an infusion preceded by an initial dose calculated as the product of
the apparent volume of distribution and the desired plasma concentration. The infusion rate is calculated as the product of steady-state
plasma concentration and clearance. A 95% block can be maintained
with an initial bolus of 0.26 mg/kg followed by an infusion at 1 µg/kg/
minute;[6] this maintains 95% block at a plasma concentration of 0.8
µg/ml.[6] Relaxant requirements are reduced during hypothermia so that
to maintain constant neuromuscular blockade, infusion rates should be
decreased during hypothermia and cardiopulmonary bypass.[27] Such an
elegant demonstration of applied pharmacokinetics is an amusing academic exercise, which, with a drug whose effects change so slowly,
is of little clinical importance.

ATRACURIUM

Atracurium is a nondepolarizing NMBD of medium duration of
action (30 to 40 minutes).

Chemistry

Structurally, atracurium is a *bis*-quaternary nitrogen compound. It
was developed by Stenlake[28] in an attempt to produce an ultra-short-
acting muscle relaxant that was independent of the liver and kidney
for termination of its action and that had minimal side effects. The
concept, described by Hofmann more than a century earlier,[29] was based
on the nonenzymatic, chemical degradation of quaternary ammonium
salts. The reaction involved was the conversion of an amide to an amine
under alkaline conditions at high temperature with the loss of water
and the formation of a tertiary base.

The Hofmann reaction of the atracurium compound occurs at body
pH and temperature because biodegradation is encouraged by incor-

porating electron-attracting substitutes. The structure of atracurium (Fig 6–4) includes ester bonds that are susceptible to hydrolysis, but the ester moiety is arranged so that the carbonyl (C=O) carbon atom facilitates breakage of the bond between the quaternary nitrogen and ester bond (Hofmann reaction). This complicated molecule has four asymmetric sites so that 16 steric isomers are possible. The commercial preparation, although a mixture of isomers, behaves as a single substance.[30] It is water soluble and stable at 5°C for 2 years.

Metabolism

In man, atracurium is broken down both by the Hofmann reaction and ester hydrolysis to several compounds (see Fig 6–4), but the contributions of each process are disputed.[28, 31–33] The amount of ester hydrolysis is species dependent, and plasma cholinesterase is not involved.[34] Recently,[35, 36] it has been argued that ester hydrolysis is more important because degradation of atracurium is severalfold faster in plasma than in buffer; dilution of plasma slows degradation; and the addition of nonspecific esterase inhibitors retards degradation towards values in buffer. It has been estimated that two thirds of atracurium is degraded by ester hydrolysis and one third by Hofmann reaction. However, although ester hydrolysis is the major metabolic pathway of atracurium degradation, Hofmann elimination provides a safety net in clinical use.[37]

The multiplicity of metabolites from atracurium degradation has raised the possibility of their toxicity. The quaternary monoacrylate, the quaternary alcohol, and monoquaternary analogues produce neuromuscular blockade when given in high doses to cats. Also, high concentrations of quaternary monoacrylate, laudanosine, quaternary alkaloid, metholaudanosine, and the monoquaternary analogue decrease blood pressure but only at concentrations that are unlikely to be found after clinical administration of atracurium.[38]

Cerebral arousal was detected in dogs who were lightly anesthetized with halothane and spinal anesthesia[39] and given atracurium in doses of 1 to 2.5 mg/kg; laudanosine was suggested as the cause. Laudanosine is excreted in the urine and bile. In dogs, it produces "awakening" of halothane anesthesia in cumulative doses of 2 to 8 mg/kg and seizure activity at 14 to 22 mg/kg.[40] Laudanosine has also been shown to increase the halothane MAC in rabbits.[41] Nevertheless, in clinical practice concentrations of laudanosine are unlikely to reach levels that produce a measurable effect,[42] although decreased renal clearance augments plasma laudanosine concentrations.[43] In one case report, an 11-year-old boy with renal failure exhibited "jerky movements of the limbs"

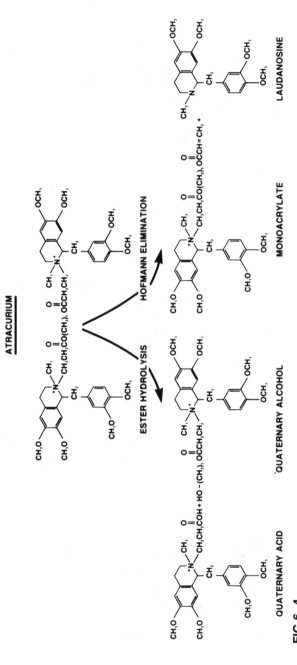

FIG 6–4.
Formula of atracurium and its main metabolic pathways.

after awakening from an anesthetic including atracurium.[44] Laudanosine was suggested as a possible cause,[43] although this seems unlikely.

The effects of laudanosine have been examined carefully and have produced largely negative or contrived results. Perhaps more attention should be given to the highly reactive acrylates.[45, 46]

Pharmacokinetics

A sensitive high-performance liquid chromatography assay has allowed plasma concentrations to be measured after bolus administration of atracurium (Fig 6–5). However, the metabolism of atracurium presented two problems before pharmacokinetic analysis could be performed. First, plasma had to be separated, acidified, and frozen rapidly to avoid further degradation. Secondly, nonenzymatic degradation of atracurium allows elimination in the tissues as well as in plasma. Thus, the pharmacokinetic model for atracurium may be better represented by Figure 6–6 where K_{10} is the elimination rate constant from the central compartment and K_{20} the elimination rate constant from the peripheral compartment.[47] However, although such a model is more "physiolog-

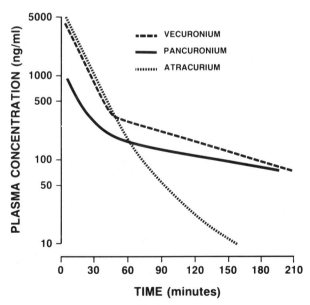

FIG 6–5.
Comparative plasma decay curves for atracurium, pancuronium, and vecuronium. (From Miller RD, Rupp SM, Fisher DM, et al: Clinical pharmacology of vecuronium and atracurium. *Anesthesiology* 1984; 61:444–453.

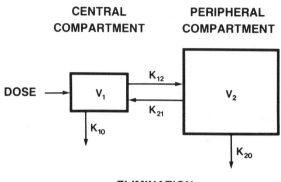

ELIMINATION

FIG 6–6.
Two-compartment open model for atracurium. (From Ward S, Neill EAM, Weatherley BC, et al: Pharmacokinetics of atracurium besylate in healthy patients (after a single IV bolus dose). *Br J Anaesth* 1983; 55:113–118. Used by permission.)

TABLE 6–2.
Pharmacokinetic Variables, Mean ± SEM, for Atracurium in Normal Patients and in Six Patients With Acute Hepatic and Renal Failure*†

		NORMAL		RENAL/HEPATIC FAILURE
Dose, mg/kg	0.31	0.59	0.76 ± 0.13	0.71 ± 0.08
n	6	6	6	6
$t_{1/2\alpha}$, min	2.27 ± 0.32	1.85 ± 0.24	2.0 ± 0.17	2.9 ± 0.06
$t_{1/2\beta}$, min	19.3 ± 0.9	20.6 ± 0.9	21.0 ± 2.0	22.0 ± 4.0
C_p (ml/min/kg)	5.5 ± 0.3	5.5 ± 0.3	5.3 ± 0.8	6.5 ± 1.5
V_1 (L/kg)	0.055 ± 0.008	0.044 ± 0.006	0.041 ± 0.016	0.076 ± 0.026
V (L/kg)	0.153 ± 0.013	0.162 ± 0.013	0.159 ± 0.021	0.207 ± 0.049

*Adapted from Ward S, Neill EAM, Weatherley BC, et al: Pharmacokinetics of atracurium besylate in healthy patients (after a single IV dose). *Br J Anaesth* 1983; 55:113–118 and Ward S, Neill EAM: Pharmacokinetics of atracurium in acute hepatic failure (with acute renal failure). *Br J Anaesth* 1983; 55:1169–1172.
†$t_{1/2\alpha}$ = distribution half-life; $t_{1/2\beta}$ = elimination half-life; C_p = plasma clearance; V_1 = volume of distribution in central compartment; V = volume of distribution.

ical," the conventional model, which presumes that elimination occurs only from the central compartment, may still be used as a "model" for predicting pharmacokinetic variables of atracurium.[48]

The pharmacokinetic profile based on these criteria and resulting from administration of either 0.3 mg/kg or 0.6 mg/kg of atracurium is shown in Table 6–2. The most obvious differences between atracurium and pancuronium or *d*-tubocurarine are the much shorter elimination half-life ($t_{1/2\beta}$) and greater plasma clearance, whereas the small volume of distribution implies limited tissue binding. Minimal changes in the pharmacokinetic profile were seen in six patients with hepatitis and renal failure to whom atracurium was given[49] (see Table 6–2). Thus it can be anticipated that atracurium would have a shorter duration of action than pancuronium. Attempts have been made to correlate the pharmacokinetic and pharmacodynamic properties. Following administration of bolus doses, a good correlation was found between plasma concentration and effect.[50] The EC50 (Table 6–3) is defined as the plasma concentration at 50% block. Unfortunately, atracurium is cleared so rapidly that bolus administration produces far from steady-state conditions, which makes comparisons with other drugs difficult. An alternative approach to kinetic dynamic modeling involves the calculation of drug concentrations in a small effect compartment[51] (Fig 6–7). It can be seen that the atracurium concentration, EC50, corresponding to 50%

TABLE 6–3.

Concentrations, Mean ± SEM, of Atracurium at 50% Neuromuscular Block Obtained Either From Plasma Decay, PC50 or From Calculation of the Concentration in the "Effect" Compartment, EC50*

	PC50, μG/ML	EC50, μG/ML
50% twitch depression	0.29 ± 0.04	0.65 ± 0.02

*Adapted from Ward S, Wright D: Combined pharmacokinetics and pharmacodynamic study of a single bolus of atracurium. *Br J Anaesth* 1983; 55:35S–38S and Weatherley BC, Williams SG, Neill EAM: Pharmacokinetics, pharmacodynamics and dose-response relationships of atracurium administered IV. *Br J Anaesth* 1983; 55:39S–45S.

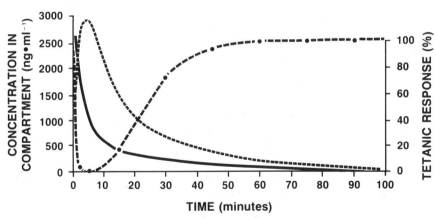

FIG 6–7.
Estimate of concentration of atracurium in the "effect" compartment *(dashed line)* from measurements of plasma concentration *(solid line)* and tetanic response *(dotted and dashed lines)*. (From Weatherley BC, Williams SG, Neill EAM: Pharmacokinetics, pharmacodynamics and dose-response relationships of atracurium administered IV. *Br J Anaesth* 1983; 55:39S–45S. Used by permission.)

block, varies considerably from that obtained from plasma decay[52] (see Table 6–3).

Neuromuscular Block

Potency

Early experiments[53] in which atracurium was administered in doses of 0.25 mg/kg demonstrated complete paralysis in cats, dogs, and monkeys. The paralysis was of medium duration, 30 minutes, and could be antagonized with anticholinesterases. A wide separation existed between neuromuscular and vagal blocking doses, and there was minimal sympathetic effect.[54] Changes in blood pressure and heart rate were not observed until doses of 0.4 mg/kg were given. Interference with renal or hepatic excretion did not prolong the effect, but the block was increased slightly during a respiratory acidosis produced by breathing 20% carbon dioxide.

Studies in man[55–59] have confirmed a similar profile despite variability in the degree of neuromuscular blockade.[57] During balanced anesthesia, the ED50 and ED95 for the adductor pollicis muscle during single twitch or train-of-four stimulation of the ulnar nerve are approximately 0.12 and 0.2 mg/kg, respectively. The dose response during 1.25 MAC anesthesia with N_2O (60%) and halothane is not affected,[60] but similar concentrations of enflurane[60] and isoflurane[61] increase the potency of atracurium (Fig 6–8). Nevertheless, the difference in potencies with different anesthetics does not vary more than 20%, which is much less than with pancuronium or d-tubocurarine.[62–64] Cumulative dose-response curves for a drug with rapid elimination like atracurium are similar but shifted to the right[65, 66] compared with those obtained using single doses. In cats, "diaphragmatic sparing" similar to other nondepolarizing relaxants has been demonstrated so that the diaphragm remains intact until the adductor pollicis is 80% paralyzed.[67]

Onset and Intubation

When equipotent doses are given the onset of action of atracurium is similar to pancuronium, d-tubocurarine, and vecuronium. The onset can be accelerated by increasing the dose (Table 6–4)[14, 56, 57, 59, 68–74] or by using the priming principle.[75–78] However, the onset is slower than that of succinylcholine, 1 mg/kg.[79, 80] Consequently, intubating conditions are less satisfactory unless appropriate time has been allowed for the block to develop. Nevertheless, at a dose of 0.6 mg/kg, patients could be intubated at between 30 to 120 seconds.[81] Intubating conditions are also dependent upon the depth of anesthesia, airway reactiv-

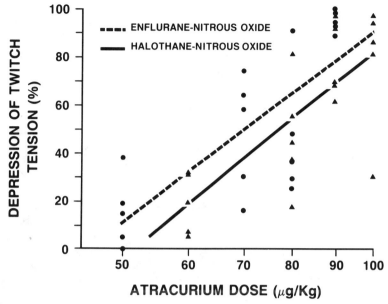

FIG 6–8.
Influence of halothane and enflurane on the potency of atracurium. (From Rupp SM, McChristian JW, Miller RD: Neuromuscular effects of atracurium during halothane-nitrous oxide and enflurane-nitrous oxide anesthesia in humans. *Anesthesiology* 1985; 63:16–19. Used by permission.)

TABLE 6–4.
Onset Time of Neuromuscular Blockade Following Administration of Atracurium During Anesthesia With N_2O-Halothane or Fentanyl*

DOSE, MG/KG	N	MEAN ONSET TIME, SEC ± SEM
0.4	40	257 ± 12
0.5	40	223 ± 9
0.6	40	220 ± 11
0.75	40	135 ± 9
1.0	40	124 ± 7

*Adapted from Mirakhur RK, Lavery GG, Clarke RSJ, et al: Atracurium in clinical anaesthesia: Effect of dosage on onset, duration and conditions for tracheal intubation. *Anaesthesia* 1985; 40:801–805.

ity, and strength of the patient. Therefore, assessment of intubating conditions is liable to error. Nevertheless, it seems that given similar anesthetic depth, intubating conditions will reflect the level of neuromuscular blockade[70, 71] (Fig 6–9). However, compared with balanced anesthesia, the addition of halothane, enflurane, and isoflurane produces little or no acceleration of the onset of blockade.[58, 60, 61]

Duration of Action

The duration of block is also related to dosage (Fig 6–10) and, when equipotent doses are administered, is similar to vecuronium but only about one third that of pancuronium and d-tubocurarine. The duration is prolonged by inhalational anesthesia—by about 10% to 20% with

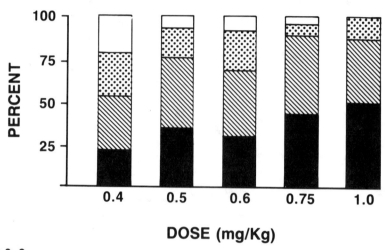

FIG 6–9.
Intubating conditions 90 seconds after administration of various doses of atracurium, 0.4 to 1.0 mg/kg. % excellent = solid black; % satisfactory = diagonal; % fair = dots; % poor = clear. (From Mirakhur RK, Lavery GG, Clarke RSJ, et al: Atracurium in clinical anaesthesia: Effect of dosage on onset, duration and conditions for tracheal intubation. *Anaesthesia* 1985; 40:801–805. Used by permission.)

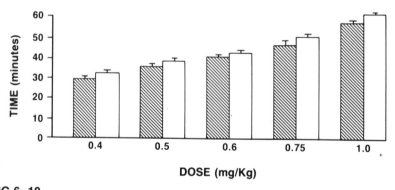

FIG 6–10.
Duration of neuromuscular blockade after administration of various doses of atracurium during fentanyl *(shaded)* or halothane anesthesia. (From Mirakhur RK, Lavery GG, Clarke RSJ, et al: Atracurium in clinical anaesthesia: Effect of dosage on onset, duration and conditions for tracheal intubation. *Anaesthesia* 1985; 40:801–805. Used by permission.)

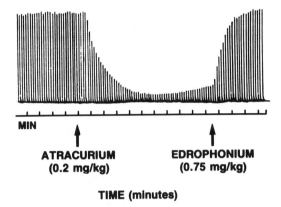

MIN

ATRACURIUM
(0.2 mg/kg)

EDROPHONIUM
(0.75 mg/kg)

TIME (minutes)

FIG 6–11.
Rapid antagonism of approximately 80% atracurium neuromuscular block with edrophonium 0.75 mg/kg. (From Baird WLM, Kerr WJ: Reversal of atracurium with edrophonium. *Br J Anaesth* 1983; 55:63S–66S. Used by permission.)

halothane[57, 60] and by 20% to 50% with enflurane[60] or isoflurane.[58, 71] Repeated doses of atracurium demonstrate little or no cumulation,[68, 82] a phenomenon reflecting its metabolism.

Recovery and Reversal

The recovery rate from 75% to 25% neuromuscular block is rapid (11 to 23 minutes)[56, 57] and similar to that of vecuronium but much more rapid than the recovery rates for pancuronium and d-tubocurarine; also, it is not altered by inhalational anesthetics.[58] This rapid rate of recovery accounts for its popularity because once recovery commences, restoration of respiration can be anticipated. Consequently, the need to reverse an atracurium neuromuscular block is often obviated.[68] When necessary, satisfactory antagonism can be achieved with either neostigmine[68, 83] or edrophonium.[84] The latter (Fig 6–11) with its more rapid action might seem more appropriate but in an intense block (>90%) may be no more rapid than neostigmine.[85, 86]

Characteristics of Neuromuscular Block

Atracurium produces similar characteristics to other nondepolarizing drugs, i.e., fade in response to train-of-four (TOF) or tetanic stimulation. The TOF fade is greater during recovery than onset of the block, and for the same decrease in first twitch height, the decrement of TOF is less than for d-tubocurarine and gallamine.[87] In this respect, atracurium resembles pancuronium, suggesting a predominant postsynaptic action at the neuromuscular junction.[88, 89]

Return of spontaneous breathing occurs more rapidly than recovery

of the small muscles of the hand.[90] Respiration is reestablished within
7 minutes of reappearance of the tetanic response at a time when there
is less than 25% recovery of the adductor pollicis force of contraction.

Cardiovascular Effects

In the development of atracurium, a wide separation between cardiovascular and neuromuscular effects was an important considera-
tion.[91] A study in which the eventual compound was used demonstrated,
in animals, an 8- to 25-fold difference in the dose required to produce
vagal blockade compared with the dose that produced muscle relaxation.[53] In cats, the 50% vagal-to-neuromuscular blocking ratio was 25:1
compared with 96:1 for vecuronium.[54] Cardiovascular effects were only
seen at high doses and were thought to result from histamine release.
This could be blocked, in dogs, with their known high potential to
release histamine, by a combination of H_1 and H_2 receptor blockade.
Similarly, the dose of atracurium required to produce ganglionic blockade in animals was 48 times the dose that produced neuromuscular
blockade compared with 9 times the dose with d-tubocurarine (Fig 6–
12).[92] Very large doses decreased the response of the nictitating membrane to preganglionic stimulation[54]—another indication of ganglionic
blockade. No changes were seen in systemic or pulmonary vasculature
or cardiac output in doses up to 0.4 mg/kg in dogs.[93]

In man, administration of atracurium is characterized by remarkable
circulatory stability,[57–59, 94] particularly when bolus doses are restricted
to less than 2 × ED95.[93, 95, 96] Such stability is also observed when it is
administered to patients with severe coronary artery disease.[96] Indeed,
a frequent complaint of the use of atracurium is bradycardia following
the use of high-dose narcotics[97] or after vagal traction,[98] an effect that
is only observed because the sympathetic stimulation of pancuronium
is missing!

Histamine Release

Hypotension and tachycardia may occur at high doses, greater than
0.4 mg/kg, during balanced[56, 99, 100] or halothane anesthesia.[83, 101] The
cardiovascular changes are dose dependent (Fig 6–13) and are associated with an increase in plasma histamine concentration. Similar
effects can be seen with d-tubocurarine and metocurine but at much
lower equivalent doses (Table 6–5).

The release of histamine in man may produce several effects
including periperhal vasodilatation and hypotension, positive
chronotropic or inotropic effects, increase in coronary perfusion,

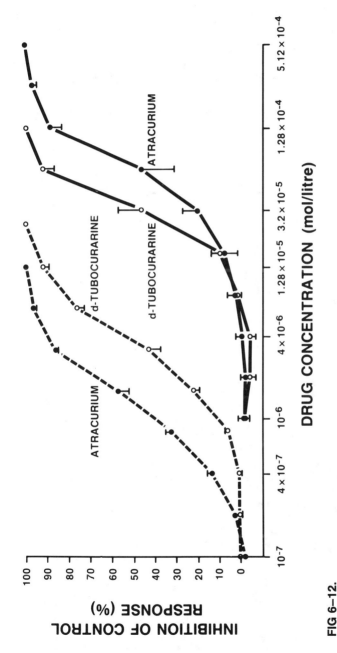

FIG 6–12.
Log dose-response curves for atracurium and *d*-tubocurarine on the response of the diaphragm to phrenic nerve stimulation *(dotted lines)* and the response of the vas deferens (ganglionic) to hypogastric nerve stimulation *(solid lines)*. (From Healey TEJ, Palmer JP: In vitro comparison between the neuromuscular and ganglionic blocking potency ratios of atracurium and tubocurarine. *Br J Anaesth* 1982; 54:1307–1311. Used by permission.)

bronchoconstriction, and skin erythema. The most frequent observation after atracurium is a cutaneous reaction in the form of a macular rash or uniform confluent erythema. The rash appears initially either along the course of the vein of administration or on the trunk, and often, but not always, it spreads peripherally. Its occurrence is dose related (Table 6–6) and is seldom associated with more widespread histamine release.[71] Cutaneous reactions have been reported frequently,[75, 96, 102–104] but few are associated with a severe systemic reaction including

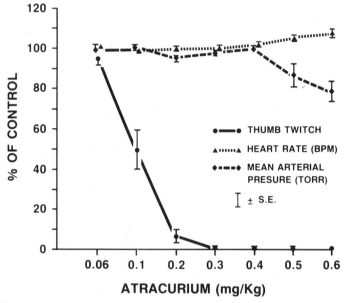

FIG 6–13.
Neuromuscular, heart rate, and blood pressure responses to atracurium at various doses (0.06 to 0.6 mg/kg). (From Savarese JJ, Basta SJ, Ali HH, et al: Neuromuscular and cardiovascular effects of BW 33A (atracurium) in patients under halothane anesthesia. *Anesthesiology* 1982; 57:A262. Used by permission.)

TABLE 6–5.
Doses of Drugs Associated With Significant Cardiovascular Changes*†

DRUG	DOSE, MG/KG	EQUIVALENT, ED95	% CONTROL BP	% CONTROL HR	% CONTROL HISTAMINE
d-Tubocurarine	0.5	1	78	116	410
Metocurine	0.5	2	79	119	212
Atracurium	0.6	3	80	108	192

*Adapted from Basta SJ, Savarese JJ, Ali HH, et al: Histamine releasing potencies of atracurium dimethyl tubocurarine and tubocurarine. *Br J Anaesth* 1983; 55:105S–106S.
†BP = mean blood pressure; HR = mean heart rate.

TABLE 6–6.
Atracurium Dosage and Incidence of
Cutaneous Reaction*

DOSE, MG/KG	N	FLUSHING, %
0.4	40	17.5
0.5	40	32.5
0.6	40	32.5
0.75	40	55.0
1.0	40	72.5

*Adapted from Mirakhur RK, Lavery GG, Clarke RSJ, et al: Atracurium in clinical anaesthesia: Effect of dosage on onset, duration and conditions for tracheal intubation. *Anaesthesia* 1985; 40:801–805.

bronchospasm[70, 105, 106] or angionecrotic edema.[107] Often when these occur, several drugs have been administered. The most likely cause of bronchospasm is from the precipitate formed by mixing thiopental and atracurium being flushed into the pulmonary circulation.[108]

The cardiovascular responses and histamine release can be decreased by slow administration over 5 minutes[104] or by pretreatment with H_1 and H_2 receptor blockade.[108, 109] However, if large doses are administered to produce a more rapid onset of action, slow injection negates the purpose.

Anaphylactoid reactions to atracurium[106, 110–112] and to all other neuromuscular blocking drugs[113] have been described. They present with severe hypotension, bronchospasm, and truncal flushing and are most likely mediated by histamine release via a direct mast cell response to the drug. Such reactions are not exaggerated forms of the frequent cutaneous histamine release, nor can they be predicted from intradermal testing.[108] Cross reactivity between several neuromuscular blocking drugs has been observed by direct binding and incubation radioimmunoassay.[114] At present, it is not possible to determine the relative incidence of life-threatening anaphylactoid reactions among the neuromuscular blocking drugs.

Intracranial and Intraocular Pressures

Several studies have confirmed that atracurium has no effect on intracranial[115–117] or intraocular pressures.[118–120] The stable cardiovascular system and unchanged cerebral perfusion, even in the presence of increased intracranial pressure (ICP),[115, 121] make it an ideal relaxant for use during neurosurgery except for its short duration of action. Similarly, for the open eye injury, good intubating conditions can be achieved by increasing the dose to 2 to 3 × ED95, yet producing a block no longer than pancuronium at 1 × ED95.

Lower Esophageal Sphincter

The increase in lower esophageal pressure observed after pancuronium is not seen after atracurium.[122] It has been suggested that to avoid regurgitation and aspiration, pancuronium may be the preferred agent either alone or as precurarization before succinylcholine. However, these observations apply only to patients with an intact lower esophageal sphincter and may not be relevant in the emergency induction of anesthesia in a patient with a full stomach.

Age

The effect of aging on the action of atracurium remains uncertain. In the very young, the potency of atracurium on a dose per square meter basis is similar for the 2-year-old child and the adult.[123] The onset time is reduced in the pediatric age group and, surprisingly, recovery time (75% to 25% block) is more rapid, except in patients under 2 months of age.[124] When given as an infusion to children aged 2 to 10 years, a stable block was achieved with a fixed infusion rate of 5 to 7 μg/kg/minute.[125] The infusion requirements are decreased by approximately 30% during halothane (0.8%) or isoflurane (1%) anesthesia.[126]

In the elderly, atracurium is not associated with the decrease in drug requirement and the slower recovery seen with vecuronium when each drug was given by infusion.[127] In part, this must be the consequence of a drug whose elimination is independent of renal and hepatic mechanisms.

Drug Interactions

The effect of many drugs including premedicants, intravenous and inhalational anesthetics, hypotensive agents, sympathomimetics and blockers, antibiotics, and azathioprine has been examined in cats.[128] Potentiation of the block was seen with inhalational anesthetics and antibiotics, whereas epinephrine antagonized the block somewhat. The influence of the inhalational anesthetics in humans has been discussed previously.

Interactions with other muscle relaxants is more complicated. It would be anticipated that atracurium would produce additive effects with other nondepolarizing NMBDs. However, using the phrenic nerve-diaphragm preparation atracurium is potentiated by d-tubocurarine and metocurine.[129] In man, atracurium is potentiated by pancuronium, *d*-tubocurarine,[134] and vecuronium[130] in a similar way to the potentiation of *d*-tubocurarine by pancuronium.[131] It is uncertain whether the mechanism is prejunctional or postjunctional. When succinylcholine is given before atracurium, the latter is potentiated, but its duration of action is not prolonged.[83] Atracurium can be used to prevent succinylcholine myalgias and fasciculations, and it will tend to decrease the potency of the succinylcholine.[132] However, the duration of action of succinylcholine is not prolonged because atracurium does not inhibit butyrlcholinesterase and, therefore, plasma cholinesterase.[133]

Special Situations

Outpatient Surgery

The short duration of action and rapid recovery produced by atracurium make it an ideal agent for many short surgical procedures[134, 135] including gynecologic surgery[13] and laparoscopy.[136] As anticipated, one study demonstrated a decrease in postoperative muscle pains when atracurium replaced succinylcholine for outpatient laparoscopy.[136] One of the interesting aspects of that study was that 30% would have preferred to have been inpatients!

Obstetric Anesthesia

Atracurium has been used to provide maintenance relaxation for cesarean section.[137] Succinylcholine was preferred to provide rapid isolation of the airway, but for maintenance atracurium was acceptable. Small quantities of the drug crossed the placenta, but umbilical-to-maternal vein ratios were between 0.03 and 0.33. Nevertheless, in one of eight infants an atracurium concentration half that associated with relaxation in adults was found. Consequently, although no problems have been reported, placental transfer may be sufficient to produce an effect in the fetus.

Renal and Hepatic Disease

The potency, duration of action, and pharmacokinetic profile[138] of atracurium are unaffected in patients with severe renal[139, 140] or hepatic disease[141] because the elimination of atracurium is independent of these organs.[49] Thus, atracurium may be indicated in such conditions, but its short duration of action may be a handicap. An alternative approach is to use pancuronium or *d*-tubocurarine and titrate their effect and antagonism with careful neuromuscular monitoring. Infusions of atracurium at doses of 0.6 mg/kg/hour for 14 to 37 hours have been used to allow intermittent positive-pressure ventilation (IPPV) in five patients with renal failure in the intensive care unit. In all patients, rapid return of spontaneous ventilation followed cessation of the infusions suggesting minimal interference with the action of atracurium in renal failure.[142]

Cardiopulmonary Bypass

The hemodynamic stability of atracurium makes it an attractive relaxant in patients with cardiovascular disease. However, care is necessary to treat the bradycardia that may follow high-dose narcotic anesthesia. Atracurium requirements decrease during hypothermic bypass,[143] but whether this reflects the action of hypothermia on atracurium metabolism or increased sensitivity of the neuromuscular junction is uncertain. Similar effects have been observed with pancuronium,[144] and with vecuronium the decreased requirement during hypothermia is greater than with atracurium.[129]

Pheochromocytoma

The use of atracurium in pheochromocytoma has met with mixed results. In one patient no problems were encountered,[145] while in another its administration was followed by hypertension[146] perhaps as a result of histamine release. Vecuronium, devoid of histamine release, would seem to be the preferred relaxant.

Myasthenia Gravis

There are several reports of the successful use of atracurium in patients with myasthenia gravis.[147–151] Requirements may vary but in most reports were about 50% of normal. Nevertheless, neuromuscular monitoring is essential. The major advantage of atracurium is that its metabolism ensures a normal rapid rate of recovery, whereas for other relaxants, including vecuronium,[152] recovery may be prolonged severely.

Malignant Hyperthermia

Altracurium does not trigger malignant hyperthermia (MH), nor does it alleviate the syndrome when triggered in susceptible Landrace pigs.[153] Thus, it would be an appropriate relaxant for patients with MH.

Myotonic Dystrophy

Myotonia is a particular challenge to anesthesiologists. Succinylcholine and anticholinesterases may produce skeletal contractions. The availability of atracurium allows both of these problems to be avoided when muscle relaxation is required.[154, 155] These patients appear to respond normally to atracurium without altered potency and with a more rapid recovery.

Burns

The patient with burns in excess of 33% surface area demonstrates resistance to atracurium commencing 6 days after the accident. The resistance appears to be maximal at 15 to 40 days and may last for more than a year.[156]

Modes of Administration

Bolus Doses

Muscle relaxation may be induced with atracurium in doses of 0.4 to 0.5 mg/kg. With a single bolus, reasonable intubating conditions will take about 2 to 3 minutes to develop. This may be accelerated by about 30 seconds if 10% of the dose is given 3 minutes before the remainder as a priming dose.[157] Surgical relaxation will last about 30 to 40 minutes when repeated doses of 0.05 to 0.1 mg/kg may be given. Reversal of the block can be antagonized with neostigmine or edrophonium, but if more than 30 minutes have elapsed since the last dose, this may be unnecessary if adequate neuromuscular activity can be demonstrated.

Infusion

An alternative technique is to start a continuous infusion at the same time as, or when some recovery has been demonstrated from, the initial bolus dose. Infusion requirements to maintain surgical relaxation vary between 0.3 to 0.5 mg/kg/hour. The drug should be diluted in normal saline rather than in the more alkaline Ringer's solution because degradation is more rapid in the latter.[158] Recovery of neuromuscular activity appears to be as rapid on stopping the infusion as after administration of a bolus dose.[159]

FAZADINIUM

Fazadinium, a synthetic muscle relaxant (Fig 6–14), was introduced into clinical practice in Great Britain in 1974 in an attempt to provide an agent with a rapid onset of action, short duration of action, and limited side effects. It was never released in North America because it is associated with tachycardia.

Chemistry

Fazadinium is an azobis-arylimidazo(1,2–a)pyridinium derivative. In animals—cats, dogs, and monkeys—fazadinium in doses of 0.2 to 0.5 mg/kg produced rapid (onset <1 minute) but brief (100% recovery within 4 minutes) paralysis. Rapid recovery, 5 to 7 minutes, also occurred after stopping a continuous infusion and was the result of breakdown to at least two metabolites. The unchanged drug and its metabolites can be found in the urine and bile.[160] However, in man, metabolism is minimal, and the duration of action using equipotent doses is similar to pancuronium.[161]

Pharmacokinetics

Modifications[162, 163] to the fluorometric assay for pancuronium allow accurate estimations of plasma fazadinium concentrations. Typical pharmacokinetic variables in normal patients[162] and in patients with renal[164] or hepatic[165] disease from one center are shown in Table 6–7. From the relatively short terminal half-life and rapid clearance, it is expected that recovery from neuromuscular blockade would occur more

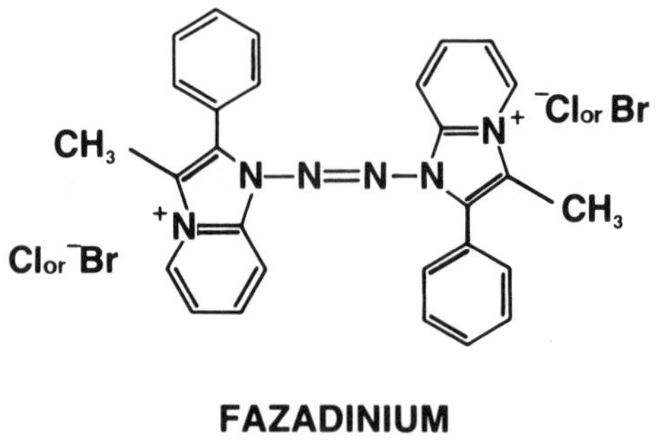

FAZADINIUM

FIG 6–14.
Structure of fazadinium.

TABLE 6–7.
Pharmacokinetic Variables, Mean ± SEM, for Fazadinium*

	V_D, L/KG	$t_{1/2\beta}$, MIN	C_p, ML/KG/MIN
Normal	0.234 ± 0.02	76.4 ± 4.7	2.1 ± 0.2
Renal failure	0.310 ± 0.01	140 ± 17	1.6 ± 0.2
Liver disease			
Cirrhosis	0.448 ± 0.15	153 ± 55	1.9 ± 0.2
Cholestasis	0.350 ± 0.08	103 ± 25	2.2 ± 0.3

*Adapted from references 162, 164, and 165.

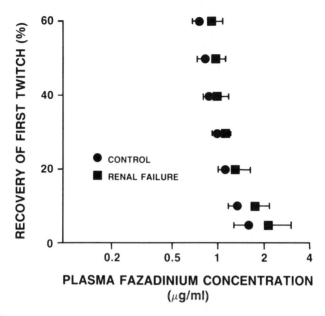

FIG 6–15.
Relationship between plasma concentration and recovery from fazadinium and neuromuscular blockade in patients with normal and abnormal renal function. (From Bevan DR, D'Souza, Rouse JM, et al: Clinical pharmacokinetics of fazadinium. *Anaesthesia* 1980; 35:873–878. Used by permission.)

rapidly after fazadinium than after pancuronium or *d*-tubocurarine but more slowly than after atracurium.

Plasma fazadinium concentrations can be plotted against neuromuscular blockade[166–169] (Fig 6–15), and the relationship is not altered in renal failure. When calculated biophase log concentrations of fazadinium are compared with simultaneous twitch depression, a hysteresis-free sigmoid relationship is obtained.[169] Such reconstructions demonstrate that fazadinium is less cumulative than pancuronium and has a more rapid onset of action.

Neuromuscular Blockade

Potency

In man, various values have been reported for the potency of fazadinium. When single stimuli and frequencies of 0.1 Hz or less are used, the ED50 is approximately 0.3 mg/kg and the ED90 about 1 mg/kg.[170] As the frequency of stimulation is increased, the ED50 and ED90 are decreased.[171, 172]

Onset

It has been suggested that the onset of block occurs more rapidly after fazadinium than after succinylcholine, pancuronium, or d-tubocurarine[173, 174] (Fig 6–16). Unfortunately, in several studies the doses chosen have not been equipotent. In particular, the dose of d-tubocurarine was small and that of pancuronium was large. Consequently, it is difficult to interpret such studies, particularly as it seems that the further development of neuromuscular block, once started, may occur at different rates with different relaxants: d-tubocurarine starts early and develops slowly, whereas pancuronium starts late but progresses rapidly.[174, 175] All are much slower than succinylcholine.

Duration of Action

Recovery from fazadinium is much quicker in cats than in man. Full recovery of single twitch activity occurs in about 40 minutes after a dose of 0.4 mg/kg during N_2O-narcotic anesthesia.[170]

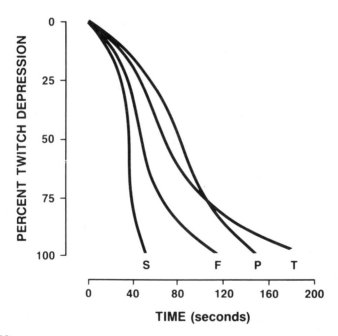

FIG 6–16.

Comparison of onset of neuromuscular block after succinylcholine *(S),* 1 mg/kg; fazadinium *(F),* 1 mg/kg; pancuronium *(P),* 0.1 mg/kg; and *d*-tubocurarine *(T),* 0.5 mg/kg. (From Blackburn CL, Morgan M: Comparison of speed of onset of fazadinium, pancuronium, tubocurarine and suxamethonium. *Br J Anaesth* 1978; 50:361–364. Used by permission.)

FAZADINIUM

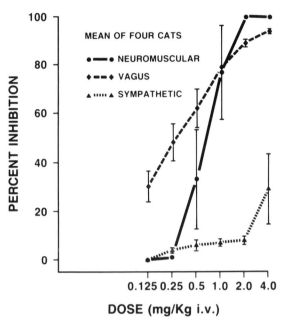

FIG 6–17.
Dose-response curves for the neuromuscular and autonomic effects of fazadinium in the cat. (From Hughes R, Payne JP, Sugai N: Studies of fazadinium bromide (AH 8165): A nondepolarizing neuromuscular blocking agent. *Can Anaesth Soc J* 1976; 23:36–47. Used by permission.)

Site of Action

In animals, fazadinium produces muscular relaxation by blocking postsynaptic cholinergic receptors. At the same concentration, fazadinium also shows evidence of stimulation of the nerve terminal as the frequency of miniature end-plate potentials is increased and repetitive activity occurs.[176, 177] The effect of fazadinium on the margin of safety of neuromuscular transmission is similar to d-tubocurarine: the twitch remains unaffected until 75% to 80% of receptors are occupied and is abolished when 90% to 95% are blocked.[177]

Cardiovascular Action

In man and animals, the tachycardia associated with fazadinium resembles that seen after gallamine. In cats, Hughes et al.[170] demonstrated vagal blockade by the inhibition of the bradycardiac response to vagal stimulation (Fig 6–17). Blockade of sympathetic mechanisms occurred only at high doses ($>2 \times$ ED95) to produce some decrease in arterial pressure.

The tachycardia is associated with an increase in cardiac output in patients with normal hearts, and this compensates for the decrease in total peripheral resistance so that arterial blood pressure is maintained.[178, 179] Patients with heart failure[180] and/or atrial fibrillation demonstrate[181] a decrease in blood pressure associated with reductions in stroke index and cardiac output. Thus, fazadinium appears to be contraindicated in patients with impaired cardiovascular function, particularly since agents without cardiovascular activity are now available.

Special Situations

Renal Failure

Although fazadinium is excreted in the urine and its clearance is decreased in renal failure,[164, 168] the duration of action of small doses, 1 mg/kg, is not prolonged.[168, 182] This is additional evidence that the decrease in plasma concentrations to levels below that necessary to cause relaxation is initially due to redistribution and will not be affected by renal or hepatic disease. However, larger or repeated doses should be given cautiously.

Mode of Administration

Intubating conditions can be achieved by about 2 minutes after administration of doses of 1 to 1.5 mg/kg. Relaxation can be maintained with additional doses of 0.25 to 0.5 mg/kg.

GALLAMINE

Gallamine, the first widely used synthetic muscle relaxant,[183, 184] contains three positively charged nitrogen atoms (Fig 6–18). It is the least potent of the relaxants used in clinical practice. Also, its cardiovascular effects limit its use so that it has been studied in less detail than other available NMBDs.

Gallamine is not metabolized but is excreted unchanged almost entirely by the kidney.[185] In dogs, nearly 85% of an injected dose of tritiated (^{3}H)-gallamine can be recovered from the urine in 24 hours.[186] In man, biliary excretion is negligible, and gallamine is excreted in the urine, but considerable individual variation exists in the rate of excretion. Following administration of a bolus dose of 2.5 mg/kg, 15% to 100% was found in the urine after 24 hours.[187]

Pharmacokinetics

Plasma concentrations of gallamine can be measured by modification of the fluorimetric method used for pancuronium.[188] Following a single dose, the plasma concentration decreases in a bi-exponential fashion. The elimination is grossly disturbed in patients with renal failure[189] but is unaffected by biliary obstruction[190] (Table 6–8). Plasma clearance of gallamine is also reduced in the elderly, and this reduction correlates with a decrease in creatinine clearance[191] (Fig 6–19).

Neuromuscular Blockade

Potency

Dose-response curves for gallamine are parallel to those for pancuronium and d-tubocurarine. The values of ED50 and ED90–95 depend on the methodology. Incremental cumulative dose-response curves during N_2O-narcotic anesthesia with single stimulation at 0.25 Hz pro-

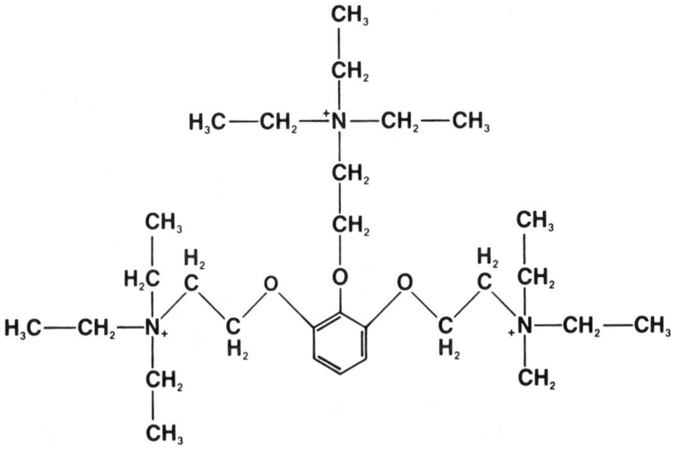

GALLAMINE

FIG 6–18.
Structure of gallamine.

TABLE 6–8.
Pharmacokinetic Variables, Mean ± SEM, for Gallamine in Normal, Cholestatic, and Renal-Failure Patients

	V_{dss}, L/KG	$t_{1/2\beta}$, MIN	C_p, ML/MIN/KG	REFERENCE
Normal	0.206 ± 0.047	134.6 ± 32.9	1.2 ± 0.3	Ramzan et al.[188]
Biliary obstruction	0.265 ± 0.023	160.1 ± 39.9	1.2 ± 0.3	Ramzan et al.[190]
Renal failure	0.284 ± 0.092	752.4	0.24 ± 0.08	Ramzan et al.[189]

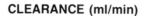

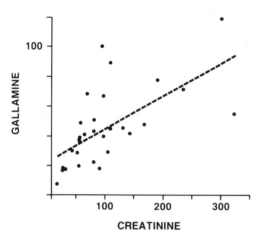

FIG 6–19.
Relationship between clearance of creatinine and gallamine in the elderly. (From Shanks CA, Fink DI, Avram MJ, et al: Gallamine administered by combined bolus and infusion. *Anesth Analg* 1982; 61:847–852. Used by permission.)

duced an ED50 of 0.76 ± 0.1 mg/kg and an ED95 of 1.9 ± 0.2 mg/kg.[192] Shanks et al.[193] produced dose-response curves using continuous infusions of relaxant and stimulation frequencies of 0.1 Hz. This produced an ED50 of 1.3 ± 0.4 mg/kg and an ED95 of 2.8 ± 0.8 mg/kg (Fig 6–20).

Onset, Duration, and Recovery

For equipotent doses, the onset of action of gallamine is similar to pancuronium and d-tubocurarine. Maximum block with an ED95 dose is achieved in 5 to 7 minutes.[190]

The time to recovery from 95% to 25% and 50% gallamine neuromuscular blockade varied widely among individuals but was similar to the recovery time for pancuronium, d-tubocurarine, and metocurine[192] (Table 6–9). Recovery of ventilation occurs when the adductor pollicis shows less than 50% return of response to single stimuli.[194]

Reversal

Gallamine is reversed rapidly by anticholinesterases. Miller et al.[195] compared the reversibility of gallamine with that of pancuronium and d-tubocurarine.[195] They found that when neostigmine, 0.25 mg, was given every 3 minutes, reversal was achieved more rapidly with d-tubocurarine and pancuronium than with gallamine (Fig 6–21).

Site of Action

The predominant action of gallamine is as a receptor antagonist. However, in common with other muscle relaxants, several additional sites have been proposed including membrane potential-dependent block of open ion channels.[196]

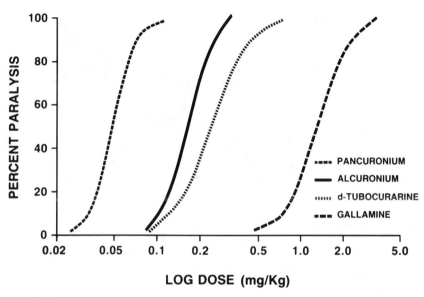

FIG 6–20.
Dose-response curves for pancuronium, alcuronium, d-tubocurarine, and gallamine derived using continuous IV infusions. (From Shanks CA, Walker JS, Ramzan MI, et al: Dose-response curves for four neuromuscular blockers using continuous IV infusions. *Br J Anaesth* 1981; 53:627–632. Used by permission.)

TABLE 6–9.
Recovery Time, Mean ± SEM, From 95% Block to 25% and 50% Twitch Height*

	RECOVERY TIME, MIN	
	25% TWITCH HEIGHT	50% TWITCH HEIGHT
Gallamine	27.0 ± 2.6	52.7 ± 7.3
Pancuronium	21.8 ± 2.9	37.4 ± 5.0
d-Tubocurarine	28.1 ± 3.8	48.4 ± 7.3
Metocurine	25.4 ± 4.8	45.6 ± 6.9

*Adapted from Donlon JV, Ali HH, Savarese JJ: A new approach to the study of four nondepolarizing relaxants in man. *Anesth Analg* 1974; 53:934–939.

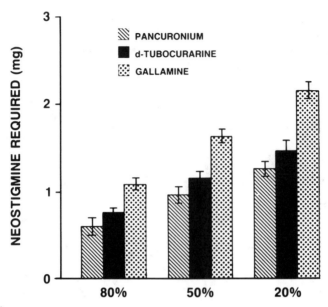

FIG 6–21.
Doses of neostigmine required to induce recovery to 80%, 50%, and 20% neuromuscular block achieved with pancuronium, d-tubocurarine, or gallamine. (From Miller RD, Way WL: Comparative antagonism of d-tubocurarine, gallamine, and pancuronium induced neuromuscular blockades by neostigmine. *Anesthesiology* 1972; 37:503–509. Used by permission.)

Cardiovascular Effects

In man, gallamine is associated with an increase in heart rate that is usually accompanied by increases in cardiac output and systemic arterial pressure[197] (Fig 6 – 22).

In cats, gallamine inhibits the bradycardic response to vagal stimulation in doses within the therapeutic range (Fig 6 – 23).[16] The vagal blocking action of gallamine occurs predominantly at the postganglionic nerve terminal.[198] In addition, gallamine, like pancuronium, augments the release of norepinephrine in vascular tissue under vagal control,[199] but this release of catecholamines probably makes only a small contribution to the cardiovascular actions of gallamine.[200]

In man, the antivagal action of gallamine in doses of 0.5 to 2 mg/kg is associated with increases in cardiac output of 25% to 50%.[197] The tachycardia is dose related and reaches its maximum at doses of 1.5 to 2 mg/kg.[201] The increase in heart rate matches the onset of neuromuscular blockade (see Fig 6 – 23) but persists during recovery from paralysis. The administration of atropine increases the heart rate further, which suggests that the vagal blocking action of gallamine is incomplete. Thus gallamine in doses of 0.3 mg/kg does not prevent the bradycardia associated with repeated doses of succinylcholine.[202, 203] Gallamine does not cause histamine release or sympathetic ganglionic blockade in the clinical dose range. Anaphylactoid reactions have been described in two patients after small precurarizing doses of gallamine.[204]

Drug Interactions

Muscle Relaxants

Combinations of gallamine with metocurine, but not d-tubocurarine or pancuronium, demonstrate potentiation in the guinea pig nerve-lumbrical preparation. The combination shows about a twofold greater potency than expected from simple addition[205] and shifts the carbachol dose-response curve about 20% further than predicted.[206] Such potentiation has not been utilized in clinical practice.

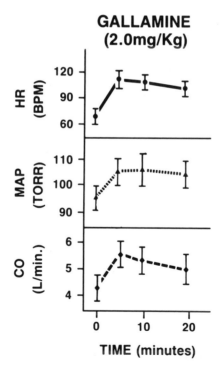

FIG 6–22.
Changes in heart rate *(HR)*, mean arterial pressure *(MAP)*, and cardiac output *(CO)* after administration of gallamine, 2 mg/kg, during nitrous oxide-oxygen-halothane anesthesia. (From Stoelting RK: Hemodynamic effects of gallamine during halothane-nitrous oxide anesthesia. *Anesthesiology* 1973; 39:645–647. Used by permission.)

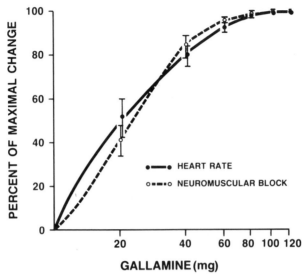

FIG 6–23.
Effect of gallamine on heart rate and neuromuscular block expressed as percent of maximal effect. (From Eisele JH, Marta JA, Davis HS: Quantitative aspects of the chronotropic and neuromuscular effects of gallamine in anesthetized man. *Anesthesiology* 1971; 35:630–633. Used by permission.)

Gallamine has 1/20,000 the action of pancuronium in inhibiting plasma butyrylcholinesterase.[207] Thus it does not prolong the action of succinylcholine when given for precurarization.

Special Situations

Renal Failure

The clearance of gallamine is reduced in renal failure more than any other muscle relaxant. Figure 6 – 24 demonstrates the combined effects of increased dose and renal failure on plasma concentrations and neuromuscular blockade. When the dose of gallamine is increased in normal subjects from 2 to 6 mg/kg, the duration of 95% paralysis is prolonged more than threefold as a result of the log-linear scale. In renal failure, rapid redistribution of gallamine (despite an increase in half-life from 2.5 to 12.5 hours) results in similar duration of 95% block but a slower recovery to 50% block after small doses. However, large or repeated doses and continuous infusions nullify the effect of redistribution and produce a prolonged neuromuscular blockade. Large doses with a half-life of 12.5 hours transpose the curve upward necessitating removal of the drug by dialysis.[191]

Mode of Administration

Gallamine is seldom used in clinical practice as a result of the tachycardia. The slow onset of action necessitated the use of succinylcholine to facilitate endotracheal intubation followed by administration of a bolus dose of gallamine, 1 to 2 mg/kg, and repeated doses of 0.25 to 0.5 mg/kg. Shanks et al.[208] demonstrated that using a bolus of 2.5 mg/kg followed by an infusion of 0.8 mg/kg/hour, a stable plasma concentration of 22 µg/ml was associated with a block of approximately 90%.[208]

Gallamine in a dose of 10 to 20 mg maintains some popularity for

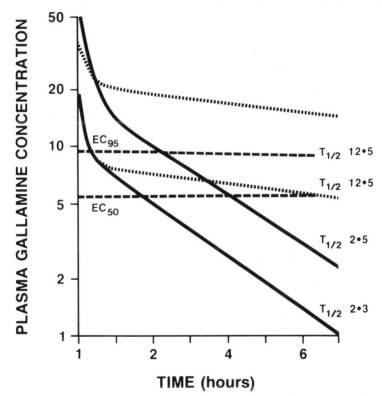

FIG 6–24.
Predicted plasma gallamine time curves from pooled data to demonstrate the effect of increasing the dose from 2 to 6 mg/kg in normal *(solid lines)* and renal failure *(dotted lines)* patients. The horizontal lines indicate plasma concentrations associated with 50% and 95% block. (Adapted from Ramzan MI, Triggs EJ, Shanks CA: Pharmacokinetic studies in man with gallamine triethiodide: I. Single and multiple clinical doses. *Eur J Clin Pharmacol* 1980; 17:135–143 and Ramzan MI, Shanks CA, Triggs EJ: Gallamine disposition in surgical patients with chronic renal failure. *Br J Clin Pharmacol* 1981; 12:141–147.)

precurarizatïon to prevent some of the complications of succinylcholine,[209] although the dose of succinylcholine needs to be increased from 1 to 1.5 mg/kg. Early reports that it might prevent the increase in intraocular pressure associated with succinylcholine[210] have not been confirmed.[211] Such small doses of nondepolarizing relaxants are not harmless. Most patients experience some weakness and are aware of heavy eyelids or blurred vision. Some develop obvious respiratory weakness, and regurgitation and aspiration has been described.

METOCURINE

Methylation of the two hydroxy (OH) groups of d-tubocurarine produces a more potent relaxant. Initially, it was called dimethyltubocurarine, but the methylated form is really O,O',N-trimethyl tubocurarine.[212] The error resulted from the belief that d-tubocurarine was a bis-quaternary compound. Thus, the methylated form has been renamed metocurine (Fig 6 – 25). Recent interest in the compound has resulted from the demonstration that it is relatively free from cardiovascular effects and because improved methods of preparation have been introduced.

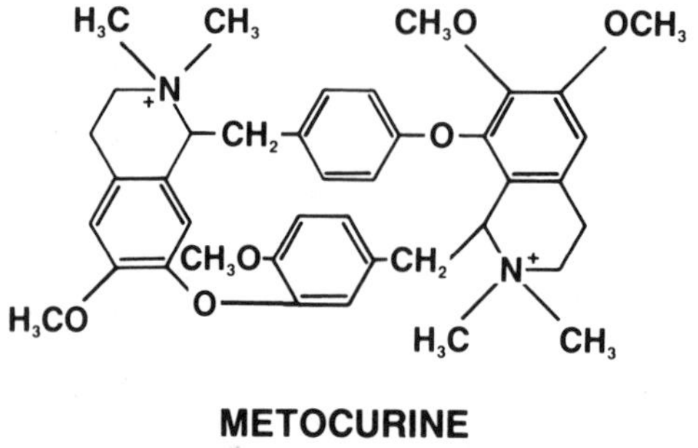

METOCURINE

FIG 6–25.
Structure of metocurine.

Metabolism and Excretion

Metocurine, like d-tubocurarine, undergoes no measurable degree of metabolism in man.[213] Within 48 hours of intravenous administration, 46% to 58% is excreted in the urine and a further 2% in the bile. Biliary excretion of metocurine is much less than d-tubocurarine (Fig 6 – 26). Total body clearance, calculated from plasma decay curves, is greater for metocurine than for d-tubocurarine, although less is recovered from the urine and bile over 48 hours. It is assumed that the remainder is distributed to storage depots within the body, e.g., cartilage mucopolysaccharides, from which it is slowly released. Protein binding of metocurine (35%) is less than for d-tubocurarine (51%).[213]

Pharmacokinetics

Pharmacokinetic variables for metocurine in man have been obtained following measurement of plasma concentrations using either radiolabeled metocurine or a radioimmunoassay.[214, 215] Metocurine is more dependent on renal excretion than d-tubocurarine, and consequently, decreased renal clearance in the elderly (Fig 6–27) is associated with a considerable increase in the terminal half-life. Typical variables for metocurine are shown in Table 6 – 10 and the relationship between serum metocurine concentration and neuromuscular block in Figure 6 – 28.

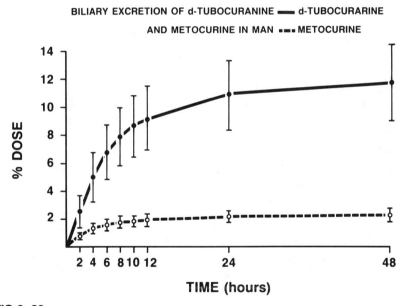

BILIARY EXCRETION OF d-TUBOCURANINE ▬▬ d-TUBOCURARINE

AND METOCURINE IN MAN ▬▪▪ METOCURINE

TIME (hours)

FIG 6–26.

Comparative biliary excretion of *d*-tubocurarine and metocurine in man. (From Meijer DKF, Weitering JG, Vermeer GA, et al: Comparative pharmacokinetics of *d*-tubocurarine and metocurarine in man. *Anesthesiology* 1979; 51:402–497. Used by permission.)

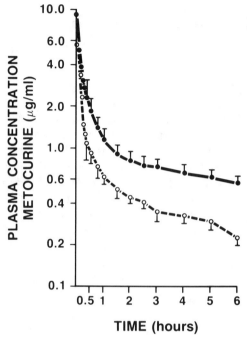

FIG 6–27.

Plasma concentration-time curves for metocurine in young *(open circles)* and elderly *(closed circles)* patients. (From Matteo RS, Backus WW, McDaniel DD, et al: Pharmacokinetics and pharmacodynamics of *d*-tubocurarine and metocurarine in the elderly. *Anesth Analg* 1985; 64:23–29. Used by permission.)

TABLE 6–10.

Comparative Pharmacokinetic Variables, Mean ± SEM, for *d*-Tubocurarine and Metocurine

		V_{dss}, L/KG	$t_{1/2\beta}$, MIN	C_p, ML/MIN/KG	REFERENCES
d-Tubocurarine	Adults	0.39 ± 0.05	346.5 ± 17.3	0.8 ± 0.2	Meijer et al.[213]
Metocurine	Adults	0.42 ± 0.08	216.6 ± 40.6	1.34 ± 1.1	Meijer et al.[213]
Metocurine	25–29 yr	0.45 ± 0.04	269 ± 56	1.1 ± 0.16	Matteo et al.[215]
	>70 yr	0.28 ± 0.03	530 ± 83	0.36 ± 0.08	Matteo et al.[215]
	Renal failure	0.35 ± 0.05	684 ± 90	0.38 ± 0.06	Brotherton and Matteo[214]

Neuromuscular Blockade

Potency

Metocurine is approximately twice as potent as *d*-tubocurarine[216, 217] although the individual response is variable. Single dose-response curves during N_2O-O_2-narcotic/thiopental anesthesia demonstrated an ED50 of 0.13 mg/kg and an ED95 of 0.29 mg/kg (Table 6–11).

Onset and Intubation

For equipotent doses, the onset of block and the associated intubating conditions with metocurine were similar to pancuronium and d-tubocurarine. Maximum block after 0.3 mg/kg was achieved in about 5 minutes.[217]

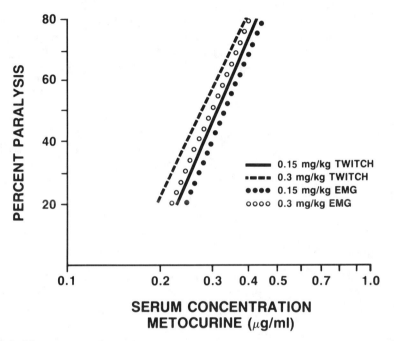

FIG 6–28.
Relationship between serum metocurine concentration and neuromuscular blockade assessed either by twitch or EMG depression during recovery from block. (From Matteo RS, Brotherton WP, Nishitatems K, et al: Pharmacodynamics and pharmacokinetics of metocurine in humans: A comparison to d-tubocurarine. *Anesthesiology* 1982; 57:183–190. Used by permission.)

TABLE 6–11.
Comparative Dose Responses of Metocurine, d-Tubocurarine, and Pancuronium During Balanced Anesthesia*

	ED50, MG/KG[†]	ED95, MG/KG[†]
Metocurine	0.13 (0.1–0.17)	0.28 (0.16–0.49)
d-Tubocurarine	0.26 (0.17–0.32)	0.51 (0.31–0.83)
Pancuronium	0.04 (0.03–0.05)	0.07 (0.04–0.12)

*Adapted from Savarese JJ, Ali HH, Antonio RP: The clinical pharmacology of metocurine: Dimethyltubocurarine, revisited. *Anesthesiology* 1977; 47:277–285.
†Mean values and 95% confidence limits.

Duration

Recovery to 25% twitch height after 0.3 mg/kg metocurine occurred in about 80 minutes, which was similar to an equipotent dose of pancuronium.[217]

Recovery and Reversal

Recovery can be accelerated with anticholinesterases. The time of recovery to 98% of control twitch height was found to be proportional to the dose of neostigmine and the depth of block at the time of reversal,[215] as had been demonstrated previously for d-tubocurarine[218] and pancuronium.[219]

Site of Action

Metocurine, a nondepolarizing neuromuscular blocking drug, has its principal site of action at the postjunctional membrane. Following administration of bolus doses, there is a good correlation between plasma concentrations and 20% to 80% recovery of neuromuscular paralysis whether the latter is assessed electromyographically or mechanically[220] (Fig 6 – 28).

Cardiovascular Action

In cats and monkeys, the separation between the neuromuscular and autonomic effects of metocurine[220] is much greater than for d-tubocurarine[16] (Fig 6 – 29). Also, it produces less histamine release.[221] Savarese, noting the difference between the autonomic and neuromuscular blocking actions of the muscle relaxants, introduced the term "autonomic margin of safety."[222] Ratios were produced by dividing the ED50 values of sympathetic block, vagal block, and histamine release by the ED95 of neuromuscular blockade (Table 6 – 12). These demonstrated the greater cardiovascular stability of metocurine.

Further studies in animals[223] and man[217, 224] confirmed that changes in heart rate and blood pressure did not occur until doses greater than the ED95 were administered (Fig 6–30). Consequently, metocurine is a better choice of relaxant for patients with cardiovascular disease than are gallamine and d-tubocurarine.[225]

Relaxant Combinations

Potentiated antagonism at the neuromuscular junction when two antagonists are employed simultaneously was first observed in man with combinations of pancuronium-metocurine and pancuronium-d-

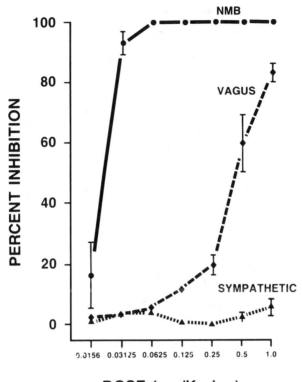

FIG 6–29.
Relationship between neuromuscular and autonomic effects of metocurine in cats. (From Hughes R, Chapple DJ: Cardiovascular and neuromuscular effects of dimethyl tubocurarine in anaesthetized cats and rhesus monkeys. *Br J Anaesth* 1976; 48:847–851. Used by permission.)

TABLE 6–12.
Autonomic Margins of Safety of Metocurine and *d*-Tubocurarine in the Cat*

DOSE RATIO	METOCURINE	*d*-TUBOCURARINE
ED50 sympathetic block / ED95 neuromuscular block	176.0	3.86
ED50 vagal block / ED95 neuromuscular block	34.0	0.83
ED50 histamine release / ED95 neuromuscular block	35.2	1.14

*Adapted from Savarese JJ: The autonomic margin of safety of metocurine and *d*-tubocurarine in the cat. *Anesthesiology* 1979; 50:40–46.

tubocurarine.[131] The mechanism of the synergism remains speculative. Addition of one relaxant in the presence of another to plasma in vitro or in vivo did not affect the unbound proportion of either.[226] Thus, the potentiation is not the result of displacement of one drug from non-specific binding sites in plasma or noncholinergic tissue by the other. An alternative suggestion is that one drug of the pair might act predominantly presynaptically and the other predominantly postsynaptically. d-Tubocurarine and presumably the structurally similar metocurine have been shown to have a preponderance of prejunctional effects[227, 228] while pancuronium acts postjunctionally.[229, 230] An alternative possibility is that the potentiation is entirely of postsynaptic origin. Waud and Waud[206] suggested that potentiation may result from asymmetry of binding of different relaxants to the alpha subunits of the nicotinic acetylcholine receptor.

Whatever the mechanism, the combination of potentiating relaxants allows the intensity of neuromuscular blockade to be maintained while diluting some of their individual side effects. For example, the combination of pancuronium-metocurine has been recommended for the

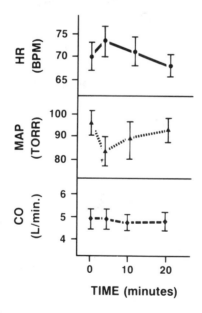

TIME (minutes)

FIG 6–30.
Changes in heart rate *(HR)*, mean arterial blood pressure *(MAP)*, and cardiac output *(CO)* after metocurine, 0.2 mg/kg. (From Stoelting RK: Hemodynamic effects of dimethyl tubocurarine during nitrous oxide-halothane anesthesia. *Anesth Analg* 1974; 53:513–515. Used by permission.)

provision of prolonged relaxation without cardiovascular effects.[231] It has also been used to maintain hemodynamic stability and prevent an increase in intraocular pressure. However, ideal intubating conditions using the mixture were not obtained for more than 4 minutes, which is unsuitable for emergency ocular surgery.[232]

Metocurine and the Burn Patient

Several studies have demonstrated resistance to nondepolarizing relaxants in the burned patient. The resistance depends on the severity of the injury and the interval between the burn and the administration of NMBD. The most likely cause of the resistance is spread of acetylcholine receptors along the muscle membrane away from the neuromuscular junction.[233] Resistance to metocurine has been observed in man.[234, 235] Repeated administration to an 8-year-old boy with a 35% body surface burn showed that during the acute phase, 12 times the normal dose and 8 times the plasma concentration of metocurine were required to achieve complete neuromuscular block. Gradually, his sensitivity returned, but it was still abnormal more than a year after the injury (Fig 6–31).

The cause of relaxant hyposensitivity in the burned patient is uncertain although disuse atrophy may be important (see Chapter 12). Resistance has also been demonstrated in several conditions including upper motor neuron lesions, thermal injury, and liver disease. Shayevitz and Matteo demonstrated in hemiplegic patients that higher plasma concentrations of metocurine were required to produce relaxation in the paralyzed limb. Surprisingly, lower concentrations but higher than normal concentrations were also required to produce relaxation on the unaffected side.[236]

Mode of Administration

Metocurine enjoyed a brief popularity as a result of the lack of cardiovascular effects. However, the introduction of atracurium and vecuronium, which have fewer cardiovascular actions, has largely replaced it for patients with compromised cardiac function.

The slow onset of maximum blockade has limited its use mainly to maintenance relaxation after facilitation of tracheal intubation with succinylcholine. Used in this fashion, doses of 0.2 to 0.3 mg/kg provide relaxation for 40 to 60 minutes. Larger doses, 0.4 mg/kg, will provide acceptable intubating conditions in most patients in 3 to 4 minutes. Metocurine has been used as the initial relaxant in a priming sequence

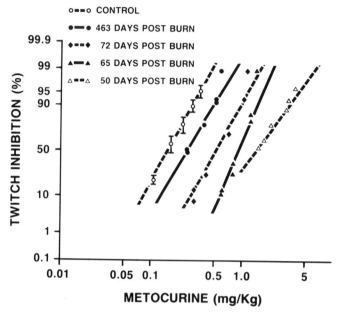

FIG 6–31.
Repeated dose-response curves in a burned patient to demonstrate that the curve is still shifted to the right more than 1 year (463 days) after the burn. (From Martyn JAJ, Matteo RS, Szyfelbein SK, et al: Unprecedented resistance to neuromuscular blocking effects of metocurine with persistence after complete recovery in a burned patient. *Anesth Analg* 1982; 61:614–617. Used by permission.)

to accelerate the onset of the main dose of pancuronium or atracurium.[237] There are no reports of a metocurine-metocurine sequence.

PANCURONIUM

Pancuronium is a long-acting nondepolarizing muscle relaxant (Fig 6–32). It was developed from a series of bis-quaternary aminosteroidal salts[238] that have no hormonal action. It represents one of the few successful examples of custom-designed drugs.

Chemistry

A bis-quaternary ammonium structure was preferred to a single nitrogen atom and quaternary nitrogen atoms rather than onium groups because of increased potency. The two quaternary groups are separated by attachment to a rigid steroid structure to maintain a constant interonium distance (1.11 nm) within the optimal range for neuromuscular blocking activity.[239] Its bulk (pachycurare) encourages nondepolarizing activity.[240] Receptor affinity was enhanced by incorporating acetylcholine moieties.[241]

In cats, pancuronium demonstrated ten times the potency of *d*-tubocurarine, and its activity was decreased at low temperatures. Little evidence of autonomic ganglionic blockade existed: the response of guinea pig ileum to stimulation was half that of *d*-tubocurarine, and when contractions of the cat nictitating membrane were induced, pancuronium showed activity only one eighth that of hexamethonium. Unlike *d*-tubocurarine, it did not release histamine or produce bronchoconstriction in the guinea pig. An atropine-like effect was not observed, but it did block the decrease in blood pressure (BP) produced by vagal stimulation. In the cat, BP and heart rate (HR) were unchanged.[242] The first use in man demonstrated that it was more potent than d-tubocurarine. A dose of 2 to 3 mg lasted for about 1 hour and produced no cardiovascular effects.[243]

Metabolism

Theoretically, pancuronium can be metabolized to 3-OH, 17-OH, and 3,17-$(OH)_2$ derivatives, but only the 3-OH compound has been identified in man.[244] This compound has one half to one third the neuromuscular blocking activity of the parent compound, whereas the 17-OH and 3,17-$(OH)_2$ metabolites have only 1% to 2% of the activity of pancuronium [244–246] (Fig 6–33). The metabolites are less potent than pancuronium in producing vagal blockade.

Several values from 20% to 87%[247, 248] for protein-binding of pancuronium have been suggested, which, in part, reflects the different

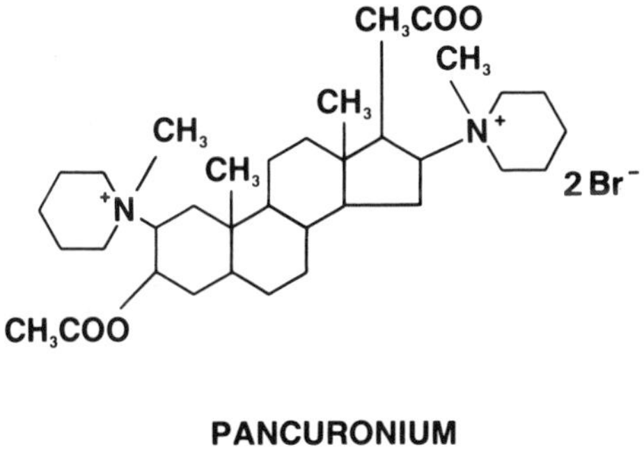

PANCURONIUM

FIG 6–32.
Structure of pancuronium.

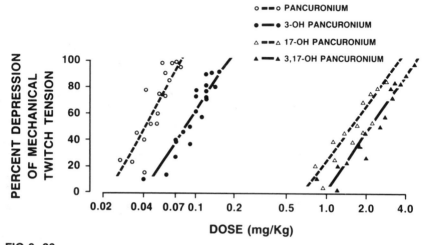

FIG 6–33.
Dose-response curves for pancuronium and its metabolites in man. (Redrawn from Miller RD, Agoston S, Booij LHD, et al: The comparative potency and pharmacokinetics of pancuronium and its metabolites in anesthetized man. *J Pharmacol Exp Ther* 1981; 207:539–543. Used by permission.)

methodology. However, the failure to demonstrate significant correlations between pancuronium dose requirements and the concentration of any of the serum protein fractions[249] suggests that protein binding is small and unimportant for its clinical activity. When drug binding was estimated by equilibrium dialysis using ³H-pancuronium, the free fraction varied from 83% to 93% and was not affected by sex, pregnancy, contraceptive use, or renal disease.[250, 251]

Pharmacokinetics

A sensitive spectrofluorimetric assay has been developed to measure pancuronium concentrations in plasma.[252] The assay also detects deacetylated metabolites, but because their concentration is low[253–255] the assay remains specific for pancuronium. Pharmacokinetic analysis using a two-compartment open model has been compared in normal patients and in those with renal and hepatic dysfunction. Typical values are shown in Figure 6–34 and Table 6–13. They demonstrate the wide scatter of pancuronium pharmacokinetics that results from difficulties with the assay, problems with the analysis, and patient variation. Similar values were found using a more specific mass spectrometry assay.[256] Nevertheless, the results demonstrate the importance of the kidney and liver in excreting the drug. In renal[251] and hepatic disease[256, 260] the duration of action may be prolonged, particularly if large doses are given. An increase in the volumes of distribution of pancuronium in renal failure, which was demonstrated in one study,[257] may have resulted from differences in fluid management during dialysis therapy in this institution. The decrease in glomerular filtration rate with age is also associated with a measurable age-related decrease in pancuronium clearance[258] (Fig 6–35).

During recovery from neuromuscular blockade, a good correlation

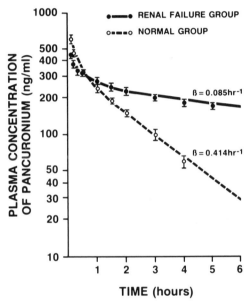

FIG 6–34.
Plasma pancuronium time curves in normal and renal failure patients. β = elimination rate constant. (Redrawn from McLeod K, Watson MJ, Rawlins MD: Pharmacokinetics of pancuronium in patients with normal and impaired renal function. *Br J Anaesth* 1976; 48:341–345. Used by permission.)

TABLE 6–13.
Mean Pharmacokinetic Variables for Pancuronium for Normal, Renal-Failure and Cholestatic Patients

	REFERENCE	$t_{1/2\beta}$, MIN	C_p, ML/MIN	V_{dss}, L/KG
Normal man	Somogyi et al.[251]	133	123	0.261
	McLeod et al.[257]	100	74	0.148
	Duvaldestin et al.[256]	114	130	0.279
Renal failure	Somogyi et al.[251]	257	53	0.296
	McLeod et al.[257]	489	20	0.236
Biliary obstruction	Duvaldestin et al.[256]	208	102	0.416
	Duvaldestin et al.[260]	270	59	0.307

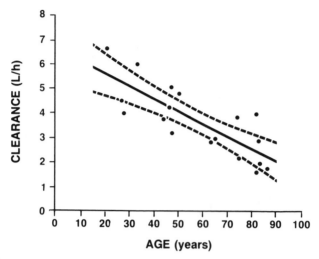

FIG 6–35.
Relationship between pancuronium clearance and age. (From McLeod K, Hull CJ, Watson MJ: Effects of aging on the pharmacokinetics of pancuronium. *Br J Anaesth* 1979; 51:435–438. Used by permission.)

exists between depression of muscle twitch and plasma concentration.[261] Moreover, a similar twitch-concentration relationship has been demonstrated during the pseudoequilibrium of a constant block produced by infusion of pancuronium.[262] However, such relationships do not hold during the temporal disequilibrium at the onset of neuromuscular blockade when the plasma concentration is much higher than at the neuromuscular junction. A pharmacodynamic model has been described[51] that allows calculation of the drug concentration at the active site—the so-called "biophase compartment"—and has been applied to *d*-tubocurarine and pancuronium[263] (Fig 6–36).

Neuromuscular Blockade

Pancuronium was introduced as a potent, nondepolarizing NMBD devoid of cardiovascular effects. Early studies demonstrated that it was about five times as potent as *d*-tubocurarine with a similar onset and duration of action and that it could be antagonized with anticholinesterases.[219, 264, 265] Administration of pancuronium was free of the hypotension and erythema associated with *d*-tubocurarine.[266]

Potency

Dose-response curves for pancuronium, *d*-tubocurarine, gallamine, or metocurine can be obtained using incremental dosing,[192] and the results are similar to those obtained with single bolus injection.[267] Cumulative dose-response curves of evoked adductor pollicis force of contraction estimate the ED50 of 0.03 to 0.04 mg/kg and ED95 of 0.05 to 0.065 mg/kg[55, 192, 245, 267, 268] (Fig 6–37). These results are similar to those obtained measuring grip strength in volunteers,[9, 265] but at doses that produce 90% paralysis of the thumb, ventilation is scarcely affected[265] (Fig 6–38).

Cumulative dose-response curves have been obtained during the course of a continuous intravenous infusion, and in general, they produce similar results if sufficient time is allowed for equilibration.[66, 193, 269] The mean effective plasma pancuronium concentrations that produced 50% and 95% paralysis are 0.20 and 0.25 μg/ml, respectively.[269] The maintenance dose required for 90% blockade was 36.9 μg/kg/hour and 60% of that was required to maintain 50% block.[66]

There is considerable individual variation in response to pancuronium, as for all relaxants. Consequently, test doses have been recommended,[219] and various ingenious dosing regimens have been suggested depending on the ptotic response to 1 mg.[270]

Onset and Intubation

When equipotent doses are used, the onset of action of pancuronium is similar to d-tubocurarine. Doses equivalent to the ED95 produce maximum effect in 3 to 4 minutes.[219, 264] Increasing the dose produces

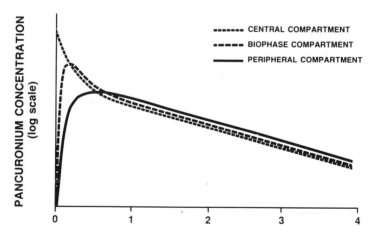

FIG 6–36.
Calculated concentrations of relaxant in central compartment, peripheral compartment, and biophase in a pharmacokinetic model for pancuronium. (From Hull CJ, Van Beem HBH, McLeod K, et al: A pharmacodynamic model for pancuronium. *Br J Anaesth* 1978; 50:1113–1122. Used by permission.)

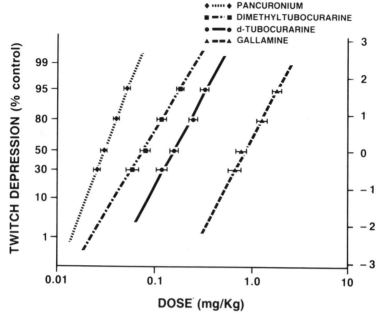

FIG 6–37.
Cumulative dose-response curves for pancuronium, metocurine, d-tubocurarine, and gallamine in man. (From Donlon JV, Ali HH, Savarese JJ: A new approach to the study of four nondepolarizing relaxants in man. *Anesth Analg* 1974; 53:934–939. Used by permission.)

an apparent acceleration of effect, but the onset is much slower than that of succinylcholine, 1 mg/kg, or fazadinium, 1 mg/kg,[173, 174] even after the use of priming doses of pancuronium[237, 271, 272] (Fig 6–39) or d-tubocurarine.[175] After doses of 0.1 mg/kg during N_2O–O_2 halothane anesthesia,[272] endotracheal intubating conditions were judged to be satisfactory in nearly all patients within 2 minutes.[127]

Duration of Action

In man, doses of 0.04 to 0.05 mg/kg recover 90% of adductor pollicis activity in about 1 hour.[219, 264] Increasing the dose prolongs the block. If a second similar dose is administered when neuromuscular activity has returned to normal, the duration of action of the second dose is much greater than the first. This is not an example of cumulation but a demonstration that, even when full recovery has occurred, 70% to 80% of the receptors may still be occupied by relaxant.[273] Consequently, the response to additional NMBD will be increased. Therefore, repeated doses are usually only 20% to 25% of the initial dose.

However, true cumulation—a progressive increase in the duration

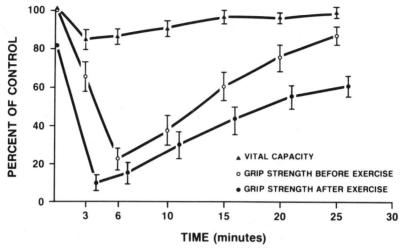

FIG 6–38.
Relationship between changes of grip strength and vital capacity after administration of 0.022 mg/kg of pancuronium in conscious volunteers. (From Foldes FF, Klonymus DH, Maisel W, et al: Studies of pancuronium with *d*-tubocurarine. *Anesthesiology* 1971; 35:496–503. Used by permission.)

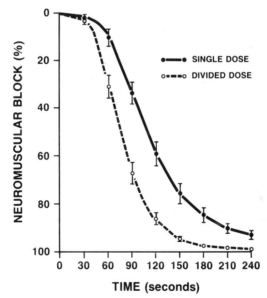

FIG 6–39.
Development of neuromuscular block after single or divided (priming) doses of pancuronium. (From Doherty, WG, Breen PJ, Donati F, et al: Accelerated onset of pancuronium with divided doses. *Can Anaesth Soc J* 1985; 32:1–4. Used by permission.)

of block after similar doses given at the same degree of recovery—has been demonstrated with pancuronium[274] (Fig 6–40). One of the advantages of the new agents, atracurium and vecuronium, is that they are almost devoid of cumulative activity.

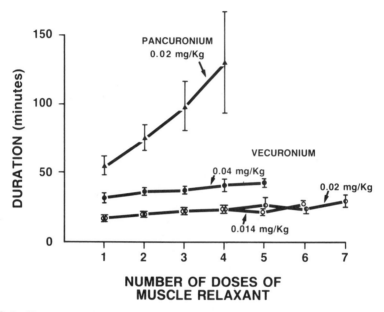

FIG 6–40.
Duration of action of repeated doses of relaxant to demonstrate cumulation with pancuronium but not with vecuronium. (Redrawn from Fahey MR, Morris RB, Miller RD, et al: Clinical pharmacology of ORG NC 45 (Novcuron): A new nondepolarizing muscle relaxant. *Anesthesiology* 1981; 55:6–11. Used by permission.)

Recovery and Reversal

Once recovery has commenced, it proceeds quite rapidly. The recovery index, recovery from 75% to 25% block, is about 24 minutes at a dose of 0.04 mg/kg and increases with higher doses of pancuronium.

Recovery can be accelerated with anticholinesterases. When neostigmine is used, time to return to control twitch height is inversely related to the degree of spontaneous recovery when the antagonist is given[219] (Fig 6–41). Recovery is accelerated more by edrophonium than neostigmine[275–278] as long as equipotent doses are given (Fig 6–42).[279]

Site of Action

The characteristics of the block produced by pancuronium are typical of a competitive neuromuscular block. During partial blockade,

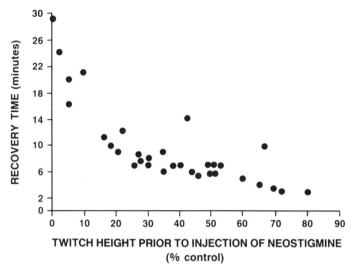

FIG 6–41.
Relationship between twitch height and rate of recovery after neostigmine. (Redrawn with permission from Katz RL: Clinical neuromuscular pharmacology of pancuronium. *Anesthesiology* 1971; 34:550–556.)

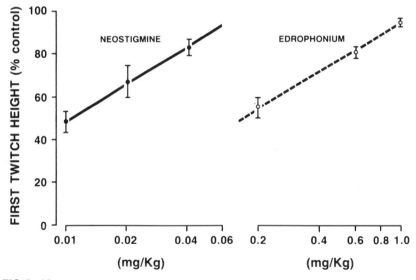

FIG 6–42.
Dose-response curves for neostigmine *(left)* and edrophonium *(right)* in the reversal of pancuronium. (From Breen PJ, Doherty WG, Donati F, et al: The potencies of edrophonium and neostigmine as antagonists of pancuronium. *Anaesthesia* 1985; 40:844–847. Used by permission.)

exercise at a fast rate causes rapid fatigue; train-of-four and tetanic stimulation demonstrate fade: tetanus also induces post-tetanic facilitation.[192] For the same degree of depression of first twitch activity, train-of-four fade for pancuronium is less than that seen after d-tubocurarine in adults[280] and children,[281] suggesting that the prejunctional activity of pancuronium is less than that of d-tubocurarine.[88]

Cardiovascular Action

Early reports of the use of pancuronium commented on the absence of hypotension.[264-266] The only cardiovascular disturbance seen was a mild tachycardia. However, it soon became apparent that when pancuronium in doses of 0.07 to 0.12 mg/kg was given during anesthesia, it was followed by increases in heart rate, blood pressure, and cardiac output[282-284]—quite different from the hypotension, tachycardia, and decreased cardiac output seen after d-tubocurarine. Heart rate and blood pressure increase further after endotracheal intubation.[285]

Despite intensive investigation, the cause of the tachycardia and hypertension remains unclear. In animals, at doses similar to those producing relaxation, pancuronium has a vagolytic effect,[16] and the site of action is probably at the postganglionic nerve terminal.[198]

Pancuronium does not block sympathetic ganglionic transmission. Indeed, it demonstrates sympathomimetic activity as a result of blocking the muscarinic receptors[199, 286, 287] that normally exert a braking effect on ganglionic transmission. Also, inhibition of muscarinic receptors at adrenergic nerve fibers facilitates transmitter release.[288] In addition, pancuronium increases release of catecholamines and decreases their reuptake by adrenergic nerves[289] (Fig 6–43). Although demonstration of a decrease in arrhythmic threshold to epinephrine after administration of pancuronium was not possible,[290] it has been suggested that the sympathomimetic effects may augment the hypertensive and tachycardic response to endotracheal intubation.[291]

In clinical doses, pancuronium has no effect on myocardial contractility in vitro,[292] but at increased doses, the force of myocardial contraction is increased, and the time to peak contraction is reduced.[293]

Pancuronium does not normally lead to an increase in circulating histamine levels although increased concentrations have been demonstrated in a patient with bronchial asthma.[294]

Intraocular and Intracranial Pressure

Pancuronium is not associated with increases in intraocular or intracranial pressure.

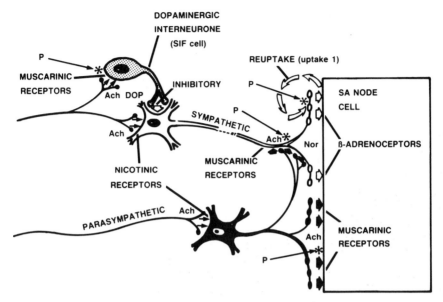

FIG 6–43.
The several possible sites of action of pancuronium *(P)* in the heart include muscarinic receptors at the sinoatrial (SA) node, noradrenergic nerve endings, and the dopaminergic interneuron. Pancuronium also blocks noradrenaline reuptake. Ach = acetylcholine; DOP = dopamine; SIF = small intensely fluorescent cells (dopaminergic interneurons). (Redrawn from *Pharmacology of Neuromuscular Function.* Bowman WC: Baltimore, University Park Press, 1980, p. 106.

Lower Esophageal Pressure

Pancuronium given in doses of 0.1 mg/kg to a group of nonobese, nonpregnant women caused an increase in barrier pressure that persisted for 5 minutes,[295] whereas atracurium had no effect,[122] and vecuronium produced a slight increase in pressure. The significance of these observations is uncertain, but if the tendency to regurgitation is influenced by barrier pressure, further investigation is required to determine the safest relaxant sequence for the patient with a full stomach.

Age

The effects of pancuronium in infants and children have been investigated incompletely. Cumulative dose-response curves during halothane anesthesia suggest that infants (<1 year old) and children respond similarly[296] (ED50, 0.04; ED95, 0.08 mg/kg) but are slightly more resistant than adults (ED50, 0.036; ED95, 0.07 mg/kg) studied in a similar fashion.[297] Recovery time (5% to 25%) seemed to be more rapid in adults

(15.6 ± 1.7 vs. 24.0 ± 2.1 minutes).[217] When given in doses of $2 \times$ ED95, maximum block was achieved in 2.5 ± 0.2 minutes and recovery to 5% control was achieved in 65 ± 6 minutes.[298]

The decline in plasma clearance of pancuronium with age suggests that the rate of recovery from a single, large, IV dose will decrease in the elderly.

Drug Interactions

Inhalational Anesthesia

Pancuronium and other nondepolarizing relaxants are potentiated by inhaled anesthetic agents in a dose-dependent fashion. Consequently, the dose requirements for pancuronium are reduced by a factor of 0.56 by 1.25 MAC of isoflurane and by a factor of 0.32 by 1.25 MAC of halothane.[299] The intensity of neuromuscular block produced by 0.02 mg/kg pancuronium increased from 44% to 77%, and the time to 90% recovery increased from 16 to 40 minutes during anesthesia with 0.5% to 1% inspired halothane concentrations.[300] Surprisingly, the potentiation was diminished in patients with renal failure.[301] Enflurane and isoflurane potentiate pancuronium to a similar but greater degree than halothane.[63] During administration of 1.25 MAC anesthesia with halothane, the ED50 for pancuronium was found to be 0.49 mg/sq m compared with 0.29 and 0.27 mg/sq m during enflurane anesthesia, respectively.

Neuromuscular Blocking Drugs

Succinylcholine, 1 mg/kg, given before pancuronium, increases the degree of twitch depression and duration of action of pancuronium.[300] Conversely, when pancuronium is given before succinylcholine, e.g., for precurarization, the duration of action of succinylcholine is prolonged by about 15%[302] because of the inhibition of plasma cholinesterase activity.[303]

Certain combinations of nondepolarizing NMBDs are synergistic in their effect on the neuromuscular junction. In particular, combinations of pancuronium and d-tubocurarine, and pancuronium and metocurine, are synergistic. Simultaneous administration increases the intensity but not the onset or duration of twitch depression[131] or the ability for reversal with neostigmine.[304] The combination has been recommended as a means to reduce unwanted hemodynamic effects without prejudicing muscle relaxation.[231] Similar synergism between pancuronium and d-tubocurarine or metocurine has been demonstrated in the rat phrenic nerve–hemidiaphragm preparation[305] and the guinea pig lumbrical muscle.[205] The cause of the potentiation is uncertain, but Waud and Waud[206] have proposed an entirely postsynaptic hypothesis. Their explanation requires that the receptor molecule contain multiple sites for acetylcholine binding. Activation of the receptor requires simultaneous acceptance of two acetylcholine molecules at distinct sites, and occupation of one of these two sites is sufficient to block the response. Thus different relaxants may act preferentially at different receptor sites.[306] A combination of two relaxants, one of which has predominant presynaptic and the other postsynaptic effects, would also lead to potentiation.[305]

Combinations of pancuronium and the new muscle relaxants atracurium and vecuronium have shown that the effect of pancuronium and vecuronium is additive but that the duration of action increases as the proportion of pancuronium increases.[307] When pancuronium and vecuronium are given alternately, the drug administered first plays a dominant role in influencing the dose requirements and duration of action of the subsequent relaxant. Thus, the duration of action of vecuronium is prolonged when preceded by pancuronium.[308] Potentiation deserves further investigation, particularly if a combination of drugs is used for the priming principle.

Other Drugs

Several other agents have been associated with abnormal reactions to pancuronium (see Chapter 12). In particular, resistance has been observed in patients receiving aminophylline[309] or diphenylhydantoin.[310]

Special Situations

Coronary Artery Bypass Surgery

The key to maintaining optimal cardiovascular function in the patient with coronary artery disease is to avoid alterations in heart rate and blood pressure and to prevent myocardial ischemia associated with an increase in rate-pressure product (RPP). Current practice is often based on a high-dose narcotic technique with fentanyl,[311] sufentanil,[312] or morphine.[313] In choosing the muscle relaxant, the bradycardia of fentanyl[314] is compensated by the cardiovascular effects of pancuronium. Sometimes this strategy fails, and pancuronium-induced increases in heart rate and RPP[315] are associated with myocardial ischemia from a deterioration in myocardial oxygen balance. The ischemia is not prevented with prophylactic nitroglycerine[315] but usually is prevented when metocurine replaces pancuronium,[316, 317] although the risk of hypotension with metocurine does exist.[318] These reports demonstrate the problems of matching the unwanted effects of one drug with those of another to produce, within the therapeutic range of each drug, a combination without side effects. Clinical anesthesia cannot be practiced with a cookbook![319] Perhaps the newer relaxants together with anticholinergic agents to counteract the narcotic bradycardia will prove superior.

Obstetric Anesthesia

Pancuronium, as a result of its cardiovascular stability, has become the most popular NMBD to provide surgical muscle relaxation for cesarean section after endotracheal intubation is facilitated with succinylcholine.[320-322] After doses of 0.05 to 0.08 mg/kg are injected into the mother, pancuronium can be detected in the umbilical vein within 2 minutes, but fetal concentrations seldom exceed 0.1 μg/ml and are less than half maternal values.[323] Effects of pancuronium on the infant have never been reported, but in adults during recovery of neuromuscular blockade a concentration of only 0.2 μg/ml is associated with 50% paralysis.[269]

Renal Failure

The duration of action and rate of recovery from pancuronium, particularly after large doses, are prolonged in renal failure[324] (Fig 6–44) because of the decrease in plasma clearance. Thus, to be used safely, the smallest possible doses together with inhalational anesthesia should be administered, and the neuromuscular junction should be monitored carefully. Fortunately, reversal of a pancuronium blockade is unaffected because the elimination of the anticholinesterases is also inhibited.[325-327] Once recovery is established, recurarization does not occur.[328] It is likely in the future that relaxants that are predominantly excreted by the kidney will be replaced by atracurium or vecuronium in patients with renal failure.

Liver Disease

Patients with chronic liver disease demonstrate resistance to pancuronium.[329-331] Pharmacokinetic studies have demonstrated that in cirrhotic patients, the resistance results from an increased volume of distribution and the prolonged paralysis from decreased plasma clearance.[330] In cholestasis, the reasons are not so clear. Two studies demonstrated an increase in terminal half-life from either a decreased plasma clearance[331] or an increased volume of distribution,[332] respectively. In addition, liver uptake of pancuronium may be reduced, which prolongs the block.[333] In patients with acute hepatitis, plasma clearance was reduced.[334] There is no evidence that resistance to pancuronium results from an increase in protein binding.[335]

Neuromuscular Disease

Myasthenia Gravis.—Myasthenic patients are sensitive to nondepolarizing relaxants so it is usually recommended that these drugs should be avoided. Nevertheless, muscle relaxation can be augmented by carefully titrated doses of pancuronium.[336] The rapid recovery from vecuronium or atracurium makes them more suitable agents.

Burns.—Burned patients show resistance to the nondepolarizing NMBDs.[337, 338] The resistance, which is associated with succinylcholine-induced hyperkalemia,[339] is not a result of increase in protein binding[340] or altered pharmacokinetic behavior[341] but is more likely to be associated with receptor multiplication,[342] which increases pancu-

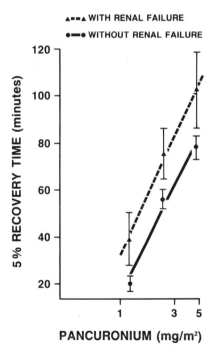

FIG 6–44.
Duration of action of pancuronium in normal patients and patients with renal failure. (From Miller RD, Stevens WC, Way WL: The effect of renal failure and hyperkalemia on the duration of action of pancuronium neuromuscular blockade in man. *Anesth Analg* 1973; 52:661–666. Used by permission.)

ronium binding sites so that higher than normal plasma concentrations are necessary to produce neuromuscular blockade.

Disuse Atrophy.—The resistance to nondepolarizing relaxants seen in burns and upper motor neuron lesions has the common feature of muscle disuse. In animals, if disuse atrophy is produced by placing one leg in a plaster cast for a month, the ED50 in the control limb increases nearly twofold.[343] This observation may provide the common link for several observations of apparent resistance to relaxants in the immobile patient.[344]

Malignant Hyperthermia.—Pancuronium is not a trigger for malignant hyperthermia.

Mode of Administration

The onset of action of pancuronium is slow. Therefore, large doses are required to produce good intubating conditions rapidly. Doses must exceed 0.15 mg/kg to produce conditions similar to those produced by administration of succinylcholine,[345] but such doses also lead to prolonged neuromuscular blockade. Therefore, pancuronium is usually given after intubation has been facilitated by succinylcholine. Initial doses of 0.03 to 0.06 mg/kg may be followed by "top-up" doses of 0.01 to 0.03 mg/kg. Alternatively, maintenance relaxation can be produced by a continuous infusion when doses of 0.4 to 0.6 μg/kg/hour will be required.[346] Ingenious researchers have attempted to provide a simple feedback control system that delivers a dose of pancuronium automatically according to the muscle response to nerve stimulation.[347]

d-TUBOCURARINE

d-Tubocurarine is the purified form of Intocostrin, the first muscle relaxant used in clinical practice.[348]

Chemistry

Until recently, it was thought that d-tubocurarine (Fig 6–45) was a bis-quaternary ammonium compound. It is now realized[349] that one of the nitrogen atoms in the molecule is tertiary, although at body pH it becomes protonated so that d-tubocurarine does possess two positively charged centers.

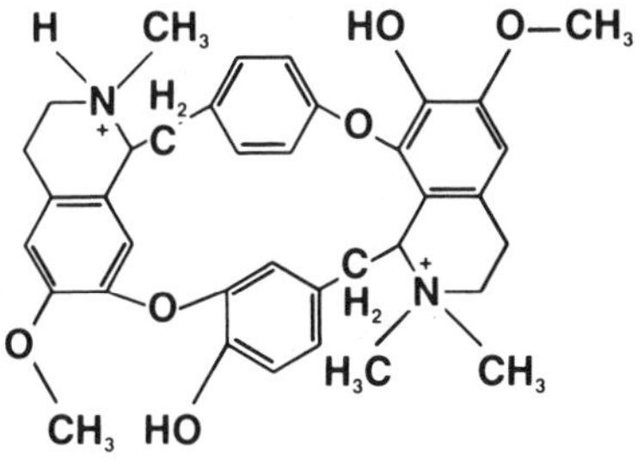

FIG 6–45.
Structure of *d*-tubocurarine.

Alternatives to d-tubocurarine are important both because of its disadvantageous actions and also because its source, *Chondodendron tomentosum* from South America, is becoming scarce.

d-Tubocurarine undergoes minimal metabolism in the body.[213] Twenty-four hours after its administration, 12% can be recovered from the bile and 44% in the urine, although the biliary proportion is increased threefold in renal failure, at least in dogs.[350] This is not a compensatory phenomenon but a passive response to elevated plasma concentrations of d-tubocurarine. The fate of the remaining relaxant is uncertain. It is assumed that after distribution, it is bound at inaccessible sites and released slowly.

Protein Binding

Several studies have reported that d-tubocurarine is 33% to 56% protein bound[335, 350–352] but that the degree of binding is not affected in renal, hepatic, or cardiac disease.[352, 353] Systematic examination of the pharmacokinetic or pharmacodynamic behavior of the relaxants in conditions of altered plasma protein has not been performed, but it is likely to be of minimal importance, particularly if binding is less than 50%.

Pharmacokinetics

The development of a radioimmunoassay for d-tubocurarine that was sensitive to 5 ng/ml and required only small volumes of biologic fluid[354] allowed the first demonstration of a correlation between plasma d-tubocurarine concentration and recovery from neuromuscular block[355] (Fig 6–46).

Previous studies in which a less sensitive spectrophotometric assay was used in humans[356] or ³H-d-tubocurarine in animals[350] described the pattern of disappearance of d-tubocurarine from plasma and its redistribution.[357, 358] These showed that the kidney was an important route of elimination[359] and encouraged rational therapeutic regimens to be based on the anticipated clearance of the drug.[360]

The following are typical pharmacokinetic values for d-tubocurarine in adults:[213, 215, 362–365] volume of distribution: 0.3 to 0.6 L/kg; plasma clearance: 1 to 3 ml/kg/minute; terminal half-life: 90 to 346 minutes.

The wide spread of values is indicative of individual variation, problems with the assay, and, unfortunately, some studies that sampled for too short a time for the variables to be calculated accurately.

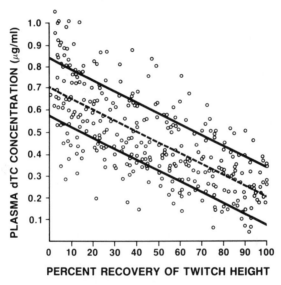

FIG 6–46.
Relationship between twitch height and plasma d-tubocurarine concentration. (From Matteo RS, Spector S, Horowitz PE: Relation of serum d-tubocurarine concentration to neuromuscular blockade. *Anesthesiology* 1974; 41:441–443. Used by permission.)

In renal failure, the plasma clearance of d-tubocurarine is reduced[361] (Fig 6–47). Similarly, as glomerular filtration deteriorates in the elderly, the clearance of d-tubocurarine is reduced. In addition, the volume of distribution is decreased, the terminal half-life is prolonged, and the recovery of neuromuscular activity is longer in the old than in the young.[215] In patients with normal renal function, the osmotic diuretic mannitol does not increase d-tubocurarine clearance or affect the pharmacokinetic variables.[362] In neonates, the terminal half-life and volume of distribution are increased.[363,364] Consequently, one might expect an increase in relaxant requirement, but the neonate's increased volume of distribution is matched by an increased sensitivity of the neuro-

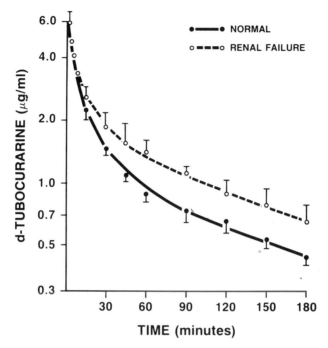

FIG 6–47.
Plasma concentration-time curves for d-tubocurarine in normal and renal failure patients. (From Miller RD, Matteo RS, Benet LZ, et al: The pharmacokinetics of d-tubocurarine in man with and without renal failure. *J Pharmacol Exp Ther* 1977; 202:1–7. Used by permission.)

muscular junction.[364] Therefore, on a mg/kg basis the d-tubocurarine requirement is unchanged. As children get older, the elimination half-life and volumes of distribution approach adult values.

Shanks et al., while attempting to determine the potency of d-tubocurarine during a constant infusion, showed that at a psuedo-steady state, 50% block was associated with a plasma concentration of 0.54 μg/ml and predicted that a concentration between 0.95 and 1.67 μg/ml would be needed for 95% block.[365]

Neuromuscular Blockade

Site of Action

The predominant site of action of d-tubocurarine is at the post-junctional membrane where the drug competes with acetylcholine at the receptor. In addition, d-tubocurarine acts at the prejunctional receptor to reduce the release of acetylcholine from nerves that are stimulated rapidly and repeatedly.[366–369] The clinical equivalent of this action is the fade in response to tetanic or train-of-four stimulation, which is the hallmark of partial nondepolarizing neuromuscular blockade. The train-of-four fade after d-tubocurarine is greater than after pancuronium.[280, 370] Consequently, it has been suggested that it has the greater prejunctional activity.[88] Others[371–373] dispute this hypothesis and suggest that the fade is indicative of postjunctional channel blockade: curare enters the open channel preventing further current flow. This too has been refuted.[374, 375]

Potency

Dose-response curves for d-tubocurarine of the force of contraction of the adductor pollicis give an ED50 of 0.26 (1.17 to 0.32) mg/kg and an ED95 of 0.51 (0.31 to 0.83) mg/kg (95% confidence limits).[217] Similar values are obtained by the cumulative and single-dose methods[192, 267] and by administering the agent using a constant-rate infusion.[11] Increasing the frequency of the nerve stimulation to more than 0.15 Hz appears to increase the drug's potency.[376] Infants and children show a sensitivity similar to adults on a mg/kg basis.[377] These studies demonstrate that d-tubocurarine is about one sixth as potent as pancuronium.[217] A similar potency ratio was obtained using grip strength as the measure of paralysis.[9] Nevertheless, the authors of all studies have described considerable individual patient variation, and some have recommended the initial use of small test doses.[378]

Onset and Intubating Conditions

The onset of neuromuscular blockade after administration of d-tubocurarine is slow. Following administration of a dose of 0.6 mg/kg, maximum block does not develop for 5.7 ± 1.1 minutes.[217] Other studies, in which equipotent doses of d-tubocurarine and pancuronium were used, showed that the onset times are similar.[9, 173] Consequently, d-tubocurarine is seldom used as an agent to facilitate intubation. The ease of intubation is dependent also on the depth of anesthesia, and authors of studies to determine cumulative dose-response effects of d-tubocurarine have often commented on the good intubating conditions when 95% block had been achieved although the vocal cords were not fully abducted.[192]

Duration

The duration of action of d-tubocurarine is similar to equipotent doses of pancuronium[217] but longer than gallamine.[379] After a dose of 0.6 mg/kg during balanced anesthesia, the twitch returns to 25% by about 80 minutes. During hyperventilation, d-tubocurarine produces a less intense and shorter neuromuscular blockade, whereas the addition of 10% CO_2 increases both the depth and duration of paralysis.[380] Surprisingly, for the same dose of d-tubocurarine, the magnitude and duration of block were found to be less in patients in London than New York.[381] There is no explanation for this finding, although it excuses the use of greater quantities of d-tubocurarine in Britain than in North America.

If a second dose of d-tubocurarine is given after recovery from an initial dose of the same magnitude, the second dose has a more prolonged effect.[382] This pseudocumulation reflects the margin of safety of the junction as 70% of receptors may still be occupied at full recovery of function.[273] Subsequent doses do demonstrate true cumulation: a progressive increase in the duration of action as a result of the gradual increase in concentration of relaxants at the sites of redistribution.

Recovery and Reversal

The rate of recovery of neuromuscular activity is similar after d-tubocurarine and pancuronium. Times of recovery from 75% to 25% block are approximately 25 to 35 minutes—much slower than atracurium and vecuronium. Recovery can be accelerated with the anticholinesterases edrophonium, neostigmine, or pyridostigmine. Edrophonium in equipotent doses is more rapid in its action.[383] When neostigmine (2.5 mg) was used, the time to recovery of twitch height was related to the degree of spontaneous recovery at the time when the reversal agent was administered[378] (Fig 6–48). To achieve rapid recovery consistently, it is more effective to modify the dose of reversal agent according to the depth of neuromuscular block.

Cardiovascular Effects

Hypotension is a common accompaniment of the administration of d-tubocurarine. In cats, autonomic blockade occurred at parasympathetic and sympathetic ganglia at similar doses to those causing neuromuscular blockade[16] (Fig 6–49). Despite the parasympathetic blockade, bradycardia is more common than tachycardia, and this may follow the concomitant sympathetic ganglionic block.[384] d-Tubocurarine is the only NMBD that produces appreciable ganglionic blockade.[385, 198]

In addition, d-tubocurarine causes histamine release at clinical doses.[385] Savarese[222] introduced the concept of the "autonomic margin of safety" to describe the separation between doses that caused muscle paralysis and sympathetic block, vagal block, or histamine release. This demonstrated that, in cats, autonomic effects and histamine release occur at clinical doses. Conversely, there was a wide separation with metocurine, suggesting that it should have less cardiovascular activity. The arrhythmogenic response to epinephrine is not modified by *d*-tubocurarine.[290]

In man, the decrease in arterial pressure is associated with only a slight increase in heart rate, systemic vascular resistance,[284] and decreased cardiac output (Fig 6–50). Muscle paralysis with *d*-tubocurarine is frequently associated with skin flushing. Recently, a dose-related increase in serum histamine concentration was demonstrated following *d*-tubocurarine administration,[386] and the increase in histamine levels correlated with the severity of the hypotension. The hypotension can be reduced by pretreatment with the antihistamine promethazine[387] or by administering *d*-tubocurarine slowly over 3 minutes.[388] Thus, in man, histamine release may be more important than ganglionic blockade as the cause of the hypotension. Histamine release may also be the reason that *d*-tubocurarine increased blood flow to the stomach but decreased perfusion to the kidney, liver, skin, spleen, intestine, and adrenal glands in cats.[389]

Other factors including preservatives[390] and direct myocardial

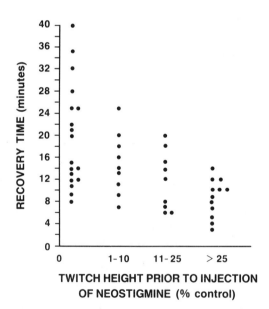

FIG 6–48.
Relationship between time to recovery of *d*-tubocurarine after neostigmine and prereversal twitch height. (From Katz RL: Neuromuscular effects of *d*-tubocurarine, edrophonium and neostigmine in man. *Anesthesiology* 1967; 28:327–336. Used by permission.)

d-TUBOCURARINE

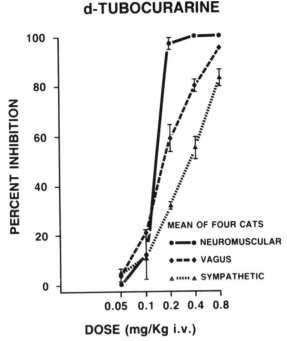

FIG 6–49.
Dose-response curves for the neuromuscular and autonomic effects of *d*-tubocurarine in cats. (From Hughes R, Chapple DJ: Effects of nondepolarizing neuromuscular blocking agents on peripheral autonomic mechanisms in cats. *Br J Anaesth* 1976; 48:59–68. Used by permission.)

depressant[391] and dopaminergic antagonist activities[392] of *d*-tubocurarine have been considered but remain unproved as etiological agents.

Intracranial and Intraocular Pressure

d-Tubocurarine does not increase intracranial pressure during N_2O-O_2-narcotic anesthesia,[393] although one report suggested that pressure may increase secondary to its cardiovascular effects.

Although d-tubocurarine does not increase intraocular pressure (IOP), its onset of action is too slow to facilitate intubation in the emergency patient with an open-eye injury. Suggestions that precurarization may prevent the increase in IOP after succinylcholine are also mistaken.[394] Careful measurement of IOP demonstrates that d-tubocurarine has no protective effect.[395]

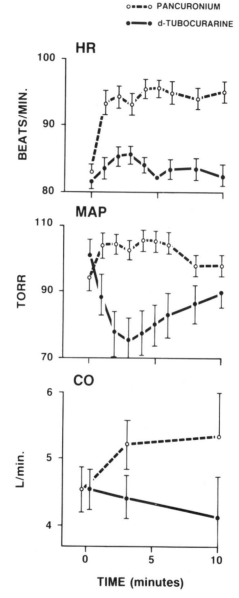

FIG 6–50.
Changes in heart rate *(HR)*, mean arterial pressure *(MAP)*, and cardiac output *(CO)* after administration of *d*-tubocurarine, 0.4 mg/kg, or pancuronium, 0.08 mg/kg, during nitrous oxide-oxygen-halothane anesthesia in man. (From Stoelting RK: The hemodynamic effects of pancuronium and d-tubocurarine in anesthetized patients. *Anesthesiology* 1972; 36:612–615. Used by permission.)

Age

There is considerable dispute whether or not sensitivity to nondepolarizing relaxants is increased in the young (see Chapter 11). Recent pharmacokinetic and pharmacodynamic studies have shown that on a milligram per kilogram basis, sensitivity to d-tubocurarine is not altered.[377] However, this is only achieved because the increased volume of distribution is matched by an increase in sensitivity of the junction.[363] Decreased glomerular filtration in infants leads to delayed elimination and a longer duration of action. The increased cardiac output and decreased circulation time cause more rapid delivery of relaxant to the junction. Consequently, the time to maximum block is age related.[175]

Following administration of a dose of d-tubocurarine, 0.3 mg/kg, recovery times are slower in the elderly than in the young (Table 6–14) as a result of decreased renal clearance (Fig 6–51).[215] However, the relationship between plasma d-tubocurarine concentration and neuromuscular block is unaffected.

TABLE 6–14.
Effect of Age on Duration of Action of d-Tubocurarine, 0.3 mg/kg IV*

RECOVERY TO TWITCH HEIGHT	YOUNG, 30–56 YR	ELDERLY, 70–87 YR	*P*
25%	43 ± 12	64 ± 22	NS
50%	65 ± 14	114 ± 34	<.02
75%	92 ± 21	158 ± 46	<.02
25%–75% recovery index	48 ± 12	94 ± 32	<.02

*Adapted from Matteo RS, et al: Pharmacokinetics and pharmacodynamics of d-tubocurarine and metocurine in the elderly. *Anesth Analg* 1976; 48:969–974. Used by permission.

Drug Interactions

Inhalational Anesthetic Agents

d-Tubocurarine is potentiated by inhalational anesthetics. Earlier studies[396] demonstrated prolonged duration of action during halothane anesthesia, and Miller and colleagues,[62–64] using carefully controlled concentrations of anesthetic, demonstrated a dose-dependent shift in the dose-response curve to d-tubocurarine (Fig 6–52).

Muscle Relaxants

Depolarizing and nondepolarizing relaxants are mutually antagonistic. When d-tubocurarine is given before succinylcholine for precurarization, the latter has decreased potency and shorter duration of action[302] so that it is recommended that the dose of succinylcholine be increased to 1.5 mg/kg. Conversely, the potency of d-tubocurarine is enhanced when administered after succinylcholine.[381]

While combinations of d-tubocurarine and metocurine are simply additive, combinations with pancuronium potentiate the block.[131] A similar potentiation of d-tubocurarine has been observed with vecuronium,[397] alcuronium,[305] and gallamine.[398]

Special Situations

Cardiovascular Disease

The unpredictable hypotensive effect of d-tubocurarine makes it unsuitable for use in patients with coronary artery disease. Indeed, the introduction of vecuronium and atracurium, which are almost devoid of cardiovascular actions, has replaced the older agents for use in patients with congenital or acquired cardiac disease. However, in certain situations, e.g., coarctation of the aorta, and in the production of deliberate hypotension, the combination of d-tubocurarine and an inhalational agent still has many adherents.

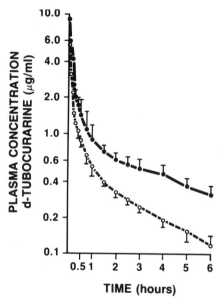

FIG 6–51.
Plasma concentration-time curves for *d*-tubocurarine after administration of 0.5 mg/kg IV in elderly *(closed circles)* and young *(open circles)* patients. (From Matteo RS, Backus WW, McDaniel DD, et al: Pharmacokinetics and pharmacodynamics of *d*-tubocurarine and metocurine in the elderly. *Anesth Analg* 1985; 64:23–29. Used by permission.)

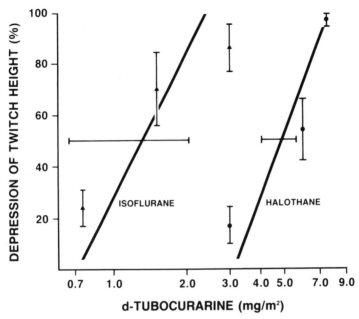

FIG 6–52.
Dose-response curves for *d*-tubocurarine in patients during isoflurane (1.5%) or halothane (0.9%) anesthesia. (From Miller RD, Way WL, Dolan WM, et al: Comparative neuromuscular effects of pancuronium, gallamine, and succinylcholine during Forane and halothane anesthesia in man. *Anesthesiology* 1971; 35:509–514. Used by permission.)

Burns

Patients with massive burns demonstrate abnormalities in response to agonist and antagonist drugs that act at the neuromuscular junction. They demonstrate a resistance to the action of d-tubocurarine that is dependent on the size of the burn and the time since the injury.[399] Although the alteration in plasma protein concentration results in a decrease in concentration of free drug, the altered pharmacokinetics are insufficient to account for the resistance.[400, 401] Rather, it is speculated that spreading of acetylcholine receptors throughout the muscle membrane is a more likely explanation to explain the the altered response to d-tubocurarine and the hyperkalemic response to succinylcholine.[402] Increased dose and serum concentrations are required to produce a given level of paralysis. The stimulus to receptor spread is unknown, but a similar resistance to d-tubocurarine has been observed during immobilization and disuse atrophy.[403]

Disuse Atrophy

Resistance to nondepolarizing relaxants has been observed in patients whose conditions predispose to disuse atrophy, such as burns and stroke,[404] and also in animals whose hind limbs have been immobilized.[405] In the experimental animal, receptor spread[406] and sprouting of the nerve terminal[407] have been demonstrated. The change in sensitivity in these animals is not limited to the immobilized limb,[408] or in man to the paralyzed side,[236] but contralateral effects also occur.

Mode of Administration

The use of d-tubocurarine is restricted to the maintenance of relaxation during anesthesia. The introduction of drugs with fewer cardiovascular effects has reduced its use considerably.

Following administration of succinylcholine to facilitate intubation, d-tubocurarine is given in an initial dose of 0.25 to 0.5 mg/kg followed by boluses of approximately one quarter to one half the initial dose.

Small doses (3 mg/70 kg) of d-tubocurarine are still used to prevent fasciculations and muscle pain after succinylcholine precurarization. Some believe that d-tubocurarine is superior to the other nondepolarizing relaxants for this purpose.[409]

VECURONIUM

Vecuronium is a nondepolarizing NMBD with an intermediate duration of action similar to that of atracurium.

Chemistry

Vecuronium was prepared by Savage and his colleagues[410] who wished to produce a relaxant with a shorter duration of action and more rapid onset than pancuronium. Demethylation of pancuronium in the 2-piperidino-substitution (Fig 6–53) produced a monoquaternary analogue that reduced the acetylcholine-like characteristics of the molecule in the area of the "A" ring of the steroid nucleus. The tertiary amine also increased the lipophilicity of the molecule, which modified its distribution within the body and encouraged hepatic metabolism. However, the acetylcholine fragments in the "D" ring preserved its neuromuscular potency.

When several similar esters were tested, 17-OH pancuronium, dacuronium, had a shorter onset of action than pancuronium but was only one fiftieth as potent.[411] The most promising compound, vecuronium, had a vagal-to-neuromuscular ratio of 6.3:1 compared with 3.4:1 for pancuronium. In cats, vecuronium was found to be less potent, but rapid deacetylation might produce a compound with a short duration of action.

Vecuronium is unstable in aqueous solution. It is prepared as a buffered lyophilized compound that has a shelf life of more than a year. The "cake" contains vecuronium, 4 mg, citric acid, 8.3 mg, disodium phosphate, 6.5 mg, and mannitol, 24.5 mg, and is dissolved in water or saline in which it is stable for 24 hours.

Metabolism

Vecuronium undergoes spontaneous deactylation to three alcohol metabolites (Fig 6–54).[246] In cats, the main metabolite, 3,17-dihydroxy derivative, has less than 2% of the neuromuscular activity of the parent compound. The most potent, 3-hydroxy derivative, has about 60% the

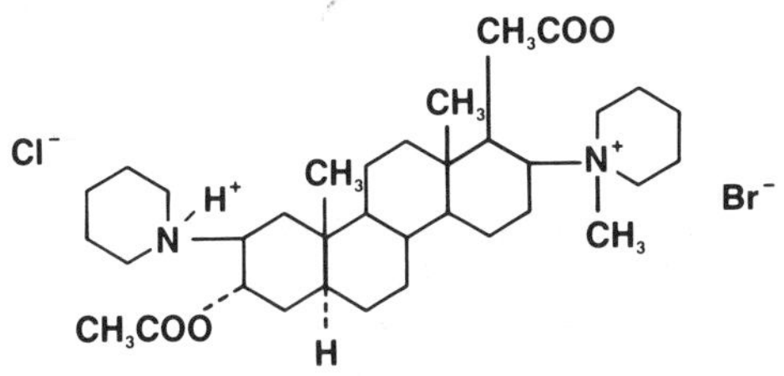

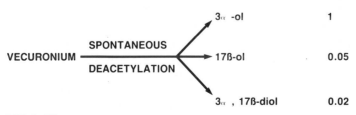

VECURONIUM

FIG 6–53.
Structure of vecuronium.

NEUROMUSCULAR POTENCY
COMPARED WITH PARENT DRUG

3α -ol	1
VECURONIUM ——SPONTANEOUS DEACETYLATION—→ 17ß-ol	0.05
3α , 17ß-diol	0.02

FIG 6–54.
Relative neuromuscular potency of hydroxy derivatives of vecuronium.

TABLE 6–15.
Median Pharmacokinetic Variables for Vecuronium Compared With Pancuronium and Atracurium*

		DISTRIBUTION VOLUME (V_{dss}), L/KG	PLASMA CLEARANCE, ML/KG/MIN	ELIMINATION HALF LIFE ($t_{1/2\beta}$, MIN
Pancuronium	Normal	0.23	1.9	145
Vecuronium	Normal	0.26	4.6	62
	Renal failure	0.24	2.5	97
	Cirrhosis	0.23	2.7	73
	Elderly	0.18	3.7	58
Atracurium	Normal	0.16	5.5	20

*Adapted from Shanks CA: Pharmacokinetics of the nondepolarizing neuromuscular relaxants applied to calculation of bolus and infusion dose regimens. *Anesthesiology* 1986; 64:72–86.

potency of vecuronium. The vagal to neuromuscular blocking ratios of the metabolites are similar to the basic compound. The quantities of metabolites produced in man are uncertain because of the difficulty in producing an accurate assay.

Pharmacokinetics

Earlier pharmacokinetic studies of vecuronium were performed with nonspecific assays that could not differentiate easily between vecuronium and its metabolites.[253, 412] Nevertheless, it was clear that the distribution and clearance of vecuronium were different from pancuronium. Median values obtained from several studies show that compared with pancuronium, $t_{1/2\beta}$ is decreased by about half, and plasma clearance is increased twofold to threefold (Table 6–15).[8] It was also realized that the values were modified little by renal failure in man[413] or animals[414] or by cirrhosis.[415] Consequently little disturbance would be expected in the elderly.[416] Surprisingly, in cats, hepatic exclusion prolonged the duration of vecuronium and all of its metabolites.[417] Cronnelly et al.[255] employed a more specific, sensitive assay using selective ion mass spectrometry to measure only the unmetabolized parent compound. The variables that they derived were similar to others, but in addition, they were able to demonstrate that plasma concentrations produced 50% neuromuscular block at steady-state levels similar to pancuronium, 88 ± 34 μg/ml, and vecuronium, 94 ± 33 μg/ml.

One puzzle remains. Why are the duration of action and rate of recovery from atracurium and vecuronium similar when their elimination half-lives (see Table 6–15) are so different? Probably the explanation lies in the relationship between plasma concentration and effect. Vecuronium has more rapid distribution within the body than atracurium. Its plasma concentration decreases through the effective range far more rapidly so that duration and recovery for vecuronium depend more on distribution than elimination[418] (Fig 6–55). However, such a phenomenon is less effective when the peripheral storage sites of vecuronium are saturated. Eventually, vecuronium demonstrates some cumulation, although this may require either very large doses or some interference with alternative routes of elimination such as the kidney.[59, 419]

Neuromuscular Blockade

Potency

Vecuronium has a potency similar to that of pancuronium. Although in rats and monkeys, it is less potent than pancuronium,[420, 421] in man, several studies have shown that it is about one third more potent. The actual values for the ED50, ED90, or ED95 depend on the method of neuromuscular stimulation, the choice of anesthesia, age, and whether dose-response curves have been obtained using single or cumulative doses of the relaxant. During balanced anesthesia and when

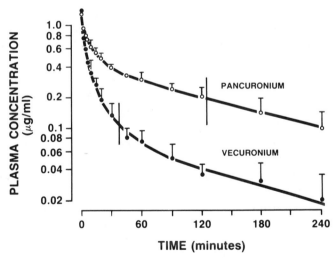

FIG 6–55.
Plasma concentrations of pancuronium and vecuronium after administration of 0.1 mg/kg IV. Plasma concentrations at 50% recovery are shown with vertical bars. (From Sohn YJ, Bencini AF, Scaf AHJ, et al: Comparative pharmacokinetics and dynamics of vecuronium and pancuronium in anesthetized patients. *Anesth Analg* 1986; 65:233–239. Used by permission.)

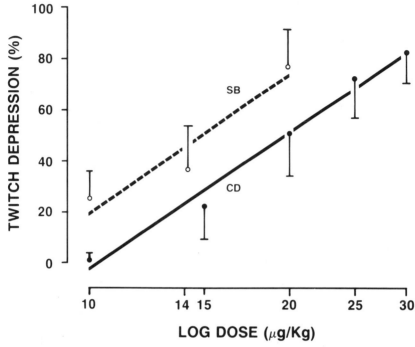

FIG 6–56.
Dose-response curves for vecuronium obtained with single bolus *(SB)* and cumulative dose *(CD)* techniques. (From Fisher DM, Fahey MR, Cronnelly R, et al: Potency determination for vecuronium: Comparisons of cumulative and single-dose techniques. *Anesthesiology* 1982; 57:309–310. Used by permission.)

single doses of vecuronium are used, the mean values for ED50 and ED95 have been found to be 23.1 and 39.6 μg/kg, respectively.[422] When cumulative doses are used, the response curve is shifted to the right (Fig 6–56).[10, 55, 423, 424] Dose-response curves obtained during anesthesia with halothane, enflurane, or isoflurane are shifted to the right,[425] although the anesthetic vapors appear to have less effect on vecuronium than on d-tubocurarine or pancuronium.[62, 64] In the elderly, the potency of vecuronium is unaltered,[426] although the amount required to maintain constant neuromuscular blockade by infusion is less than in the young.[427] Requirements in pediatric patients are discussed in Chapter 11.

Onset

When equipotent doses are used, the onset of action of vecuronium is similar to that of atracurium and pancuronium. After a single dose equivalent to 1 × ED95 is given, maximum blockade is not achieved for 5 to 6 minutes,[10, 59, 69, 427–433] although subsequent doses produce their neuromuscular effect more rapidly. In part, this may explain the shift of the dose-response curves during cumulative administration, which may result from giving repeated doses before maximum block has been attained.[55] Complete block of the adductor pollicis is achieved more rapidly as the dose is increased.[10, 59, 427] As the dose was increased from 50 to 400 μg/kg, the onset time decreased from over 3 minutes to 90 seconds[433] (Fig 6–57). Bencini and Newton[432] observed that ventilation stopped earlier after administration of vecuronium than after giving pancuronium. After pancuronium was given, spontaneous respiration continued until the force of contraction of the adductor pollicis was reduced by 50%, whereas after vecuronium was given, it ceased at 20% to 40% block. It is not certain why ventilation should cease before total paralysis of the hand muscles,[434] particularly as the force of diaphragmatic contraction by indirect stimulation is unaffected at these doses.[435]

The Priming Principle

Attempts have been made to accelerate the onset of action of vecuronium by using the priming principle.[436–439] This refers to the administration of a small, subparalyzing dose several minutes before the principal dose is given. It has been shown that for vecuronium, priming doses should not exceed 0.01 mg/kg if respiratory depression[440] and aspiration[441] are to be avoided, and a priming dose should be followed 3 to 4 minutes later by a 0.1-mg/kg dose.[438] If the relaxant is given in this fashion, the onset of maximal block can be reduced by

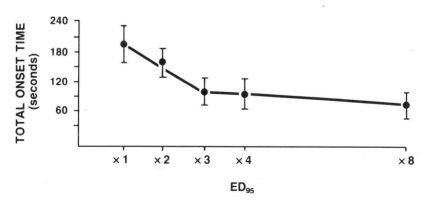

FIG 6–57.
Onset times for vecuronium with increasing multiples of the ED95. (From Jones RM, Casson WR, Lethbridge JR: Influence of dose on onset times of vecuronium-induced neuromuscular blockade. *Br J Anaesth* 1985; 57:828P–829P. Used by permission.)

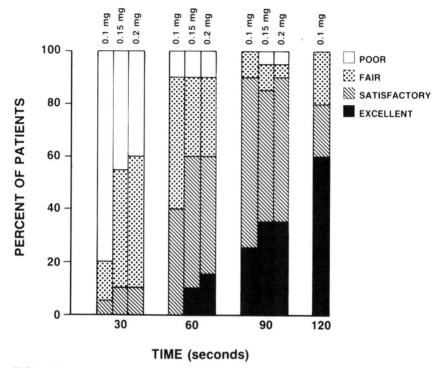

FIG 6–58.
Intubating conditions 30 to 120 seconds after administration of various doses of vecuronium, 0.1 to 0.2 mg/kg. (From Mirakhur RK, Ferres CJ, Clarke RSJ, et al: Clinical evaluation of ORG NC 45. *Br J Anaesth* 1983; 55:119–124. Used by permission.)

about 25%, and intubating conditions are improved, but they do not equal those produced by succinylcholine.[441]

Intubating Conditions

The rapid production of excellent intubating conditions produced by succinylcholine, 1 to 1.5 mg/kg, cannot be matched by vecuronium (Fig 6–58). Nevertheless, by a combination of deep anesthesia, large doses (2 to 3 × ED95), and priming, acceptable conditions can be achieved by about 2 minutes in most patients.[428, 429, 431, 433, 442] Intubating conditions are not better than after an equivalent dose of pancuronium, but they can be achieved without the latter's prolonged duration of action.[81, 443] When very large doses (6 × ED95) are given, satisfactory to excellent conditions can be achieved in all patients using atracurium or vecuronium. Both have the disadvantage of prolonged action, 70 to 90 minutes, but when vecuronium is used, the hypotension and tachycardia seen after administration of atracurium are not observed.[73]

Duration

For equipotent doses, the duration of action of vecuronium is only about one third that of pancuronium.[59, 428] Recovery of adductor pollicis to 90% of control values occurs in about 20 minutes after giving 43 μg/kg (1 × ED90), and this is prolonged to 52 minutes when the dose is increased to 130 μg/kg (3 × ED90);[59] these results are similar to those achieved with atracurium. The rate of recovery is more rapid than after giving pancuronium. The recovery index (time from 25% to 75% recovery of adductor pollicis) is approximately 10 to 15 minutes.[10, 59, 429, 431] The recovery rate is prolonged only slightly as the dose of vecuronium is increased. The duration of action of vecuronium is increased during anesthesia with halothane or enflurane by approximately 30% to 50%.[424, 431] After repeated doses of vecuronium are given to controls only minimal increases in duration of action and recovery index exist.[424, 431, 442, 445, 446] Thus, in contrast to pancuronium, cumulation does not occur.

Recovery and Reversal

Recovery of neuromuscular activity can be accelerated with anticholinesterases and, from the same degree of block, can be achieved with smaller doses of neostigmine when neostigmine antagonizes vecuronium rather than pancuronium.[428] However, when the relaxants were administered by continuous infusion, the doses of neostigmine required to antagonize pancuronium and vecuronium were similar.[447] This suggests that the more rapid apparent recovery results from faster spontaneous recovery and not from enhanced removal of vecuronium from the receptor by neostigmine. The more rapid antagonism of neuromuscular blockade by edrophonium makes it particularly suitable to reverse the action of vecuronium.[448] Edrophonium is effective (Fig 6–59), and its dose should be adjusted according to the degree of neuromuscular activity. Lee et al.[449] recommended that light blocks (Tl > 50%) require only 10 mg edrophonium, while more intense blocks (75% to 80% or >95%) need 0.3 or 0.5 mg/kg, respectively.[449] Edrophonium is less effective than neostigmine in antagonizing intense (>90%) blockade.[85] Anticholinesterases can be omitted safely if spontaneous activity has recovered so that no weakness can be detected by single twitch, train-of-four, or 50 Hz tetanic stimulation of the adductor pollicis.[428, 445]

Site of Action

Like other nondepolarizing muscle relaxants, the action of vecuronium is not restricted to the postjunctional membrane. In cats, vecuronium has biphasic prejunctional actions, suppressing post-tetanic and postdrug repetition at high doses and stimulating them at low dosage.[450] In man, prejunctional activity is suggested by fade in response to TOF stimulation. During recovery from the block, the degree of fade is similar to that seen with pancuronium but greater than with gallamine.[444, 451]

Cardiovascular Effects

One of the critical factors leading to the development of vecuronium was its lack of cardiovascular actions in a wide variety of animals even at high doses.[389, 452] This lack of cardiovascular activity has been confirmed in man. No evidence of action at the autonomic ganglia or sympathetic nervous system exists,[285] and serum histamine concentrations are not increased at doses up to 0.2 mg/kg.[453] Rare anaphylactoid reactions have been described,[113] but cardiovascular problems encountered following administration of vecuronium usually result from the absence of sympathetic stimulation that is expected after pancuronium.

VECURONIUM

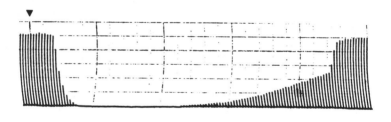

EDROPHONIUM

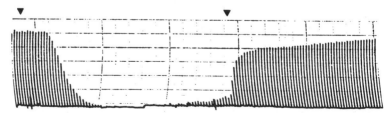

FIG 6–59.
Reversal of vecuronium, 40 µg/kg, with edrophonium, 0.5 mg/kg, at approximately 90% and 50% block of adductor pollicis.

For example, during halothane or enflurane anesthesia,[454] or when vecuronium was given in doses up to 0.28 mg/kg to patients for coronary artery bypass grafting during halothane anesthesia, no changes were observed in heart rate or blood pressure.[455, 456] However, when vecuronium was given following large doses of narcotics, the patients exhibited a continuing decrease in heart rate and blood pressure.[457, 458] Indeed three such patients had either severe bradycardia or asystole when vecuronium was given after administration of large doses of sufentanil.[459] Clearly, narcotic-induced bradycardia is not counteracted by vecuronium. Similarly, bradycardia resulting from manipulation during strabismus surgery—occulocardiac reflex—is not modified by vecuronium.[22]

Drug Interactions

Interactions between vecuronium and several drugs have been described. These include inhalational and local anesthetic agents, induction agents, and antibiotics. In cats, dose-response curves reflected an increase in potency during anesthesia when clinical concentrations of halothane, enflurane, isoflurane,[456] and nitrous oxide were used, but the response was unaffected by nitrous oxide and cyclopropane.[460] Vecuronium is also potentiated by althesin, etomidate, ketamine, methohexital, propanidid, and thiopental. No effect was observed with diazepam, morphine, or fentanyl, but the response to benzodiazepines is variable. The drug is also potentiated by streptomycin but not penicillin, and a specific delayed potentiation is seen 1 hour after administration of metronidazole.[460]

Anesthetic Vapors

In man, a similar potentiation with the inhalational vapors has been described (Fig 6–60),[425] although it appears to be less pronounced than with d-tubocurarine[62] or pancuronium.[64] The potentiation by anesthetic vapors is associated with prolonged duration of the block and slower recovery; the 25% to 75% recovery index increases from 14 to 21 minutes.[461] The steady-state vecuronium requirement to maintain steady block by infusion is also increased by about 30 to 40 seconds during halothane (0.5% end tidal [ET]) anesthesia.[462]

Muscle Relaxants

Following succinylcholine the action of vecuronium is potentiated. Single doses produce a more intense and longer lasting block,[10, 463, 464] and the dose response curve to vecuronium is shifted to the left. The

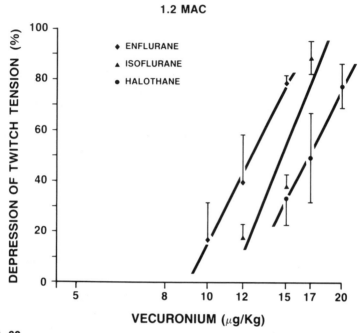

FIG 6–60.
Dose-response curves for vecuronium during nitrous oxide (0.6 MAC) and 0.6 MAC halothane, enflurane, or isoflurane. (From Rupp SM, Miller RD, Gencarelli PJ: Vecuronium-induced neuromuscular blockade during enflurane, isoflurane, and halothane anesthesia in humans. *Anesthesiology* 1984; 60:102–105. Used by permission.)

effect is short lasting, and 10 minutes after the administration of succinylcholine, the response to vecuronium returns to normal.[465, 466] Vecuronium has only 1/20 the anticholinesterase activity of pancuronium,[467] and thus is not expected to prolong the duration of action of succinylcholine if used for precurarization.

When nondepolarizing neuromuscular blocking drugs are mixed or given sequentially, their effect may be different from simple addition.[308] If pancuronium and vecuronium are given alternately, the drug administered first modifies the activity of the second. When pancuronium was given first, it reduced the dose requirements and prolonged the action of vecuronium. Conversely, the earlier administration of vecuronium increased dose requirements and reduced the duration of action of pancuronium.[308, 469] The incentive to study other relaxant combinations with vecuronium is small because when used alone, its properties are so attractive that any addition might be deleterious. However, investigation of its use as a priming dose before other relaxants is worth investigation. Studies in animals and man have demonstrated that combinations of vecuronium and pancuronium are simply additive. Equipotent mixtures affect neither the dose responses[470, 424] nor the onset or duration of action or recovery of neuromuscular blockade.[307] However, mixtures of vecuronium and d-tubocurarine[470, 471] or atracurium[130] demonstrate potentiation, which suggests that the actions of vecuronium and pancuronium at the neuromuscular junction are similar to each other but different from those of d-tubocurarine and atracurium. Differences may result from a different site of action—prejunctional or postjunctional—or from different activity at the same site (see Chapter 3).

Age

Few studies have been made with vecuronium in infants and children. The shorter duration of action, compared with pancuronium, has been confirmed in children aged 1 to 13 years.[473-475] It has also been shown that, in common with other relaxants, the onset of action is more rapid in infants than in children, which is quicker than in adults. However, the duration of action is prolonged, and the rate of recovery in infants is reduced presumably as a result of impaired elimination, although pharmacokinetic studies are necessary to confirm this. Dose-response curves show similar sensitivity at all ages, although one study suggested that adolescents (aged 10 to 17 years) were more sensitive than younger children (aged 2 to 9 years).[474] Further investigations are required.

Intracranial and Intraocular Pressure

Several studies have confirmed that vecuronium does not, like succinylcholine[487] or d-tubocurarine,[488] produce an increase in intracranial pressure.[489, 490] No increases were observed when it was given in the presence of normal or elevated intracranial pressure. Thus, the absence of cardiovascular and intracranial effects makes it an appropriate agent for use during neurosurgical procedures.

Similarly, no increase in intraocular pressure was detected after administration to healthy patients.[120, 491] Thus, it is an ideal relaxant for the patient with an open-eye injury. If rapid relaxation is required for the patient with a full stomach, large doses will be necessary together with priming, deep anesthesia, and lidocaine (Xylocaine) pharyngeal spray in an attempt to match the conditions produced by succinylcholine.

Special Situations

Outpatient Surgery

The short duration of action and rapid recovery following administration of vecuronium make it an ideal muscle relaxant for short intra-abdominal operations such as laparoscopy[442, 476, 477] and day care surgery.[478] An initial dose of 0.05 to 0.06 mg/kg usually provides acceptable conditions for intubation and surgery with balanced or inhalational anesthesia. Often, antagonism of the block is unnecessary, and the problems of succinylcholine are avoided.

Cardiovascular Disease

The lack of cardiovascular effects makes vecuronium the most suitable NMBD during anesthesia for the patient with compromised cardiovascular function.[479] Treatment of bradycardia may be necessary when vecuronium is given with narcotics or during procedures that cause vagal stimulation. Accumulating evidence indicates that if bradycardia is treated, the use of vecuronium during cardiac surgery avoids the hypertensive and tachycardic response of pancuronium and pancuronium-metocurine mixtures and the reduction in systemic vascular resistance (SVR) with atracurium.[480] During hypothermic cardiopulmonary bypass, the requirement for vecuronium decreases.[481]

Obstetric Anesthesia

Vecuronium, in common with other NMBDs, crosses the placenta, but only small quantities are found in fetal blood. Following administration of a dose of 0.05 to 0.08 mg/kg during cesarean section, mean venous cord concentration was 40 μg/kg compared with 390 μg/ml in the mother. The slow onset of action of vecuronium suggests it should be used only for maintenance relaxation following intubating after succinylcholine. Used in this way, it is a satisfactory muscle relaxant.[482, 483]

Renal and Hepatic Disease

Because vecuronium is an ionized, water-soluble compound, some excretion in the urine would be expected. However, the duration of action is only slightly increased in anephric animals[484] and man.[419] In pharmacokinetic studies with a small number of subjects only small, nonsignificant, increases in elimination half-life ($t_{1/2\beta}$) and decreases in plasma clearance were detected.[413] With larger numbers it was possible to demonstrate a small (20%) increase in duration of action of single boluses in renal failure. More importantly, some evidence of cumulation after repeated doses was observed but was of minimal clinical significance (Fig 6–61). The potency of vecuronium was unaltered in renal failure.[419]

Vecuronium and its metabolites are excreted in the bile, and exclusion of the liver from the circulation in cats produced a marked prolongation of action.[417] After vecuronium was given to cirrhotic patients, there was an increase in the elimination half-life, decrease in clearance, and a twofold prolongation of neuromuscular blockade.[415]

Thus, in patients with renal failure, the action of vecuronium is altered minimally, whereas with severe liver disease, prolonged action should be anticipated.

Myasthenia Gravis

The short duration of action and rapid recovery from vecuronium in the normal patient suggest that it might be useful in the myasthenic patient. In addition, if neuromuscular activity is allowed to recover spontaneously, then neostigmine can be avoided, and this would avoid the possibility of cholinergic symptoms in the patient already receiving

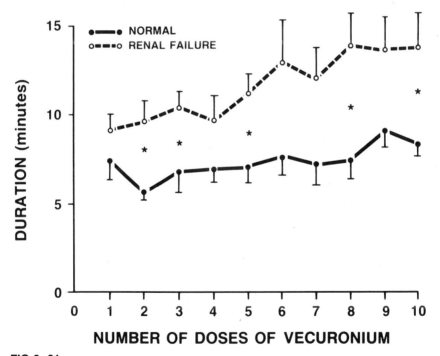

FIG 6–61.
Durations of action of repeated small doses of vecuronium, (0.01 mg/kg) in normal and renal failure patients. Renal failure is associated with a progressive increasing duration of block, cumulation, and a more prolonged block at each dose. * = significant differences at the time interval. (From Bevan DR, Donati, F, Gyasi H, et al: Vecuronium in renal failure. *Can Anaesth Soc J* 1984; 31:491–496. Used by permission.)

anticholinesterases. It has been shown that with doses of one fourth to one half normal and by titrating the effect with neuromuscular monitoring, such an approach is successful.[485] However, the rate of recovery may be prolonged grossly in the myasthenic patient—25% to 75% recovery times increasing up to 140 minutes.[152] Thus, in myasthenia, atracurium is a more appropriate agent.

Tetanus

The lack of cardiovascular effects of vecuronium have allowed its successful use by infusion to control the muscle spasms of tetanus. In one case, the infusion was continued at a rate of 4 mg/hour for 19 hours. When the infusion was stopped, spontaneous ventilation recommenced within $1\frac{1}{2}$ hours.[486]

Pheochromocytoma

The lack of cardiovascular effects and particularly the absence of histamine release and sympathetic stimulation make vecuronium an ideal drug to produce relaxation in patients with pheochromocytoma.[492]

Mode of Administration

Vecuronium may be given by intermittent bolus doses or by continuous infusion. The initial bolus dose required to achieve satisfactory intubation conditions in 2 to 3 minutes is 2 to 3 × ED95 (0.1 to 0.15 mg/kg), which may be followed either by supplementary boluses of 1 to 2 mg (0.01 to 0.02 mg/kg) or by infusion. Maintenance doses for infusions vary, but to maintain 50% blockade required a mean dose of 1 μg/kg/minute and doses of 1 to 1.7 μg/kg/minute were required to maintain 90% blockade.[8, 66, 427, 428, 493] Clearly, the variability of response and rapid recovery from vecuronium emphasizes the importance of neuromuscular monitoring to achieve adequate relaxation. Long-term infusions result in saturation of peripheral storage sites for vecuronium so that recovery after stopping an infusion may be slower than after a bolus injection.[494] Closed-loop systems have been described to provide automatic adjustment of the infusion rate according to the required neuromuscular blockade.[495]

REFERENCES

1. Lund I, Stovner J: Experimental and clinical experiences with a new muscle relaxant RO 4–3816, diallyl-nor-toxiferine. *Acta Anaesthesiol Scand* 1962; 62:85–97.
2. Parkin JE: Determination of alcuronium chloride in biological fluids by high performance liquid chromatography. *J Chromatogr* 1981; 225:240–242.
3. Raaflaub J, Frey P: Zur pharmacokinetik von diallyl-nor-toxiferin bein menschen. *Arzneimittelforschung* 1972; 22:73–78.
4. Buzello W, Agoston S: Comparative clinical pharmacokinetics of tubocurarine, gallamine, alcuronium and pancuronium. *Anaesthetist* 1978; 27:313–318.
5. Walker JS, Triggs EJ, Shanks CA: Clinical pharmacokinetics of alcuronium chloride in man. *Eur J Clin Pharmacol* 1980; 17:449–457.
6. Walker JS, Shanks CA, Brown KF: Alcuronium kinetics and plasma concentration-effect relationship. *Clin Pharmacol Ther* 1983; 33:510–516.
7. Stephens D, Ho PC, Holloway AM, et al: Pharmacokinetics of alcuronium in elderly patients undergoing total hip replacement or aortic reconstructive surgery. *Br J Anaesth* 1984; 56:465–471.
8. Shanks CA: Pharmacokinetics of the nondepolarizing neuromuscular relaxants applied to calculation of bolus and infusion dose regimens. *Anesthesiology* 1986; 64:72–86.
9. Lund I, Stovner J: Dose-response curves for d-tubocurarine, alcuronium and pancuronium. *Acta Anaesthesiol Scand (Suppl)* 1970; 37:238–242.
10. Krieg N, Crul JF, Booij LHDJ: Relative potency of ORG NC 45, pancuronium, alcuronium and tubocurarine in anaesthetized man. *Br J Anaesth* 1980; 52:783–787.
11. Shanks CA, Walker JS, Ramzan MI, et al: Dose-response curves for four neuromuscular blockers using continuous i.v. infusion. *Br J Anaesth* 1981; 53:627–632.
12. Keens SJ, Hunter JM, Snowdon SL, et al: Potentiation of alcuronium neuromuscular blockade by volatile anaesthetic agents. *Br J Anaesth* 1986; 58:803P.
13. Woolmer DF, Gibbs JM, Smeele PQ: Clinical comparison of atracurium and alcuronium in gynaecological surgery. *Anaesth Intensive Care* 1985; 13:33–37.
14. Lin LPS, Homi J: A comparison of atracurium and alcuronium during halothane anaesthesia by measurement of the train-of-four response of the adductor pollicis muscle and clinical observation. *Br J Anaesth* 1985; 57:1067–1072.
15. Astley BA, Hughes R, Payne JP: Recovery from neuromuscular blockade following alcuronium administration. *Br J Anaesth* 1983; 55:1164P.
16. Hughes R, Chapple DJ: Effects of non-depolarizing neuromuscular blocking agents on peripheral autonomic mechanisms in cats. *Br J Anaesth* 1976; 48:59–68.

17. Kennedy BR, Kelman GR: Cardiovascular effects of alcuronium in man. *Br J Anaesth* 1970; 42:625–629.

18. Foldes FF, Brown IM, Lunn JN, et al: The neuromuscular effects of diallylnortoxiferine in anesthetized subjects. *Anesth Analg* 1963; 42:177–181.

19. Baraka A: A comparative study between diallyl-nor-toxiferine and tubocurarine. *Br J Anaesth* 1967; 39:624–628.

20. Hunter AR: Diallyl toxiferine. *Br J Anaesth* 1964; 36:466–469.

21. Harrison GA: The cardiovascular effects and some relaxant properties of four relaxants in patients about to undergo cardiac surgery. *Br J Anaesth* 1972; 44:485–489.

22. Karhunen U, Nilsson E, Brander P: Comparison of four nondepolarizing neuromuscular blocking drugs in the suppression of the oculocardiac reflex during strabismus surgery in children. *Br J Anaesth* 1985; 57:1209–1212.

23. Chan CS, Yeung ML: Anaphylactic reaction to alcuronium. *Br J Anaesth* 1972; 44:103–105.

24. Balamoutsos NG, Tsakona H, Kanakoudes PS, et al: Alcuronium and intraocular pressure. *Anesth Analg* 1983; 62:521–523.

25. Harrop-Griffiths AW, Grounds RM, Moore M: Intubating conditions following pre-induction priming with alcuronium. *Anaesthesia* 1986; 41:282–286.

26. Black AMS, Hutton R, El-Hassan KM, et al: Priming and the onset of neuromuscular blockade with alcuronium. *Br J Anaesth* 1986; 58:827–833.

27. Buzello W, Schluermann D, Pollmaechert T, et al: Modification of d-tubocurarine and alcuronium-induced neuromuscular blockade by hypothermic cardiopulmonary bypass. *Anesthesiology* 1985; 62:201–204.

28. Stenlake JB, Waigh RB, Urwin J, et al: Atracurium: Conception and inception. *Br J Anaesth* 1983; 55:3S–10S.

29. Hofmann, AW: Beitrage zur Kenntriss der fluchtragen organischen Basen. *Ann Chem* 1851; 78:253–259.

30. Amaki Y, Waud BE, Waud DR: Atracurium-receptor kinetics: Simple behavior of a mixture. *Anesth Analg* 1985; 64:777–780.

31. Merrett RA, Thompson CW, Webb FW: In vitro degradation of atracurium in human plasma. *Br J Anaesth* 1983; 55:61–66.

32. Nigrovic V, Auen M, Wajskol A: Enzymatic hydrolysis of atracurium in vivo. *Anesthesiology* 1985; 62:606–609.

33. Nigrovic V, Pandya JB, Auen M, et al: Inactivation of atracurium in human and rat plasma. *Anesth Analg* 1985; 64:1047–1052.

34. Neill EAM, Chapple DJ, Thompson CW: Metabolism and kinetics of atracurium: An overview. *Br J Anaesth* 1983; 55:23S–26S.

35. Cook DR, Stiller R, Ingram M: In vitro degradation of atracurium. *Anesth Analg* 1986; 65:539–547.

36. Fisher DM, Canfell PC, Fahey MR, et al: Elimination of atracurium in humans: Contribution of Hofmann elimination and ester hydrolysis ver-

sus organ-based elimination. *Anesthesiology* 1986; 65:6–12.
37. Stiller RL, Cook DR, Chakravorti S: In vitro degradation of atracurium in human plasma. *Br J Anaesth* 1985; 57:1085–1088.
38. Chapple DJ, Clark JS: Pharmacological action of breakdown products of atracurium and related substances. *Br J Anaesth* 1983; 55:11S–16S.
39. Lanier WL, Milde JH, Michenfelder JD: The cerebral effects of pancuronium and atracurium in halothane-anesthetized dogs. *Anesthesiology* 1985; 63:589–597.
40. Hennis PJ, Fahey MR, Canfell PC, et al: Pharmacology of atracurium during isoflurane anesthesia in normal and anephric patients. *Anesth Analg* 1986; 65:743–746.
41. Shi WZ, Fahey MR, Fisher DM, et al: Laudanosine (a metabolite of atracurium) increases the minimal alveolar concentration of halothane in rabbits. *Anesthesiology* 1985; 63:584–588.
42. Ingram MDM, Sclabassi RJ, Cook DR, et al: Cardiovascular and electroencephalographic effects of laudanosine in "nephrectomized" cats. *Br J Anaesth* 1986; 58:14S–18S.
43. Fahey MR, Rupp SM, Canfell C, et al: Effect of renal failure on laudanosine excretion in man. *Br J Anaesth* 1985; 57:1049–1051.
44. Duncan PW: A problem with atracurium. *Anesthesia* 1983; 38:597.
45. Nigrovic V, Koechel DA: Atracurium—More information needed. *Anesthesiology* 1984; 60:606–607.
46. Nigrovic V, Klaunig JE, Smith SL, et al: Comparative toxicity of atracurium and metocurine in isolated rat hepatocytes. *Anesth Analg* 1983; 65:1107–1111.
47. Ward S, Neill EAM, Weatherley BC, et al: Pharmacokinetics of atracurium besylate in healthy patients (after a single IV bolus dose). *Br J Anaesth* 1983; 55:113–118.
48. Hull CJ: A model for atracurium? *Br J Anaesth* 1983; 55:95–96.
49. Ward S, Neill EAM: Pharmacokinetics of atracurium in acute hepatic failure (with acute renal failure). *Br J Anaesth* 1983; 55:1169–1172.
50. Ward S, Wright D: Combined pharmacokinetic and pharmacodynamic study of a single bolus of atracurium. *Br J Anaesth* 1983; 55:35S–38S.
51. Sheiner LB, Stanski DR, Vorch S, et al: Simultaneous modelling of pharmacokinetics and pharmacodynamics: Application to d-tubocurarine. *Clin Pharmacol Ther* 1979; 25:358.
52. Weatherley BC, Williams SG, Neill EAM: Pharmacokinetics, pharmacodynamics and dose-response relationships of atracurium administered I.V. *Br J Anaesth* 1983; 55:39S–45S.
53. Hughes R, Chapple DJ: The pharmacology of atracurium: A competing neuromuscular blocking agent. *Br J Anaesth* 1981; 53:31–44.
54. Sutherland GA, Squire IB, Gibb AJ, et al: Neuromuscular blocking and autonomic effects of vecuronium and atracurium in the anaesthetized cat. *Br J Anaesth* 1983; 55:1119–1126.
55. Gramstad L, Lilleaasen P: Dose-response relation for atracurium, ORG NC 45 and pancuronium. *Br J Anaesth* 1982; 54:647–651.

56. Basta SJ, Ali HH, Savarese JJ, et al: Clinical pharmacology of atracurium besylate (BW33A): A new non-depolarizing muscle relaxant. *Anesth Analg* 1982; 61:723–729.
57. Katz RL, Stirt J, Murray AL, et al: Neuromuscular effects of atracurium in man. *Anesth Analg* 1982; 61:730–734.
58. Sokoll MD, Gergis SD, Mehta M, et al: Safety and efficacy of atracurium (BW33A) in patients receiving balanced or isoflurane anesthesia. *Anesthesiology* 1983; 58:450–455.
59. Robertson EN, Booij LHD, Fragen RJ, et al: Clinical comparison of atracurium and vecuronium (ORG NC 45). *Br J Anaesth* 1983; 55:125–129.
60. Rupp SM, McChristian JW, Miller RD: Neuromuscular effects of atracurium during halothane-nitrous oxide and enflurane-nitrous oxide anesthesia in humans. *Anesthesiology* 1985; 63:16–19.
61. Rupp SM, Fahey MR, Miller RD: Neuromuscular blocking effects of atracurium during N_2O-fentanyl or isoflurane anesthesia. *Anesthesiology* 1982; 57:A257.
62. Miller RD, Eger EI, Way WL, et al: Comparative neuromuscular effects of Forane and halothane alone and in combination with d-tubocurarine in man. *Anesthesiology* 1971; 35:38–42.
63. Fogdall RP, Miller RD: Neuromuscular effects of enflurane, alone and combined with d-tubocurarine, pancuronium and succinylcholine in man. *Anesthesiology* 1975; 42:173–178.
64. Miller RD, Way WL, Dolan WM, et al: Comparative neuromuscular effects of pancuronium, gallamine, and succinylcholine during Forane and halothane anesthesia in man. *Anesthesiology* 1971; 35:509–514.
65. Gibson FM, Mirakhur RK, Lavery GG, et al: Potency of atracurium: A comparison of single dose and cumulative dose techniques. *Anesthesiology* 1985; 62:657–659.
66. Gramstad L, Lilleaasen P: Neuromuscular blocking effects of atracurium, vecuronium and pancuronium during bolus and infusion administration. *Br J Anaesth* 1985; 57:1052–1059.
67. Tran DQ, Amaki Y, Ohta Y, et al: Simultaneous in vivo measurement of NM block on three muscles. *Anesthesiology* 1982; 57:A276.
68. Payne JP, Hughes R: Evaluation of atracurium in anaesthetized man. *Br J Anaesth* 1981; 53:45–54.
69. Gramstad L, Lilleaasen P, Minsaas B: Onset time and duration of action for atracurium, ORG NC 45 and pancuronium. *Br J Anaesth* 1982; 54:827–830.
70. Foldes FF, Nagashima H, Boros M, et al: Muscular relaxation with atracurium, vecuronium and Duador under balanced anaesthesia. *Br J Anaesth* 1983; 55:97S–103S.
71. Mirakhur RK, Lavery GG, Clarke RSJ, et al: Atracurium in clinical anaesthesia: Effect of dosage on onset, duration and conditions for tracheal intubation. *Anaesthesia* 1985; 40:801–805.
72. Scott RPF, Savarese JJ, Basta SJ, et al: Clinical pharmacology of atracurium given in high dose. *Br J Anaesth* 1986; 58:834–838.

73. Lennon RL, Olson RD, Gronert GA: Atracurium or vecuronium for rapid sequence endotracheal intubation. *Anesthesiology* 1986; 64:510–513.
74. Healey TEJ, Pugh ND, Kay B, et al: Atracurium and vecuronium: Effect of dose on the time of onset. *Br J Anaesth* 1986; 58:620–624.
75. Gergis SD, Sokoll MD, Mehta M, et al: Intubation conditions after atracurium and suxamethonium. *Br J Anaesth* 1983; 55:83S–86S.
76. Weinberg G, Stirt JA, Longnecker DE: Single versus divided doses of atracurium: Does 0.05 + 0.10 equal 0.15? *Anesthesiology* 1986; 64:111–113.
77. Naguib M, Gyasi HK, Abdulatif M, et al: Rapid tracheal intubation with atracurium: A comparison of priming intervals. *Can Anaesth Soc J* 1986; 33:150–156.
78. Naguib M, Abdullatif M, Absood GH: The optimal priming dose for atracurium. *Can Anaesth Soc J* 1986; 33:453–457.
79. Scott RPF, Goat VA: Atracurium: Its speed of onset. A comparison with suxamethonium. *Br J Anaesth* 1982; 54:909–911.
80. Stirt JA, Katz RL, Schehl DC, et al: Atracurium for intubation in man: A clinical and myographic study. *Anaesthesia* 1984; 39:1214–1221.
81. Schiller DJ, Feldman SA: Comparison of intubating conditions with atracurium, vecuronium and pancuronium. *Anaesthesia* 1984; 39:1188–1191.
82. Ali HH, Savarese JJ, Basta SJ, et al: Evaluation of cumulative properties of three new non-depolarizing neuromuscular blocking drugs BW A444U, atracurium and vecuronium. *Br J Anaesth* 1983; 55:107S–111S.
83. Stirt JA, Murray AL, Katz RL, et al: Atracurium during halothane anesthesia in humans. *Anesth Analg* 1983; 62:207–210.
84. Baird WLM, Kerr WJ: Reversal of atracurium with edrophonium. *Br J Anaesth* 1983; 55:63S–66S.
85. Rupp SM, McChristian JW, Miller RD, et al: Neostigmine and edrophonium antagonism of varying intensity neuromuscular blockade induced by atracurium, pancuronium or vecuronium. *Anesthesiology* 1986; 64:711–717.
86. Casson WR, Jones RM: Profound atracurium induced neuromuscular blockade: A comparison of evoked reversal with edrophonium or neostigmine. *Anaesthesia* 1986; 41:382–385.
87. Calvey TN, Macmillan RR, West DM, et al: Electromyographic assessment of neuromuscular blockade induced by atracurium. *Br J Anaesth* 1983; 55:57S–62S.
88. Bowman WC: Prejunctional and postjunctional cholinoceptors at the neuromuscular junction. *Anesth Analg* 1980; 59:935–943.
89. Kemmotsu O, Sokell MD, Gergis SD: Site of action of BW33A at the rat neuromuscular junction. *Anesthesiology* 1982; 57:A289.
90. Hackett GH, Hughes R, Payne JP: Recovery of spontaneous breathing following neuromuscular blockade with atracurium. *Br J Anaesth* 1986; 58:494–497.
91. Stenlake JB: Atracurium: A contribution to anaesthetic practice. *Pharm J* 1982; 229:116–120.

92. Healey TEJ, Palmer JP: In vitro comparison between the neuromuscular and ganglion blocking potency ratios of atracurium and tubocurarine. *Br J Anaesth* 1982; 54:1307–1311.

93. Moyers JR, Carter JG, Davies LR, et al: Circulatory effects of BW33A in the dog. *Anesthesiology* 1982; 57:A285.

94. Hilgenberg JC, Stoelting RK, Harris WA: Haemodynamic effects of atracurium during enflurane-nitrous oxide anaesthesia in man. *Br J Anaesth* 1983; 55:81S.

95. Hilgenberg JC, Stoelting RK: Haemodynamic effects of atracurium in the presence of potent inhalational agents. *Br J Anaesth* 1986; 58:70S–74S.

96. Philbin DM, Machaj VR, Tomichek RC, et al: Haemodynamic effects of bolus injections of atracurium in patients with coronary artery disease. *Br J Anaesth* 1983; 55:131S–134S.

97. Hunter JM: Bradycardia after the use of atracurium. *Br Med J* 1983; 287:759.

98. Carter ML: Bradycardia after the use of atracurium. *Br Med J* 1983; 287:247–248.

99. Hughes R, Payne JP: Clinical assessment of atracurium using the single twitch and tetanic responses of the adductor pollicis. *Br J Anaesth* 1983; 55:47S–52S.

100. Barnes PK, Thomas VJE, Boyd I, et al: Comparison of the effects of atracurium and tubocurarine on heart rate and arterial pressure in anaesthetized man. *Br J Anaesth* 1983; 55:91S–94S.

101. Savarese JJ, Basta SJ, Ali HH, et al: Neuromuscular and cardiovascular effects of BW 33A (atracurium) in patients under halothane anesthesia. *Anesthesiology* 1982; 57:A262.

102. Barnes PK, deRenzy-Martin N, Thomas VJE, et al: Plasma histamine levels following atracurium. *Anaesthesia* 1986; 41:821–824.

103. Goudsouzian NG, Young ET, Moss J, et al: Histamine release during the administration of atracurium or vecuronium in children. *Br J Anaesth* 1986; 58:1229–1233.

104. Basta SJ, Savarese JJ, Ali HH, et al: Histamine releasing potencies of atracurium dimethyl tubocurarine and tubocurarine. *Br J Anaesth* 1983; 55:105S–106S.

105. Sale JP: Bronchospasm following the use of atracurium. *Anaesthesia* 1983; 38:511–512.

106. Siler JN, Mager JG, Wyche MQ: Atracurium: Hypotension, tachycardia and bronchospasm. *Anesthesiology* 1985; 62:645–646.

107. Srivastava S: Angioneurotic oedema following atracurium. *Br J Anaesth* 1984; 56:932.

108. Moss J, Roson CE: Histamine release by narcotics and muscle relaxants in humans. *Anesthesiology* 1983; 59:330–339.

109. Scott RPF, Savarese JJ, Basta SJ, et al: Atracurium: Clinical strategies for preventing histamine release and attenuating the haemodynamic response. *Br J Anaesth* 1985; 57:550–553.

110. Mercer JD: A severe anaphylactoid reaction to atracurium. *Anaesth Intensive Care* 1984; 12:262–269.

111. Lavery GG, Boyle MM, Mirakhur RK: Probable histamine liberation with atracurium. *Br J Anaesth* 1985; 57:811–813.
112. Tetzlaff JE, Gellman MD: Anaphylactoid reaction to atracurium. *Can Anaesth Soc J* 1986; 33:647–650.
113. Fisher MM, Munro E: Life-threatening reactions to muscle relaxants. *Anesth Analg* 1983; 62:559–564.
114. Harle DG, Baldo BA, Fisher MM: Cross-reactivity of metocurine, atracurium, vecuronium and fazadinium with IgE antibodies from patients unexposed to these drugs but allergic to other myoneural blocking drugs. *Br J Anaesth* 1985; 57:1073–1076.
115. Giffin JP, Litwak B, Cottrell JE: Intracranial pressure, mean arterial pressure and heart rate after rapid paralysis with atracurium in cats. *Can Anaesth Soc J* 1985; 32:618–621.
116. Minton MD, Stirt JA, Bedford RF, et al: Intracranial pressure after atracurium in neurosurgical patients. *Anesth Analg* 1985; 64:1113–1116.
117. Rosa G, Orfei P, Sanfilippo M, et al: The effects of atracurium besylate (Tracrium) on intracranial pressure and cerebral perfusion pressure. *Anesth Analg* 1986; 65:381–384.
118. Tattersall MP, Manus NJ, Jackson DM: The effect of atracurium or fazadinium on intra-ocular pressure: A comparative study during induction of general anaesthesia. *Anaesthesia* 1985; 40:805–807.
119. Lavery GG, McGalliard JN, Mirakhur RK, et al: The effects of atracurium on intraocular pressure during steady state anaesthesia and rapid sequence induction: A comparison with succinylcholine. *Can Anaesth Soc J* 1986; 33:437–442.
120. Schneider MJ, Stirt JA, Finholt DA: Atracurium, vecuronium, and intraocular pressure in humans. *Anesth Analg* 1986; 65:877–882.
121. Haigh JD, Nemato EM, Bleyaerst AL: Comparison of the effects of succinylcholine and atracurium on intracranial pressure in monkeys with intracranial hypertension. *Can Anaesth Soc J* 1986; 33:421–426.
122. Hunt PCW, Cotton BR, Smith G: Comparison of the effects of pancuronium and atracurium on the lower esophageal sphincter. *Anesth Analg* 1984; 63:65–68.
123. Brandom BW, Rudd GD, Cook DR: Clinical pharmacology of atracurium in paediatric patients. *Br J Anaesth* 1983; 55:117S–121S.
124. Meretoja OA, Kalli I: Spontaneous recovery of neuromuscular function after atracurium in pediatric patients. *Anesth Analg* 1986; 65:1042–1046.
125. Cook DR, Brandom BW, Woelfel SK, et al: Atracurium infusion in children during fentanyl, halothane, and isoflurane anesthesia. *Anesth Analg* 1984; 63:201.
126. Brandom BW, Cook DR, Woelfel SK, et al: Atracurium infusion requirements in children during halothane, isoflurane, and narcotic anesthesia. *Anesth Analg* 1985; 64:471–476.
127. d'Hollander AA, Luyckx C, Barvais L, et al: Clinical evaluation of atracurium besylate requirement for a stable muscle relaxation during sur-

gery: Lack of age-related effects. *Anesthesiology* 1983; 59:237–240.

128. Chapple DJ, Clark JS, Hughes R: Interaction between atracurium and drugs used in anaesthesia. *Br J Anaesth* 1983; 55:17S–22S.

129. Duncalf D, Chaudhry I, Aoki T, et al: Potentiation of pancuronium, vecuronium and atracurium by d-tubocurarine or metocurine. *Anesthesiology* 1983; 59:A292.

130. Black TE, Healey TEJ, Kay B, et al: The interaction of atracurium and vecuronium. *Br J Anaesth* 1985; 57:344P.

131. Lebowitz PW, Ramsey FM, Savarese JJ, et al: Potentiation of neuromuscular blockade in man produced by combinations of pancuronium and metocurine or pancuronium and d-tubocurarine. *Anesth Analg* 1980; 59:604–609.

132. Manchikanti L, Grow JB, Colliver JA, et al: Atracurium pretreatment for succinylcholine-induced fasciculations and postoperative myalgia. *Anesth Analg* 1985; 64:1010–1014.

133. Foldes FF, Deery A: Protein binding of atracurium and other short-acting neuromuscular blocking agents and their interaction with human cholinesterases. *Br J Anaesth* 1983; 55:31S–34S.

134. Pearce AC, Williams JP, Jones RM: Atracurium for short surgical procedures in day patients. *Br J Anaesth* 1984; 56:973–976.

135. Gyasi HK, Naguib M, Adu-Gyamfi Y: Atracurium for short surgical procedures: A comparison with succinylcholine. *Can Anaesth Soc J* 1985; 32:613–617.

136. Sleigh JW, Matheson KH, Boys JE: The use of atracurium besylate for laparoscopy. *Anaesthesia* 1984; 39:277–279.

137. Flynn PJ, Frank M, Hughes R: Use of atracurium in caesarean section. *Br J Anaesth* 1984; 56:599–605.

138. deBros FM, Lai A, Scott R, et al: Pharmacokinetics and pharmacodynamics of atracurium during isoflurane anesthesia in normal and anephric patients. *Anesth Analg* 1986; 65:743–746.

139. Hunter JM, Jones RS, Utting JE: Use of atracurium in patients with no renal function. *Br J Anaesth* 1982; 54:1251–1258.

140. Mongin-Long D, Chabrol B, Baude C, et al: Atracurium in patients with renal failure. *Br J Anaesth* 1986; 58:44S–48S.

141. Gyasi HK, Naguib M: Atracurium and severe hepatic disease: A case report. *Can Anaesth Soc J* 1985; 32:161–164.

142. Griffiths RB, Hunter JM, Jones RS: Atracurium infusions in patients with renal failure on an ITU. *Anaesthesia* 1986; 41:375–381.

143. Flynn PJ, Hughes R, Walton B: Use of atracurium in cardiac surgery involving cardiopulmonary bypass with induced hypothermia. *Br J Anaesth* 1984; 56:967–972.

144. Futter M, Whalley DG, Wynands JE, et al: Pancuronium requirements during hypothermic cardiopulmonary bypass in man. *Anaesth Intensive Care* 1983; 11:216–219.

145. Stirt JA, Bram RE, Ross WT, et al: Atracurium in a patient with pheochromocytoma. *Anesth Analg* 1985;64:547–550.

146. Forrest AL: Atracurium and pheochromocytoma. *Anesth Analg* 1986; 65:211.
147. Ward S, Wright DJ,: Neuromuscular blockade in myasthenia gravis with atracurium besylate. *Anaesthesia* 1984; 39:51–53.
148. Bell CF, Florence AM, Hunter JM, et al: Atracurium in the myasthenic patient. *Anaesthesia* 1984; 39:961–968.
149. Baraka A, Dajani A: Atracurium in myasthenics undergoing thymectomy. *Anesth Analg* 1984; 63:1127–1130.
150. Macdonald AM, Keen RI, Pugh ND: Myasthenia gravis and atracurium. *Br J Anaesth* 1984; 56:651–654.
151. Ramsey FM, Smith GD: Clinical use of atracurium in myasthenia gravis. *Can Anaesth Soc J* 1985; 32:642–645.
152. Buzello W, Noeldge G, Krieg N, et al: Vecuronium for muscle relaxation in patients with myasthenia gravis. *Anesthesiology* 1986; 64:507–509.
153. Morrell DF, Harrison GG: The screening of atracurium in MHS swine. *Br J Anaesth* 1986; 58:444–446.
154. Stirt JA, Stone DJ, Weinberg G, et al: Atracurium in a child with myotonic dystrophy. *Anesth Analg* 1985; 64:369–370.
155. Nightingale P, Healey TEJ, McGuinness K: Dystrophia myotonica and atracurium. *Br J Anaesth* 1985; 57:1131–1135.
156. Dwersteg JF, Pavlin EG, Heinbach DM: Patients with burns are resistant to atracurium. *Anesthesiology* 1986; 65:517–520.
157. Gerber HR, Romppainen J, Schwina W: Potentiation of atracurium by pancuronium and d-tubocurarine. *Can Anaesth Soc J* 1986; 33:563–570.
158. Fisher DM, Canfell C, Miller RD: Stability of atracurium administered by infusion. *Anesthesiology* 1984; 61:347–348.
159. Madden AP, Hughes R, Payne JP: Recovery from neuromuscular blockade after infusion of atracurium. *Br J Anaesth* 1982; 54:226P–227P.
160. Bolger L, Brittain RT, Jack D, et al: Short-lasting, competitive neuromuscular blocking activity in a series of azobis-arylimidazo-(1,2-a)-pyridinium dihalides. *Nature* 1972; 238:354–355.
161. Simpson BR, Savege TM, Foley ET, et al: An azobis-arylimidazo-pyridinium derivative: A rapidly acting non-depolarizing muscle-relaxant. *Lancet* 1972; 1:516–519.
162. Duvaldestin P, Henzel D, Demetriou M, et al: Pharmacokinetics of fazadinium in man. *Br J Anaesth* 1978; 50:773–777.
163. D'Souza J, Caldwell J, Dring LG, et al: ^{125}I-labelled rose bengal in the quantitative estimation of fazadinium and other quaternary ammonium compounds in biological fluids. *J Pharm Pharmacol* 1979; 31:416–418.
164. Duvaldestin P, Bertrand JC, Concina D, et al: Pharmacokinetics of fazadinium in patients with renal failure. *Br J Anaesth* 1979; 51:943–947.
165. Duvaldestin P, Saada J, Henzel D, et al: Fazadinium pharmocokinetics in patients with liver disease. *Br J Anaesth* 1980; 52:789–793.
166. d'Hollander AA, Duvaldestin P, Henzel D, et al: Relationship between

decay of plasma concentration of fazadinium and recovery from its neuromuscular blocking effect. *Br J Anaesth* 1981; 53:853–857.

167. Bevan DR, D'Souza J, Rouse JM, et al: Clinical pharmacokinetics of fazadinium. *Anaesthesia* 1980; 35:873–878.

168. Bevan DR, D'Souza J, Rouse JM, et al: Clinical pharmacokinetics and pharmacodynamics of fazadinium in renal failure. *Eur J Clin Pharmacol* 1981; 20:293–298.

169. Hull CJ, English MJM, Sibbald A: A pharmacodynamic model for fazadinium. *Br J Anaesth* 1980; 52:632P–633P.

170. Hughes R, Payne JP, Sugai N: Studies of fazadinium bromide (AH 8165): A new non-depolarizing neuromuscular blocking agent. *Can Anaesth Soc J* 1976; 23:36–47.

171. Camu F, d'Hollander AA: Neuromuscular blockade of fazadinium bromide (AH 8165) in renal failure patients. *Acta Anaesthesiol Scand* 1978; 22:221–226.

172. Hussain SZ, Healey TEJ, Birmingham AT: Comparative potency and speed of onset of fazadinium and d-tubocurarine. *Acta Anaesthesiol Scand* 1979; 23:331–335.

173. Blackburn CL, Morgan M: Comparison of speed of onset of fazadinium, pancuronium, tubocurarine and suxamethonium. *Br J Anaesth* 1978; 50:361–364.

174. Minsaas B, Stovner J: Artery-to-muscle onset time for neuromuscular blocking drugs. *Br J Anaesth* 1980; 52:403–407.

175. Donati F, Walsh CM, Lavelle PA, et al: Onset of pancuronium and d-tubocurarine blockade with priming. *Can Anaesth Soc J* 1986; 33:571–577.

176. Post EL, Sokoll MD, Gergis SD, et al: Actions of a new muscle relaxant (AH 8165) on neuromuscular transmission. *Anesthesiology* 1975; 42:240–244.

177. Waud BE: Kinetic analysis of the AH 8165–receptor interaction at the mammalian neuromuscular junction. *Anesthesiology* 1977; 46:94–96.

178. Patschke E, Bruckner JB, Tarnow J, et al: The influence of AH 8165, a new non-depolarizing relaxant on the haemodynamics in man. *Anaesthetist* 1974; 23:430–434.

179. Coleman AJ, Walling PT, Downing JW, et al: The effect of carbon dioxide on the neuromuscular and haemodynamic effects of AH 8165, a new nondepolarizing muscle relaxant. *Br J Anaesth* 1975; 47:365–369.

180. Pinaud M, Rochedreux A, Dixneuf B, et al: Effects hemodynamiques compares du fazadinium et du pancuronium chez l'homme, in *Curares et Curarisation*. Paris, Arnette, 1980, p 323.

181. Pinaud M, Arnould F, Souron R, et al: Influence of cardiac rhythm on the haemodynamic effects of fazadinium in patients with heart failure. *Br J Anaesth* 1983; 55:507–512.

182. Camu F, d'Hollander A: Neuromuscular blockade of fazadinium bromide (AH 8165) in renal failure patients. *Acta Anaesthesiol Scand* 1978; 22:221–226.

183. Bovet D, Depierre F, Lestrange Y: Proprietes curarisantes des ethers phenoliques a fonctions ammonium quaternaires. *Comptes Rendus Hebdomadaires des Seances de l'Academie des Sciences.* 1947; 225:74–76.

184. Huguenard P, Boue A: Un nouveau curarisant francais de synethese. *Anesth et Analgesie* 1950; 7:1–17.

185. Churchill Davidson HC, Way WL, de Jong RH: The muscle relaxants and renal excretion. *Anesthesiology* 1965; 28:540–546.

186. Feldman SA, Cohen EN, Golling RC: The excretion of gallamine in the dog. *Anesthesiology* 1969; 30:593–598.

187. Agoston S, Vermeer GA, Kersten UW, et al: A preliminary investigation of the renal and hepatic elimination of gallamine triethiodide in man. *Br J Anaesth* 1978; 50:345–351.

188. Ramzan MI, Triggs EJ, Shanks CA: Pharmacokinetic studies in man with gallamine triethiodide: I. Single and multiple clinical doses. *Eur J Clin Pharmacol* 1980; 17:135–143.

189. Ramzan MI, Shanks CA, Triggs EJ: Gallamine disposition in surgical patients with chronic renal failure. *Br J Clin Pharmacol* 1981; 12:141–147.

190. Ramzan MI, Shanks CA, Triggs EJ: Pharmacokinetics and pharmacodynamics of gallamine triethiodide in patients with total biliary obstruction. *Anesth Analg* 1981; 60:289–309.

191. Lowenstein E, Goldfine C, Flacke WE: Administration of gallamine in the presence of renal failure: Reversal of neuromuscular blockade by peritoneal dialysis. *Anesthesiology* 1970; 33:556–558.

192. Donlon JV, Ali HH, Savarese JJ: A new approach to the study of four nondepolarizing relaxants in man. *Anesth Analg* 1974; 53:934–939.

193. Shanks CA, Walker JS, Ramzan MI, et al: Dose-response curves for four neuromuscular blockers using continuous i.v. infusion. *Br J Anaesth* 1981; 53:627–632.

194. Pitt GM, Payne JP: Recovery of respiration after neuromuscular block by gallamine. *Br J Anaesth* 1985; 57:831P.

195. Miller RD, Larson CP, Way WL: Comparative antagonism of d-tubocurarine, gallamine, and pancuronium induced neuromuscular blockades by neostigmine. *Anesthesiology* 1972; 37:503–509.

196. Colquhoun D, Sheridan RE: Modes of action of gallamine at the neuromuscular junction. *Br J Pharmacol* 1979; 66:78–79P.

197. Stoelting RK: Hemodynamic effects of gallamine during halothane-nitrous oxide anesthesia. *Anesthesiology* 1973; 39:645–647.

198. Lee Son S, Waud DR: Effects of non-depolarizing neuromuscular blocking agents on the cardiac vagus nerve in the guinea pig. *Br J Anaesth* 1980; 52:981–987.

199. Vercruysse P, Bossuyt P, Hanegreefs G: Gallamine and pancuronium inhibit pre- and post-junctional muscarinic receptors in canine saphenous veins. *J Pharmacol Exp Ther* 1979; 209:225–230.

200. Brown BR, Crout JR: The sympathomimetic effect of gallamine on the

heart. *J Pharmacol Exp Ther* 1970; 172:266–271.

201. Eisele JH, Marta JA, Davis HS: Quantitative aspects of the chronotropic and neuromuscular effects of gallamine in anesthetized man. *Anesthesiology* 1971; 35:630–633.

202. Wisborg K, Christensen V, Viby-Mogensen J: Halothane anaesthesia and suxamethonium: II. The significance of preoperative gallamine administration. *Acta Anaesthesiol Scand* 1977; 21:266–271.

203. Viby-Mogensen J, Wisborg K, Sorensen O: Effects of atropine and gallamine in patients receiving suxamethonium. *Br J Anaesth* 1980; 52:1137–1142.

204. Harrison JF, Bird AG: Anaphylaxis to precurarising doses of gallamine triethiodide. *Anaesthesia* 1986;41:600–604.

205. Waud BE, Waud DR: Quantitative examination of the interaction of competitive neuromuscular blocking agents on the indirectly elicited muscle twitch. *Anesthesiology* 1984; 61:420–427.

206. Waud BE, Waud DR: Interaction among agents that block end-plate depolarization competitively. *Anesthesiology* 1985; 63:4–15.

207. Foldes FF: Enzymes of acetylcholine metabolism, in Foldes FF: *Enzymes in Anesthesiology*. New York, Springer-Verlag, 1978, pp 91–168.

208. Shanks CA, Fink DI, Avram MJ, et al: Gallamine administered by combined bolus and infusion. *Anesth Analg* 1982; 61:847–852.

209. Cullen DJ: The effect of pretreatment with nondepolarizing muscle relaxants on the neuromuscular blocking action of succinylcholine. *Anesthesiology* 1971; 35:572–578.

210. Miller RD, Way WL: Inhibition of succinylcholine-induced increased intraocular pressure by nondepolarizing muscle relaxants. *Anesthesiology* 1968; 29:123–126.

211. Meyers EF, Krupin T, Johnson M, et al: Failure of nondepolarizing neuromuscular blockers to inhibit succinylcholine-induced increased intraocular pressure, a controlled study. *Anesthesiology* 1978; 48:149–151.

212. Sobell HM, Sakore, TD, Tavale SS, et al: Stereochemistry of curare alkaloid: O,O′,N-trimethyl-d-tubocurarine. *Proc Natl Acad Sci USA* 1972; 69:2212–2215.

213. Meijer DKF, Weitering JG, Vermeer GA, et al: Comparative pharmacokinetics of d-tubocurarine and metocurine in man. *Anesthesiology* 1979; 51:402–407.

214. Brotherton WP, Matteo RS: Pharmacokinetics and pharmacodynamics of metocurine in humans with and without renal failure. *Anesthesiology* 1981; 55:273–276.

215. Matteo RS, Backus WW, McDaniel DD, et al: Pharmacokinetics and pharmacodynamics of d-tubocurarine and metocurine in the elderly. *Anesth Analg* 1985; 64:23–29.

216. Hughes R, Ingram GS, Payne JP: Studies on dimethyl tubocurarine in anaesthetized man. *Br J Anaesth* 1976; 48:969–974.

217. Savarese JJ, Ali HH, Antonio RP: The clinical pharmacology of metocurine: Dimethyltubocurarine, revisited. *Anesthesiology* 1977; 47:277–285.

218. Katz RL: Neuromuscular effects of d-tubocurarine, edrophonium, and neostigmine in man. *Anesthesiology* 1967; 28:327–336.

219. Katz RL: Clinical neuromuscular pharmacology of pancuronium. *Anesthesiology* 1971; 34:550–556.

220. Hughes R, Chapple DJ: Cardiovascular and neuromuscular effects of dimethyl tubocurarine in anaesthetized cats and rhesus monkeys. *Br J Anaesth* 1976; 48:847–851.

221. McCullough LS, Stone WA, Delaunois AL, et al: The effects of dimethyltubocurarine iodide on cardiovascular parameters, postganglionic sympathetic activity and histamine release. *Anesth Analg* 1972; 51:554–559.

222. Savarese JJ: The autonomic margin of safety of metocurine and d-tubocurarine in the cat. *Anesthesiology* 1979; 50:40–46.

223. Antonio RP, Philbin DM, Savarese JJ: Comparative haemodynamic effects of tubocurarine and metocurine in the dog. *Br J Anaesth* 1979; 51:1007–1010.

224. Stoelting RK: Hemodynamic effects of dimethyl tubocurarine during nitrous oxide-halothane anesthesia. *Anesth Analg* 1974; 53:513–515.

225. Zaidan JR, Kaplan JA: Cardiovascular effects of metocurine in patients with aortic stenosis. *Anesthesiology* 1982; 56:395–397.

226. Martyn JAJ, Leibel WS, Matteo RS: Competitive nonspecific binding does not explain the potentiating effects of muscle relaxant combinations. *Anesth Analg* 1983; 62:160–163.

227. Standaert FG: The action of d-tubocurarine on the motor nerve terminal. *J Pharmacol Exp Ther* 1964; 143:181–186.

228. Glavinovic MI: Presynaptic action of curare. *J Physiol (Lond)* 1979; 290:499–506.

229. Galindo A: Curare and pancuronium compared: Effects on previously undepressed mammalian myoneural junctions. *Science* 1972; 178:753–755.

230. Su PC, Su WL, Rosen AD: Pre- and post-synaptic effects of pancuronium at the neuromuscular junction of the mouse. *Anesthesiology* 1979; 50:199–204.

231. Lebowitz PW, Ramsey FM, Savarese JJ, et al: Combination of pancuronium and metocurine: Neuromuscular and hemodynamic advantages over pancuronium alone. *Anesth Analg* 1981; 60:12–17.

232. Cunningham AJ, Kelly CP, Farmer J, et al: The effect of metocurine and metocurine-pancuronium combination on intraocular pressure. *Can Anaesth Soc J* 1982; 29:617–621.

233. Martyn J: Clinical pharmacology and drug therapy in the burned patient. *Anesthesiology* 1986; 65:67–75.

234. Martyn JAJ, Matteo RS, Szyfelbein SK, et al: Unprecedented resistance to neuromuscular blocking effects of metocurine with persistence after complete recovery in a burned patient. *Anesth Analg* 1982; 61:614–617.

235. Martyn JAJ, Goudsouzian NG, Matteo RS, et al: Metocurine require-

ments and plasma concentrations in burned paediatric patients. *Br J Anaesth* 1983; 55:263–268.

236. Shayevitz JR, Matteo RS: Decreased sensitivity to metocurine in patients with upper motoneuron disease. *Anesth Analg* 1985; 64:767–772.

237. Mehta MP, Choi WS, Gergis SD, et al: Facilitation of rapid endotracheal intubation with divided doses of nondepolarizing neuromuscular blocking drugs. *Anesthesiology* 1985; 62:392–395.

238. Buckett WR, Hewitt CL, Savage DS: Pancuronium bromide and other steroidal neuromuscular blocking agents containing acetylcholine fragments. *J Med Chem* 1973; 16:1116–1124.

239. Ing HR, Wright WM: The curariform action of quaternary ammonium salts. *Proc R Soc Lond Biol* 1931; 109:337–353.

240. Bovet D: Some aspects of the relationship between chemical constitution and curare-like activity. *Ann NY Acad Sci* 1951; 54:407–432.

241. Martin-Smith M: *Drug Design.* New York, Academic Press, 1971, vol 2, pp 454–530.

242. Buckett WR, Marjoribanks EB, Marwick FA, et al: The pharmacology of pancuronium bromide (ORG NA97), a new potent steroidal neuromuscular blocking agent. *Br J Pharmacol* 1968; 32:671–682.

243. Baird WLM, Reid AM: The neuromuscular blocking properties of a new steroid compound, pancuronium bromide. *Br J Anaesth* 1967; 39:775–780.

244. Agoston S, Vermeer GA, Kersten UW, et al: The fate of pancuronium bromide in man. *Acta Anaesthesiol Scand* 1973; 17:267–275.

245. Miller RD, Agoston S, Booij LHD, et al: The comparative potency and pharmacokinetics of pancuronium and its metabolites in anesthetized man. *J Pharmacol Exp Ther* 1978; 207:539–543.

246. Marshall IG, Gibb AJ, Durant NN: Neuromuscular and vagal blocking actions of pancuronium bromide, its metabolites, and vecuronium bromide (ORG NC 45) and its potential metabolites in the anaesthetized cat. *Br J Anaesth* 1983; 55:703–714.

247. Waser PG: Localization of [^{14}C] pancuronium by wholebody-autoradiography in normal and pregnant mice. *Naunyn Schmiedebergs Arch Pharmacol* 1973; 279:339–412.

248. Thompson JM: Pancuronium binding by serum proteins. *Anaesthesia* 1976; 31:219–227.

249. Stovner J, Theodorsen L, Bjelke E: Sensitivity to gallamine and pancuronium with special reference to serum proteins. *Br J Anaesth* 1971; 43:953–958.

250. Wood M, Stone WJ, Wood AJJ: Plasma binding of pancuronium: Effects of age, sex, and disease. *Anesth Analg* 1983; 62:29–32.

251. Somogyi AA, Shanks CA, Triggs EJ: The effect of renal failure on the disposition and neuromuscular blocking action of pancuronium bromide. *Eur J Clin Pharmacol* 1977; 12:23–29.

252. Agoston S, Crul JF, Kersten UW, et al: Relationship of the serum concentration of pancuronium to its neuromuscular activity in man. *Anesthesiology* 1977; 47:509–512.

253. Kersten UW, Meijer DK, Agoston S: Fluorimetric and chromatographic determination of pancuronium bromide and its metabolites in biological materials. *Clin Chim Acta* 1973; 44:59–66.
254. Buzello W: Der Stoffwechsil von Pancuronium beim menschen. *Anaesthetist* 1975; 24:13–18.
255. Cronnelly R, Fisher DM, Miller RD, et al: Pharmacokinetics and pharmacodynamics of vecuronium (ORG NC 45) and pancuronium in anesthetized humans. *Anesthesiology* 1983; 58:405–408.
256. Duvaldestin P, Agoston S, Henzel D, et al: Pancuronium pharmacokinetics in patients with liver cirrhosis. *Br J Anaesth* 1978; 50:1131–1136.
257. McLeod K, Watson MJ, Rawlins MD: Pharmacokinetics of pancuronium in patients with normal and impaired renal function. *Br J Anaesth* 1976; 48:341–345.
258. McLeod K, Hull CJ, Watson MJ: Effects of ageing on the pharmacokinetics of pancuronium. *Br J Anaesth* 1979; 51:435–438.
259. Somogyi AA, Shanks CA, Triggs EJ: Disposition kinetics of pancuronium bromide in patients with total biliary obstruction. *Br J Anaesth* 1977; 49:1103–1108.
260. Duvaldestin P, Saada J, Berger JL, et al: Pharmacokinetics, pharmacodynamics and dose-response relationships of pancuronium in control and elderly subjects. *Anesthesiology* 1982; 56:36–40.
261. Agoston S, Crul JF, Kersten UW, et al: Relationship of the serum concentration of pancuronium to its neuromuscular activity in man. *Anesthesiology* 1977; 47:509–512.
262. Shanks CA, Somogyi AA, Triggs EJ: Plasma concentrations of pancuronium during predetermined intensities of neuromuscular blockade. *Br J Anaesth* 1978; 50:235–239.
263. Hull CJ, Van Beem HBH, McLeod K, et al: A pharmacodynamic model for pancuronium. *Br J Anaesth* 1978; 50:1113–1122.
264. Norman J, Katz RL, Seed RF: The neuromuscular blocking action of pancuronium in man during anaesthesia. *Br J Anaesth* 1970; 42:702–709.
265. Foldes FF, Klonymus DH, Maisel W, et al: Studies of pancuronium in conscious and anesthetized man. *Anesthesiology* 1971; 35:496–503.
266. McDowall SA, Clarke RSJ: A clinical comparison of pancuronium with d-tubocurarine. *Anaesthesia* 1969; 24:581–590.
267. Donlon JV, Savarese JJ, Ali HH, et al: Human dose-response curves for neuromuscular blocking drugs: A comparison of two methods of construction and analysis. *Anesthesiology* 1980; 53:161–166.
268. Engbaek J, Ording H, Pedersen T, et al: Dose-response relationships and neuromuscular blocking effects of vecuronium and pancuronium during ketamine anaesthesia. *Br J Anaesth* 1984; 56:953–957.
269. Shanks CA, Somogyi AA, Triggs EJ: Dose-response and plasma concentration-response relationships of pancuronium in man. *Anesthesiology* 1979; 51:111–118.

270. Lee C, Yang E, Katz RL: Predetermination of dose requirement of pancuronium. *Anesth Analg* 1980; 59:722–726.

271. Doherty WG, Breen PJ, Donati F, et al: Accelerated onset of pancuronium with divided doses. *Can Anaesth Soc J* 1985; 32:1–4.

272. Bevan JC, Donati F, Bevan DR: Attempted acceleration of the onset of action of pancuronium: Effect of divided doses in infants and children. *Br J Anaesth* 1985; 57:1204–1208.

273. Paton WDM, Waud DR: The margin of safety of neuromuscular transmission. *J Physiol* 1967; 191:59–90.

274. Fahey MR, Morris RB, Miller RD, et al: Clinical pharmacology of ORG NC 45 (Norcuron): A new nondepolarizing muscle relaxant. *Anesthesiology* 1981; 55:6–11.

275. Bevan DR: Reversal of pancuronium with edrophonium. *Anaesthesia* 1979; 34:614–619.

276. Kopman AF: Edrophonium antagonism of pancuronium-induced neuromuscular blockade in man: A reappraisal. *Anesthesiology* 1979; 51:139–142.

277. Ferguson A, Egerszegi P, Bevan DR: Neostigmine, pyridostigmine, and edrophonium as antagonists of pancuronium. *Anesthesiology* 1980; 53:390–394.

278. Cronnelly R, Morris RB, Miller RD: Edrophonium: Duration of action and atropine requirement in anesthetized man. *Anesthesiology* 1982; 57:261–266.

279. Breen PJ, Doherty WG, Donati F, et al: The potencies of edrophonium and neostigmine as antagonists of pancuronium. *Anaesthesia* 1985; 40:844–847.

280. Williams NE, Webb SN, Calvey TN: Differential effects of myoneural blocking drugs on neuromuscular transmission. *Br J Anaesth* 1980; 52:1111–1115.

281. Robbins R, Donati F, Bevan DR, et al: Differential effects of myoneural blocking drugs on neuromuscular transmission in infants. *Br J Anaesth* 1984; 56:1095–1099.

282. Loh L: The cardiovascular effect of pancuronium bromide. *Anaesthesia* 1970; 25:356–363.

283. Kelman GR, Kennedy BR: Cardiovascular effects of pancuronium in man. *Br J Anaesth* 1971; 43:335–338.

284. Stoelting RK: The hemodynamic effects of pancuronium and d-tubocurarine in anesthetized patients. *Anesthesiology* 1972; 36:612–615.

285. Barnes PK, Brindle-Smith G, White WD, et al: Comparison of the effects of ORG NC 45 and pancuronium bromide on heart rate and arterial pressure in anaesthetized man. *Br J Anaesth* 1982; 54:435–439.

286. Gardiner RW, Tserdos EJ, Jackson DB: Effect of gallamine and pancuronium on inhibitory transmission in cat sympathetic ganglia. *J Pharm Exp Ther* 1978; 204:46–53.

287. Vercruysse P, Hanegreefs G, Vanhoutte PM: Influence of skeletal muscle relaxants on the prejunctional effects of acetylcholine in adrenergi-

cally-innervated blood vessels. *Arch Int Pharmacodyn Ther* 1978; 232:350–352.

288. Domenech S, Garcia RC, Sasiain JMR, et al: Pancuronium bromide: An indirect sympathomimetic agent. *Br J Anaesth* 1976; 48:1143–1148.

289. Docherty JR, McGrath JC: Sympathomimetic effects of pancuronium bromide on the cardiovascular system of the pitted rat: A comparison with the effects of drugs blocking the neural uptake of noradrenaline. *Br J Pharmacol* 1978; 64:589–599.

290. Schick LM, Chapin JC, Munson ES, et al: Pancuronium, d-tubocurarine, and epinephrine-induced arrhythmias during halothane anesthesia in dogs. *Anesthesiology* 1980; 52:207–209.

291. Cummings MF, Russell WJ, Frewin DB: Effects of pancuronium and alcuronium on the changes in arterial pressure and plasma catecholamine concentrations during tracheal intubation. *Br J Anaesth* 1983; 55:619–623.

292. Duke PC, Fung H, Gartner J: The myocardial effects of pancuronium. *Can Anaesth Soc J* 1975; 22:680–686.

293. Iwatsuki N, Hashimoto Y, Amaha K, et al: Inotropic effects of non-depolarizing muscle relaxants in isolated canine heart muscle. *Anesth Analg* 1980; 59:717–721.

294. Buckland RS, Avery AF: Histamine release following pancuronium: A case report. *Br J Anaesth* 1973; 45:518–521.

295. Cotton BR, Smith G: The lower oesophageal sphincter and anaesthesia. *Br J Anaesth* 1984; 56:37–46.

296. Goudsouzian NG, Ryan JF, Savarese JJ: The neuromuscular effects of pancuronium in infants and children. *Anesthesiology* 1974; 41:95–98.

297. Goudsouzian NG, Martyn JJA, Liu LMP, et al: The dose response effect of long-acting nondepolarizing neuromuscular blocking agents in children. *Can Anaesth Soc J* 1984; 31:246–250.

298. Goudsouzian NG, Liu LMP, Cote CJ: Comparison of equipotent doses of non-depolarizing muscle relaxants in children. *Anesth Analg* 1981; 60:862–866.

299. Miller RD, Way WL, Dolan WM, et al: The dependence of pancuronium and d-tubocurarine-induced neuromuscular blockade on alveolar concentrations of halothane and forane. *Anesthesiology* 1972; 37:573–581.

300. Katz RL: Modification of the action of pancuronium by succinylcholine and halothane. *Anesthesiology* 1971; 35:602–606.

301. Bennett MJ, Hahn JF: Potentiation of the combination of pancuronium and metocurine by halothane and isoflurane in humans with and without renal failure. *Anesthesiology* 1985; 62:759–764.

302. Ferguson A, Bevan DR: Mixed neuromuscular block: The effect of precurarization. *Anaesthesia* 1981; 36:661–666.

303. Stovner J, Oftedal N, Holmboe J: The inhibition of cholinesterases by pancuronium. *Br J Anaesth* 1975; 47:949–954.

304. Frankel DZN: Neostigmine reversal of d-tubocurarine and pancuronium bromide combinations in man. *Can Anaesth Soc J* 1982; 29:395–397.

305. Pollard BJ, Jones RM: Interactions between tubocurarine, pancuronium and alcuronium demonstrated in the rat phrenic nerve-hemidiaphragm preparation. *Br J Anaesth* 1983; 55:1127–1131.

306. Taylor P: Are neuromuscular blocking agents more efficacious in pairs? *Anesthesiology* 1985; 63:1–3.

307. Pandit SK, Ferres CJ, Gibson FM, et al: Time course of action of combination of vecuronium and pancuronium. *Anaesthesia* 1986; 41:151–154.

308. Rashkovsky OM, Agoston S, Ket JM: Interaction between pancuronium bromide and vecuronium bromide. *Br J Anaesth* 1985; 57:1063–1066.

309. Azar I, Kumar D, Betcher AA: Resistance to pancuronium in an asthmatic patient treated with aminophylline and steroids. *Can Anaesth Soc J* 1982; 29:380–382.

310. Callanan DC: Development of resistance to pancuronium in adult respiratory distress syndrome. *Anesth Analg* 1985; 64:1126–1128.

311. Stanley TH, Webster CR: Anesthetic requirements and cardiovascular effects of fentanyl-oxygen and fentanyl-diazepam-oxygen anesthesia in man. *Anesth Analg* 1978; 57:411–417.

312. de Lange S, Boscoe MJ, Stanley TH, et al: Comparison of sufentanil-O_2 and fentanyl O_2 for coronary artery surgery. *Anesthesiology* 1982; 56:112–118.

313. Lowenstein E, Hallowell P, Levine FH: Cardiovascular responses to large doses of intravenous morphine in man. *N Engl J Med* 1969; 281:1389–1393.

314. Liu W, Bidwal AV, Stanely TH, et al: Cardiovascular dynamics after large doses of fentanyl and fentanyl plus N_2O in the dog. *Anesth Analg* 1976; 55:168–172.

315. Thomson IR, Mutch AC, Culligan JD: Failure of intravenous nitroglycerin to prevent intraoperative myocardial ischemia during fentanyl-pancuronium anesthesia. *Anesthesiology* 1984; 61:385–393.

316. Thomson IR, Putnins CL: Adverse effects of pancuronium during high-dose fentanyl anesthesia for coronary artery bypass grafting. *Anesthesiology* 1985; 62:708–713.

317. Thomson IR, Putnins CL, Friesen RM: Hyperdynamic cardiovascular responses to anesthetic induction with high-dose fentanyl. *Anesth Analg* 1986; 65:91–95.

318. Heinonen J, Yrjola H: Comparison of haemodynamic effects of metocurine and pancuronium in patients with coronary artery disease. *Br J Anaesth* 1980; 52:931–937.

319. Savarese JJ: The name of the game: No anesthesia by cookbook. *Anesthesiology* 1985; 62:703–705.

320. Speirs I, Sim AW: The placental transfer of pancuronium bromide. *Br J Anaesth* 1972; 44:370–373.

321. Booth PN, Watson MJ, McLeod K: Pancuronium and the placenta barrier. *Anaesthesia* 1977; 32:320–325.

322. Neeld JB, Seabrook PD Jr, Chastain GM, et al: A clinical comparison of

pancuronium and tubocurarine for cesarean section anesthesia. *Anesth Analg* 1974; 53:7–12.

323. Abouleish E, Wingard LB, de la Vega S, et al: Pancuronium in caesarean section and its placental transfer. *Br J Anaesth* 1980; 52:531–536.

324. Miller RD, Stevens WC, Way WL: The effect of renal failure and hyperkalemia on the duration of action of pancuronium neuromuscular blockade in man. *Anesth Analg* 1973; 52:661–666.

325. Cronnelly R, Stanski DR, Miller RD, et al: Renal function and the pharmacokinetics of neostigmine in anesthetized man. *Anesthesiology* 1979; 51:222–226.

326. Cronnelly R, Stanski DR, Miller RD, et al: Pyridostigmine kinetics with and without renal function. *Clin Pharm Ther* 1980; 28:78–81.

327. Morris RB, Cronnelly R, Miller RD, et al: Pharmacokinetics of edrophonium and neostigmine when antagonizing a d-tubocurarine neuromuscular block in man. *Anesthesiology* 1981; 54:394–402.

328. Bevan DR, Archer D, Donati F, et al: Antagonism of pancuronium in renal failure: No recurarization. *Br J Anaesth* 1982; 54:63–68.

329. Nana A, Cardan E, Leitersdorfer T: Pancuronium bromide: Its use in asthmatics and patients with liver disease. *Anaesthesia* 1972; 27:154–158.

330. Ward ME, Adu-Gyamfi Y, Strunin L: Althesin and pancuronium in chronic liver disease. *Br J Anaesth* 1975; 47:1199–1204.

331. Duvaldestin P, Agoston A, Henzel D, et al: Pancuronium pharmacokinetics in patients with liver cirrhosis. *Br J Anaesth* 1978; 50:1131–1136.

332. Westra P, Vermeer GA, de Lange AR, et al: Hepatic and renal disposition of pancuronium and gallamine in patients with extrahepatic cholestasis. *Br J Anaesth* 1981; 53:331–338.

333. Westra P, Keulemans GTP, Houwertjes MC, et al: Mechanism underlying the prolonged duration of action of muscle relaxants caused by extrahepatic cholestasis. *Br J Anaesth* 1981; 53:217–226.

334. Ward S, Judge S, Corall I: Pharmacokinetics of pancuronium bromide in liver failure. *Br J Anaesth* 1982; 54:227P.

335. Duvaldestin P, Henzel D: Binding of tubocurarine, fazadinium, pancuronium and ORG NC 45 to serum protein in normal man and in patients with cirrhosis. *Br J Anaesth* 1982: 54:513–516.

336. Blitt CD, Wright WA, Peat J: Pancuronium and the patient with myasthenia gravis. *Anesthesiology* 1975; 42:624–626.

337. Yamashita M, Shiga T, Matsuki A, et al: Unusual resistance to pancuronium in severely burned patients: Case reports. *Can Anaesth Soc J* 1982; 29:630–631.

338. Martyn JAJ, Liu LMP, Szyfelbein SK, et al: Neuromuscular effects of pancuronium in burned children. *Anesthesiology* 1983; 59:561–564.

339. Tolmine JD, Joyce TH, Mitchell GD: Succinylcholine danger in the burned patient. *Anesthesiology* 1967; 28:467–470.

340. Leibel WS, Martyn JAJ, Szyfelbein SK, et al: Elevated plasma binding

cannot account for burn related d-tubocurarine hyposensitivity. *Anesthesiology* 1981; 54:378–382.

341. Martyn JAJ, Matteo RS, Greenblatt DJ, et al: Pharmacokinetics of d-tubocurarine in patients with thermal injury. *Anesth Analg* 1982, 61:241–246.

342. Gronert GA, Theyr RA: Pathophysiology of succinylcholine hyperkalemia. *Anesthesiology* 1975; 43:89–99.

343. Gronert GA: Disease atrophy with resistance to pancuronium. *Anesthesiology* 1981; 55:547–549.

344. Callanan DL: Development of resistance to pancuronium in adult respiratory distress syndrome. *Anesth Analg* 1985; 64:1126–1128.

345. Brown EM, Krishnaprasad D, Smiler BG: Pancuronium for rapid induction technique for tracheal intubation. *Can Anaesth Soc J* 1979; 26:489–491.

346. Asbury AJ, Linkins DA: Clinical automatic control of neuromuscular blockade. *Anaesthesia* 1986; 41:316–320.

347. Shanks CA: Design of therapeutic regimens. *Clin Anaesthetist* 1985; 3:283–291.

348. Griffith HR, Johnson GE: The use of curare in general anesthesia. *Anesthesiology* 1942; 3:418–420.

349. Everett AJ, Lowe LA, Wilkinson S: Revision of the structures of (+)-tubocurarine chloride and (+)-chondrocurine. *J Chem Soc* 1970; 10:1020–1021.

350. Cohen EN, Brewer HW, Smith D: The metabolism and elimination of d-tubocurarine-^{3}H. *Anesthesiology* 1967; 2:308–317.

351. Wood M, Wood AJJ: Changes in plasma drug binding and alpha$_1$-acid glycoprotein in mother and newborn infant. *Clin Pharmacol Ther* 1981; 29:522–526.

352. Walker JS, Shanks CA, Brown KF: Determinants of d-tubocurarine plasma protein in health and disease. *Anesth Analg* 1983; 62:870–874.

353. Ghoneim MM, Kramer E, Barrow R, et al: Binding of d-tubocurarine to plasma proteins in normal man and patients with hepatic and renal disease. *Anesthesiology* 1973; 39:410–415.

354. Horowitz PE, Spector S: Determination of serum d-tubocurarine concentration by radioimmunoassay. *J Pharmacol Exp Ther* 1973; 185:94–100.

355. Matteo RS, Spector S, Horowitz PE: Relation of serum d-tubocurarine concentration to neuromuscular blockade. *Anesthesiology* 1974; 41:441–443.

356. Cohen EN, Paulson WJ, Ebert B: Studies of d-tubocurarine with measurements of concentration in human blood. *Anesthesiology* 1957; 18:300–309.

357. Kalow W: The distribution, destruction and elimination of muscle relaxants. *Anesthesiology* 1969; 20:505–518.

358. Gibaldi M, Levy G, Hayton W: Kinetics of the elimination and neuromuscular blocking effect of d-tubocurarine in man. *Anesthesiology* 1972; 36:213–218.

359. Kalow W: Urinary excretion of d-tubocurarine in man. *J Pharmacol Exp Ther* 1953; 109:74–89.
360. Ryan AR: Tubocurarine administration based upon its disappearance and accumulation curves in anaesthetized man. *Br J Anaesth* 1964; 36:287–294.
361. Miller RD, Matteo RS, Benet LZ, et al: The pharmacokinetics of d-tubocurarine in man with and without renal failure. *J Pharmacol Exp Ther* 1977; 202:1–7.
362. Matteo RS, Nishitateno K, Pua EK, et al: Pharmacokinetics of d-tubocurarine in man: Effect of an osmotic diuretic on urinary excretion. *Anesthesiology* 1980; 52:335–338.
363. Fisher DM, O'Keeffe C, Stanski DR, et al: Pharmacokinetics and pharmacodynamics of d-tubocurarine in infants, children and adults. *Anesthesiology* 1982; 57:203–208.
364. Matteo RS, McDaniel DD, Lieberman IG, et al: Pharmacokinetics of d-tubocurarine in neonates, infants and children. *Anesthesiology* 1982; 57:A269.
365. Ramzan MI, Shanks CA, Triggs EJ: Pharmacokinetics of tubocurarine administered by combined i.v. bolus and infusion. *Br J Anaesth* 1980; 52:893–899.
366. Bearni L, Bianchi C, Ledda F: The effect of tubocurarine on acetylcholine release from motor nerve terminals. *J Physiol (Lond)* 1964; 74:172–183.
367. Standaert FG: The action of d-tubocurarine on the motor nerve terminal. *J Pharmacol Exp Ther* 1964; 143:181–186.
368. Glavinovic MI: Presynaptic action of curare. *J Physiol (Lond)* 1979; 290:499–506.
369. Hubbard JI, Wilson DF, Miyamoto M: Reduction of transmitter release by d-tubocurarine. *Nature* 1969; 223:531–533.
370. Cashman JN, Jones RM, Vella LM: Fade characteristics and onset times following administration of pancuronium, tubocurarine and a mixture of both agents. *Br J Anaesth* 1985; 57:488–492.
371. Dreyer F: Acetylcholine receptor. *Br J Anaesth* 1982; 54:115–130.
372. Peper K, Bradley RJ, Dreyer D: The acetylcholine receptor in skeletal muscle. *Ann Rev Physiol* 1982; 44:319–335.
373. Standaert FG: Site of action of muscle relaxants. *American Society of Anesthesiologists, Review Course Lectures, Las Vegas, Nevada*, 1982; pp 226(1–3).
374. Magleby KL, Pallotta BS, Terror DA: The effect of (+)-tubocurarine on neuromuscular transmission during repetitive stimulation in the rat, mouse and frog. *J Physiol (Lond)* 1981; 312:97–113.
375. Gibb AJ, Marshall IG: Pre- and post-junctional effects of tubocurarine and other nicotinic antagonists during repetitive stimulation in the rat. *J Physiol (Lond)* 1984; 351:275–297.
376. Ali HH, Savarese JJ: Stimulus frequency and dose-response curve to d-tubocurarine in man. *Anesthesiology* 1980; 52:36–39.

377. Goudsouzian NG, Donlon JV, Savarese JJ, et al: Re-evaluation of dosage and duration of action of d-tubocurarine in the pediatric age group. *Anesthesiology* 1975; 43:416–425.

378. Katz RL: Neuromuscular effects of d-tubocurarine, edrophonium and neostigmine in man. *Anesthesiology* 1967; 28:327–336.

379. Walts LF, Dillon JB: Durations of action of d-tubocurarine and gallamine. *Anesthesiology* 1968; 29:499–504.

380. Katz RL, Wolf CE: Neuromuscular and electromyographic studies in man: Effects of hyperventilation, carbon dioxide inhalation and d-tubocurarine. *Anesthesiology* 1964; 25:781–787.

381. Katz RL, Newman J, Seed RF, et al: A comparison of the effects of suxamethonium and tubocurarine in patients in London and New York. *Br J Anaesth* 1969; 45:1041–1047.

382. Walts LF, Dillon JB: d-Tubocurarine cumulation studies. *Anesth Analg* 1968; 47:696–701.

383. Morris RB, Cronnelly R, Miller RD, et al: Pharmacokinetics of edrophonium and neostigmine when antagonizing d-tubocurarine neuromuscular block in man. *Anesthesiology* 1981; 54:399–402.

384. Guyton AC, Reeder RC: Quantitative studies on the autonomic action of curare. *J Pharmacol Exp Ther* 1950; 98:188–194.

385. McCullough LS, Reier CE, Delaunois AL, et al: The effects of d-tubocurarine on spontaneous post-ganglionic sympathetic activity and histamine release. *Anesthesiology* 1970; 33:328–334.

386. Moss J, Roscow CE, Savarese JJ, et al: Role of histamine in the hypotensive action of d-tubocurarine in humans. *Anesthesiology* 1981; 55:19–25.

387. Stoelting RK, Longnecker DE: Effect of promethazine on hypotension following d-tubocurarine use in anesthetized patients. *Anesth Analg* 1972; 51:509–513.

388. Stoelting RK, McCammon RL, Hilgenberg JC: Changes in blood pressure with varying rates of administration of d-tubocurarine. *Anesth Analg* 1980; 59:697–699.

389. Saxena PR, Dhasmana KM, Prakash O: A comparison of systemic and regional hemodynamic effects of d-tubocurarine, pancuronium, and vecuronium. *Anesthesiology* 1983; 59:102–108.

390. Stoelting RK: Blood pressure response to d-tubocurarine and its preservatives in anesthetized patients. *Anesthesiology* 1971; 35:315–317.

391. Johnstone M, Mahmoud AA, Mrozinski RA: Cardio-vascular effects of tubocurarine in man. *Anaesthesia* 1978; 33:587–593.

392. Nelson SH, Steinsland OS: d-Tubocurarine as a dopaminergic antagonist in the rabbit ear artery. *Anesthesiology* 1983; 59:98–101.

393. Stullken EH, Sokoll MD: Anesthesia and subarachnoid intracranial pressure. *Anesth Analg* 1975; 54:494–498.

394. Miller RD, Way WL, Hickey RF: Inhibition of succinylcholine-induced increased intraocular pressure by non-depolarizing muscle relaxant. *Anesthesiology* 1968; 29:123–126.

395. Cook JH: The effect of suxamethonium on intraocular pressure. *Anaesthesia* 1981; 35:359–365.

396. Katz RL, Gissen AJ: Neuromuscular and electromyographic effects of halothane and its interaction with d-tubocurarine in man. *Anesthesiology* 1967; 28:564–567.

397. Mirakhur RK, Gibson FM, Ferres CJ: Vecuronium and d-tubocurarine combination: Potentiation of effect. *Anesth Analg* 1985; 64:711–714.

398. Ghoneim MM, Urgene RB, Dretchen K, et al: The interaction between d-tubocurarine and gallamine during halothane anaesthesia. *Can Anaesth Soc J* 1972; 19:66–74.

399. Martyn JAJ, Szyfelbein SK, Ali HH, et al: Increased d-tubocurarine requirement following major thermal injury. *Anesthesiology* 1980; 52:352–355.

400. Leibel WS, Martyn JAJ, Szyfelbein SK, et al: Elevated plasma binding cannot account for burn-related d-tubocurarine hyposensitivity. *Anesthesiology* 1981; 54:378–382.

401. Martyn JAJ, Matteo RS, Lebowitz PW, et al: Pharmacokinetics of d-tubocurarine in patients with thermal injury. *Anesth Analg* 1982; 61:241–246.

402. Gronert GA: A possible mechanism of succinylcholine-induced hyperkalemia. *Anesthesiology* 1980; 53:356.

403. Gronert GA, Matteo RS, Perkins S: Canine gastrocnemius disuse atrophy: Resistance to paralysis by dimethyltubocurarine. *J Appl Physiol* 1984; 57:1502–1056.

404. Graham DH: Monitoring neuromuscular block may be unreliable in patients with upper-motor-neuron lesions. *Anesthesiology* 1980; 52:74–75.

405. Gronert GA: Disuse atrophy with resistance to pancuronium. *Anesthesiology* 1981; 55:547–549.

406. Fischbach GD, Robbins N: Effect of chronic disease on rat soleus neuromuscular junction and postsynaptic membrane. *J Neurophysiol* 1971; 34:562–569.

407. Snider WD, Harris GL: A physiological correlate of disuse-induced sprouting at the neuromuscular junction. *Nature* 1979; 281:69–71.

408. Waud BE, Amaki Y, Waud DR: Disuse and d-tubocurarine sensitivity in isolated muscles. *Anesth Analg* 1985; 64:1178–1182.

409. Erkola O, Salmenpera A, Kumoppamaki R: Nondepolarizing muscle relaxants in precurarisation. *Acta Anaesthesiol Scand* 1983; 27:427–432.

410. Savage DS, Sleigh T, Carlyle I: The emergence of ORG NC 45, 1- [(2 beta, 3 alpha, 5, 16 beta, 17 beta)-3,17-bis(acetyloxy)-2-(1-piperidinyl)-androstan-16-yl]-1-methyl-piperidinium bromide, from the pancuronium series. *Br J Anaesth* 1980; 52:3S–9S.

411. Norman J, Katz RL: Some effects of the steroidal muscle relaxant, dacuronium bromide, in anaesthetized patients. *Br J Anaesth* 1971; 43:313–317.

412. Paanakker JE, Van de Laar GLM: Determination of ORG NC 45 (a my-

oneural blocking agent) in human plasma using high performance normal phase liquid chromatography. *J Chromatog* 1980; 183:459–466.

413. Fahey MR, Morris RB, Miller RD, et al: Pharmacokinetics of ORG NC45 (Norcuron) in patients with and without renal failure. *Br J Anaesth* 1981; 53:1049–1053.

414. Bencini AF, Scaf AHJ, Agoston S, et al: Disposition of vecuronium bromide in the cat. *Br J Anaesth* 1985; 57:782–788.

415. Lebrault C, Berger JL, d'Hollander AA, et al: Pharmacokinetics and pharmacodynamics of vecuronium (ORG NC 45) in patients with cirrhosis. *Anesthesiology* 1985; 62:601–605.

416. Rupp SM, Fisher DM, Miller RD, et al: Pharmacokinetics and pharmacodynamics of vecuronium in the elderly. *Anesthesiology* 1983; 59:A270.

417. Bencini AF, Houwertjes MC, Agoston S: Effects of hepatic uptake of vecuronium bromide and its putative metabolites on their neuromuscular blocking actions in the cat. *Br J Anaesth* 1985; 57:789–795.

418. Sohn YJ, Bencini AF, Scaf AHJ, et al: Comparative pharmacokinetics and dynamics of vecuronium and pancuronium in anesthetized patients. *Anesth Analg* 1986; 65:233–239.

419. Bevan DR, Donati F, Gyasi H, et al: Vecuronium in renal failure. *Can Anaesth Soc J* 1984; 31:491–496.

420. Durant NN, Houwertjes MC, Crul JF: Comparison of the neuromuscular blocking properties of ORG NC 45 and pancuronium in the rat, cat and rhesus monkey. *Br J Anaesth* 1980; 52:723–729.

421. Marshall RJ, McGrath JC, Miller RD, et al: Comparison of the cardiovascular actions of ORG NC 45 with those produced by other non-depolarizing neuromuscular blocking agents in experimental animals. *Br J Anaesth* 1980; 52:21S–32S.

422. Gibson FM, Mirakhur RK, Clarke RSJ, et al: Comparison of cumulative and single bolus dose techniques for determining the potency of vecuronium. *Br J Anaesth* 1985; 57:1060–1062.

423. Fisher DM, Fahey MR, Cronnelly R, et al: Potency determination for vecuronium (ORG NC 45): Comparison of cumulative and single-dose techniques. *Anesthesiology* 1982; 57:309–310.

424. Ferres CJ, Mirakhur RK, Pandit SK, et al: Dose-response studies with pancuronium, vecuronium and their combination. *Br J Clin Pharmacol* 1984; 18:947–951.

425. Rupp SM, Miller RD, Gencarelli PJ: Vecuronium-induced neuromuscular blockade during enflurane, isoflurane and halothane anesthesia in humans. *Anesthesiology* 1984; 60:102–105.

426. O'Hara D, Fragen RJ, Shanks CA: The effects of age on the dose-response curves for vecuronium in adults. *Anesthesiology* 1985; 63:542–544.

427. d'Hollander A, Massaux F, Nevelsteen M, et al: Age-dependent dose-response relationships of ORG NC 45 in anaesthetized patients. *Br J Anaesth* 1982; 54:653–657.

428. Fahey MR, Morris RB, Miller RD, et al: Clinical pharmacology of ORG NC 45 (Norcuron). *Anesthesiology* 1981; 55:6–11.
429. Agoston S, Salt P, Newton D: The neuromuscular blocking action of ORG NC 45, a new pancuronium derivative, in anaesthetized patients. *Br J Anaesth* 1980; 52:53S–59S.
430. Kerr WJ, Baird WLM: Clinical studies on ORG NC 45: Comparison with pancuronium. *Br J Anaesth* 1982; 54:1159–1165.
431. Mirakhur RK, Ferres CJ, Clarke RSJ, et al: Clinical evaluation of ORG NC 45. *Br J Anaesth* 1983; 55:119–124.
432. Bencini A, Newton DEF: Rate of onset of good intubating conditions, respiratory depression and hand muscle paralysis after vecuronium. *Br J Anaesth* 1984; 56:959–965.
433. Jones RM, Casson WR, Lethbridge JR: Influence of dose on onset times of vecuronium-induced neuromuscular blockade. *Br J Anaesth* 1985; 57:828P–829P.
434. Norman J, Read J, du Boulay M: Hand and respiratory muscle paralysis produced by ORG NC 45 in man. *Br J Anaesth* 1980; 52:956P.
435. Donati F, Antzaka C, Bevan DR: Potency of pancuronium at the diaphragm and the adductor pollicis muscle in humans. *Anesthesiology* 1986; 65:1–5.
436. Schwartz S, Ilias W, Lackner F, et al: Rapid tracheal intubation with vecuronium: The priming principle. *Anesthesiology* 1985; 62:388–391.
437. Kunjappen VE, Brown EM, Alexander GD: Rapid sequence induction using vecuronium. *Anesth Analg* 1986; 65:503–506.
438. Taboada JA, Rupp SM, Miller RD: Refining the priming principle for vecuronium during rapid-sequence induction of anesthesia. *Anesthesiology* 1986; 64:243–247.
439. Clarke RSJ, Gibson FM, Mirakhur RK, et al: Effect of "priming" on intubating conditions after vecuronium: A pilot study. *Br J Anaesth* 1985; 57:827P–828P.
440. Engbaek J, Howardy-Hensen P, Ording H, et al: Precurarization with vecuronium and pancuronium in awake, healthy volunteers: The influence on neuromuscular transmission and pulmonary function. *Acta Anaesthesiol Scand* 1985; 29:117–120.
441. Musich J, Walts LF: Pulmonary aspiration after a priming dose of vecuronium. *Anesthesiology* 1986; 64:517–519.
442. Williams A, Gyasi H, Melloni C, et al: Clinical experience with ORG NC 45 (Norcuron) as the sole muscle relaxant. *Can Anaesth Soc J* 1982; 29:567–572.
443. Harrison P, Feldman SA: Intubating conditions with ORG NC 45. *Anaesthesia* 1981; 36:874–877.
444. Ali HH, Savarese JJ, Basta SJ, et al: Comparative patterns of recovery of three new nondepolarizing relaxants: BW A444U, BW 33A (atracurium) and ORG NC 45 (vecuronium). *Anesthesiology* 1982; 57:A263.
445. Crul JF, Booij LHDJ: First clinical experiences with ORG NC 45. *Br J Anaesth* 1980; 52:49S–52S.

446. Buzello W, Noeldge G: Repetitive administration of pancuronium and vecuronium (ORG NC 45, Norcuron) in patients undergoing long lasting operations. Br J Anaesth 1982; 54:1151–1157.
447. Gencarelli PJ, Miller RD: Antagonism of ORG NC 45 (vecuronium) and pancuronium neuromuscular blockade by neostigmine. Br J Anaesth 1982; 54:53–56.
448. Baird WLM, Bowman WC, Kerr WJ: Some actions of ORG NC 45 and of edrophonium in the anaesthetized cat and in man. Br J Anaesth 1982; 54:375–385.
449. Lee C, Yang E, Tran BK, et al: Optimal dose of edrophonium for the reversal of Norcuron. Anesth Analg 1983; 62:271–272.
450. Baker T, Aguero A, Staree A, et al: Prejunctional effects of vecuronium in the cat. Anesthesiology 1986; 65:480–484.
451. Power SJ, Darowski MJ, Gallagher IJ, et al: Fade profiles during spontaneous offset of neuromuscular blockade: Gallamine and vecuronium compared. Br J Anaesth 1986; 58:1328P.
452. Fitzal S, Gilly H, Ilias W: Comparative investigations on the cardiovascular effects of ORG NC 45 and pancuronium in dogs. Br J Anaesth 1983; 55:641–646.
453. Basta SJ, Savarese J, Ali HH, et al: Vecuronium does not alter serum histamine within the clinical dose range. Anesthesiology 1983; 59:A273.
454. Gregoretti SM, Sohn TJ, Sia RL: Heart rate and blood pressure changes after ORG NC 45 (vecuronium) and pancuronium during halothane and enflurane anesthesia. Anesthesiology 1982; 56:392–395.
455. Morris RB, Cahalan MK, Miller RD, et al: The cardiovascular effects of vecuronium (ORG NC 45) and pancuronium in patients undergoing coronary artery bypass grafting. Anesthesiology 1983; 58:438–440.
456. Lee C, Tran BK, Durant N, et al: Vecuronium, isoflurane, and hypotensive anesthesia in the cat. Anesthesiology 1983; 59:A271.
457. Ferres CJ, Carson IW, Clarke RSJ, et al: Comparison of the haemodynamic effects of vecuronium and pancuronium in patients undergoing coronary artery bypass grafting. Br J Anaesth 1983; 55:915P.
458. Salmenpera M, Peltola K, Takkunen O, et al: Cardiovascular effects of pancuronium and vecuronium during high-dose fentanyl anesthesia. Anesth Analg 1983; 62:1059–1064.
459. Starr NJ, Sethna DH, Estafanous FG: Bradycardia and asystole following the rapid administration of sufentanil with vecuronium. Anesthesiology 1986; 64:521–523.
460. McIndewar IC, Marshall RJ: Interactions between the neuromuscular blocking drug ORG NC 45 and some anaesthetic, analgesic and antimicrobial agents. Br J Anaesth 1981; 53:785–792.
461. Duncalf A, Nagashima H, Hollinger I, et al: Relaxation with ORG NC 45 during enflurane anesthesia. Anesthesiology 1981; 55:A203.
462. Swen J, Gencarelli PJ, Koot HWJ: Vecuronium infusion dose requirements during fentanyl and halothane anesthesia in humans. Anesth Analg 1985; 64:411–414.

463. Krieg N, Hendrickx HHL, Crul JF: Influence of suxamethonium on the potency of ORG NC 45 in anaesthetized patients. *Br J Anaesth* 1981; 53:259–261.

464. d'Hollander AA, Agoston S, De Ville A, et al: Clinical and pharmacological actions of a bolus injection of suxamethonium: Two phenomena of distinct duration. *Br J Anaesth* 1983; 55:131–134.

465. Fisher DM, Miller RD: Interaction of succinylcholine and vecuronium during N₂O-halothane anesthesia. *Anesthesiology* 1983; 59:A278.

466. d'Hollander A, Agoston S, Barvais L, et al: Evaluation of vecuronium requirements for stable mechanical effect: Comparison with or without previous succinylcholine administration. *Anesth Analg* 1985; 64:319–322.

467. Bowman WC: Non-relaxant properties of neuromuscular blocking drugs. *Br J Anaesth* 1982; 54:147–160.

468. van Poorten JF, Dhasmana KM, Kuypers RSM, et al: Verapamil and reversal of vecuronium neuromuscular blockade. *Anesth Analg* 1984; 63:155–157.

469. Kay B, Chestnut RJ, Sum Ping J, et al: Effect of vecuronium after pancuronium. *Br J Anaesth* 1986; 58:1327P.

470. Duncalf D, Chaudhry I, Aoki T, et al: Potentiation of pancuronium, vecuronium and atracurium by d-tubocurarine or metocurine. *Anesthesiology* 1983; 59:A292.

471. Mirakhur RJ, Gibson FM, Ferres CJ: Vecuronium and d-tubocurarine combination: Potentiation of effect. *Anesth Analg* 1985; 64:711–714.

472. Ferres CJ, Crean PM, Mirakhur RK: The evaluation of ORG NC 45 (vecuronium) in paediatric patients. *Anaesthesia* 1983; 38:943–947.

473. Fisher DM, Miller RD: Neuromuscular effects of vecuronium (ORG NC 45) in infants and children during N₂O, halothane anesthesia. *Anesthesiology* 1983; 58:519–523.

474. Goudsouzian NG, Martyn JJA, Liu LMP, et al: Safety and efficacy of vecuronium in adolescents and children. *Anesth Analg* 1983; 82:1083–1088.

475. Meistelman C, Loose JP, SaintMaurice C, et al: Clinical pharmacology of vecuronium in children. *Br J Anaesth* 1986; 58:996–1000.

476. Fragen RJ, Shanks CA: Neuromuscular recovery after laparoscopy. *Anesth Analg* 1984; 63:51–54.

477. Caldwell JE, Braidwood JM, Simpson DS: Vecuronium bromide in anaesthesia for laparoscopic sterilization. *Br J Anaesth* 1985; 57:765–769.

478. Pearce AC, Hodge M, Jones RM: Vecuronium in day-stay surgery. *Br J Anaesth* 1984; 56:794P–795P.

479. Stoelting RK: Choice of muscle relaxants in patients with heart disease. *Semin Anesthesia* 1985; 4:7–8.

480. Heinonen J, Salmenpera M, Suomicouri M: Contribution of muscle relaxant to the haemodynamic course of high dose fentanyl anaesthesia: A comparison of pancuronium, vecuronium and atracurium. *Can Anaesth Soc J* 1986; 33:597–605.

481. Buzello W, Schluermann D, Pollmaecher T, et al: Unequal effects of cardiopulmonary bypass-induced hypothermia on neuromuscular blockade from constant infusion of alcuronium, d-tubocurarine, pancuronium, and vecuronium. Anesthesiology 1987; 66:842–846.
482. Demetriou M, Depoix JP, Diakite B, et al: Placental transfer of ORG NC 45 in women undergoing caesarean section. Br J Anaesth 1982; 54:643–645.
483. Baraka A, Noueihed R, Sinno H, et al: Succinylcholine-vecuronium (ORG NC 45) sequence for cesarean section. Anesth Analg 1983; 62:909–913.
484. Durant NN, Houwertjes MC, Agoston S: Renal elimination of ORG NC 45 and pancuronium. Anesthesiology 1979; 51:S266.
485. Hunter JM, Bell CF, Florence AM, et al: Vecuronium in the myasthenic patient. Anaesthesia 1985; 40:848–853.
486. Powles AB, Ganta R: Use of vecuronium in the management of tetanus. Anaesthesia 1985; 40:879–881.
487. Cottrell JE, Hartung J, Griffin JP, et al: Intracranial and hemodynamic changes after succinylcholine administration in cats. Anesth Analg 1983; 62:1006–1009.
488. Tarkkanen L, Laitmen L, Johansson G: Effects of d-tubocurarine on intracranial pressure and thalamic electrical impedance. Anesthesiology 1974; 40:247–251.
489. Rosa G, Sanfilippo M, Vilardi V, et al: Effects of vecuronium bromide on intracranial pressure and cerebral perfusion pressure. Br J Anaesth 1986; 58:437–440.
490. Giffin JP, Hartung J, Cottrell JE, et al: Effect of vecuronium on intracranial pressure, mean arterial pressure and heart rate in cats. Br J Anaesth 1986; 58:441–443.
491. Jantzen JP, Hackett GH, Erdmann K, et al: Effect of vecuronium on intraocular pressure. Br J Anaesth 1986; 58:433–436.
492. Gencarelli PJ, Roizen MF, Miller RD, et al: ORG NC 45 (Norcuron) and pheochromocytoma: A report of three cases. Anesthesiology 1981; 55:690–693.
493. d'Hollander AA, Czerucki R, Deville A: Stable muscle relaxation during abdominal surgery using combined intravenous bolus and demand infusion: Clinical appraisal with ORG NC 45. Can Anaesth Soc J 1982; 29:136–141.
494. Noeldge G, Hinsken H, Buzello W: Comparison between the continuous infusion of vecuronium and the intermittent administration of pancuronium and vecuronium. Br J Anaesth 1984; 56:473–477.
495. de Vries JJ, Ros HH, Booij LHD: Infusion of vecuronium controlled by a closed-loop system. Br J Anaesth 1986; 58:1100–1103.

7

Depolarizing Agents: Succinylcholine

Thirty-five years after its introduction,[1, 2] succinylcholine still enjoys widespread popularity, despite the lack of understanding of the mechanisms of its action at the neuromuscular junction, the varying nature of the block, the growing list of associated complications, and the introduction of several short-acting nondepolarizing alternatives. None of these has curtailed the use of an agent with unique properties: the production of profound relaxation with rapid onset and short duration of action.

STRUCTURE

Succinylcholine consists of two acetylcholine molecules joined back-to-back (Fig 7–1). Like acetylcholine, it depolarizes the postsynaptic membrane at the neuromuscular junction.[3, 4] Rapid depolarization, by either acetylcholine or succinylcholine, causes the membrane potential to exceed the threshold necessary for a muscle action potential to be generated and produces a contraction. The depolarized end-plate region and its immediate surroundings become a zone of inexcitability. This blocks the propagation to muscle fibers of muscle action potentials evoked by nerve stimulation.[5] The continuing presence of acetylcholine or succinylcholine varies the threshold.[4, 6] The block following acetylcholine is short-lived because acetylcholine is metabolized rapidly (within milliseconds) by acetylcholinesterase.[7] However, after administration of succinylcholine, the block persists because of the slower metabolism of succinylcholine by plasma cholinesterase. End-plate de-

247

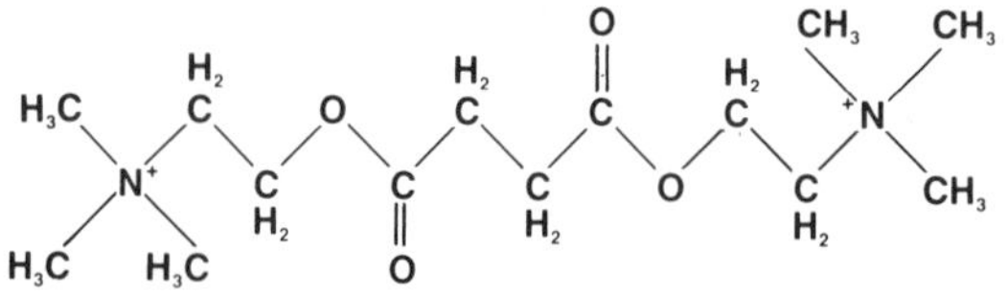

SUCCINYLCHOLINE

FIG 7–1.
Structure of succinylcholine.

polarization gradually diminishes, but it persists for as long as succinylcholine remains.[3]

Decamethonium is another depolarizing muscle relaxant that enjoyed only brief popularity,[8] despite the loyalty of some practitioners.[9] The characteristics of its block are similar to succinylcholine, but it has a slower onset of action, a longer duration, and its action cannot be antagonized. It has been replaced by shorter-acting nondepolarizing relaxants whose effects are more controllable.

METABOLISM

Succinylcholine is hydrolyzed rapidly by an enzyme produced in the liver, plasma cholinesterase (PCHE), to succinylmonocholine and choline. Succinylmonocholine is hydrolyzed more slowly to succinate and choline[7] and has weaker neuromuscular blocking effects than succinylcholine but it too produces both phase I and II blocks.

The maximum rate of succinylcholine hydrolysis, estimated from studies with continuous infusions in man,[10–12] is about 100 μg/minute/kg. Thus, if the half-life of succinylcholine is about 3 minutes, about 70% of a 100-mg bolus is metabolized within 1 minute. The biosynthesis of PCHE in the liver is controlled by two allelic genes, E_1^u and E_1^u, and the enzyme has a half-life of 5 to 12 days.[13, 14]

REDUCED PLASMA CHOLINESTERASE ACTIVITY

Plasma cholinesterase activity is determined by the rate of hydrolysis of the substrate benzoylcholine[15] or the thiocholine esters of propionic[16] or butyric acids. The duration of action of succinylcholine has been correlated with PCHE activity in adults[17, 18] (Fig 7–2) and children.[19] The action of PCHE is reduced by physiologic variation, inherited abnormalities, or acquired and iatrogenic disease[13] (Table 7–1).

Physiologic Variation

Plasma cholinesterase activity is greater in men than women.[13] During pregnancy, it is reduced by about 25%,[20] and this may decrease further in the postpartum period.[21] Concentrations at birth are approximately half those of the adult,[22] and normal values are not reached until 6 months postpartum. However, these reductions in PCHE do not result in prolonged action of succinylcholine[23, 24] unless liver disease is superimposed, e.g., from toxemia of pregnancy[25] or trophoblastic disease.[26]

Acquired Disease

Several chronic diseases are associated with decreased PCHE activity and prolonged duration of action of succinylcholine. These include carcinoma, collagen diseases, myocardial infarction, and chronic debilitating diseases.

Iatrogenic Causes

Many therapeutic procedures, including cardiopulmonary bypass[27] and plasmaphoresis,[28, 29] lead to a reduction in PCHE activity. Several

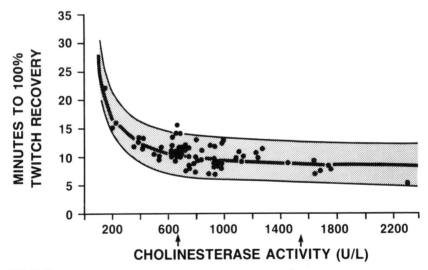

FIG 7–2.
Time to 100% return of twitch tensions after succinylcholine (1 mg/kg) vs. plasma cholinesterase activity. (Redrawn from Viby-Mogensen J: Correlation of succinylcholine duration of action with plasma cholinesterase activity in subjects with genotypically normal enzyme. *Anesthesiology* 1980; 53:517–520. Used by permission.)

TABLE 7–1.
Decreased Plasma Cholinesterase
Activity

Inherited
  Cholinesterase variants

Acquired
  Hepatic disease
  Uremia
  Malnutrition
  Carcinoma
  Acute infection
  Burns

Iatrogenic
  Plasmapheresis
  Extracorporeal circulation
  Anticholinergic drugs
  Alkylating anticancer drugs
  Burns
  Contraceptive pill
  Echothiophate
  Esmolol
  Monoamine oxidase inhibitors
  Pancuronium
  Propranolol

drugs inhibit the enzyme's activity. The effect of some, e.g., antichol-inergic agents,[30] pancuronium,[31] and propranolol,[32] is small, resulting in only a slight prolongation of action of succinylcholine; the effect of others, e.g., anticancer drugs,[33, 34] anticholinesterases,[31, 35–38] and echothiopate[39–42] is prolonged paralysis. The new, short-acting, intra-venous β-blocking drug esmolol inhibits PCHE in vitro but has a min-imal effect in vivo,[43] so that a measurable interaction with succinylcholine is unlikely.

Inherited Disorders

Inherited variants of PCHE may be identified by distinct inhibition profiles of the rates of hydrolysis of benzoylcholine with varying con-centrations of dibucaine[44] fluoride or chloride.[13] At present four allelic genes are recognized, although this list is not exhaustive: the normal gene E_1^u, the atypical gene E_1^a, the silent gene E_1^s, and the fluoride resistant gene E_1^f.[45] An abnormal gene is present in about 4% of the population.

The duration of neuromuscular block is prolonged to 2 to 3 hours in patients homozygous for E_1^{a46-47} or E_1^s,[48] whereas it is prolonged only slightly and in fewer than half the heterozygotes.[49, 50] Abnormal phenotypes, such as E_1^a, or E_1^f, may show variable responses.[51] When twitch activity begins to recover, it has the appearance of phase II block (Fig 7–3), but it cannot be antagonized completely with neostigmine or edrophonium.[52-55] Safe management includes respiratory support until spontaneous ventilation is restored. Plasma cholinesterase is stable so that whole blood[56] or plasma is a potential store. However, the possible risks of transfusion may exceed those of ventilation for 2 to 3 hours. When available, purified human serum cholinesterase is effective.[57]

The use of succinylcholine in patients known to possess atypical or reduced PCHE activity is not absolutely contraindicated. When in doubt, small test doses (20 to 200 μg/kg) may be used in the diagnosis[58] and additional doses titrated as small boluses[59] or by infusion.[40] Small doses (5 to 10 mg/70 kg) in a homozygous subject have a short duration of action (20 to 30 minutes) but a slower onset (2 to 7 minutes)[60] so that the pharmacodynamic profile resembles atracurium or vecuronium, and the unique advantages of succinylcholine are lost.

INCREASED PLASMA CHOLINESTERASE ACTIVITY

The activity of PCHE is increased in several states[13] (Table 7–2). These observations are of minimal clinical importance, although careful studies demonstrate a reduction in the duration of action of succinylcholine. In obesity (Fig 7–4) the increase in PCHE[61] activity is matched by an increase in extracellular fluid (ECF) so that succinylcholine requirements may increase. Succinylcholine dosage in the obese person should be based on total and not lean body weight.

Plasma cholinesterase can be separated into four isoenzymes, C1 through C4. In addition, a fifth slow-moving component has been found in some individuals who have been labeled C5 positive. Sera that contain the C5 + component usually have increased PCHE activity.[62]

PHYSIOLOGIC ROLE OF PLASMA CHOLINESTERASE

An unequivocal physiologic role has not been established for PCHE. Various suggestions have been made including transmission of slow nerve conduction, lipid metabolism, and choline homeostasis. Pharmacologically, it is of considerable importance in the metabolism of ester-type local anesthetics (procaine, chloroprocaine) and esmolol, as well as succinylcholine.

SUCCINYLCHOLINE APNEA

ATTEMPTED REVERSAL WITH ANTICHOLINESTERASES

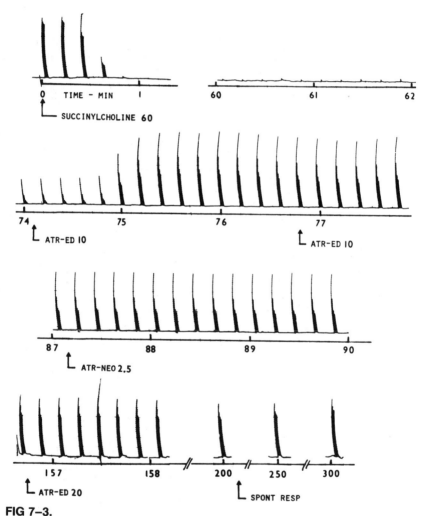

FIG 7–3.
Failure to antagonize neuromuscular blockade with atropine (ATR) and edrophonium (ED) or neostigmine (NEO) after succinylcholine in a patient homozygous for $E_1{}^a E_1{}^a$. (From Bevan DR, Donati F: Succinylcholine apnoea: Attempted reversal with anticholinesterases. *Can Anaesth Soc J* 1983; 30:536–539. Used by permission.)

TABLE 7–2.
Some Causes of
Increased Plasma
Cholinesterase Activity

Inherited
   C5 and other variants

Acquired
   Alcoholism
   Anxiety states
   Asthma
   Hypertension
   Obesity

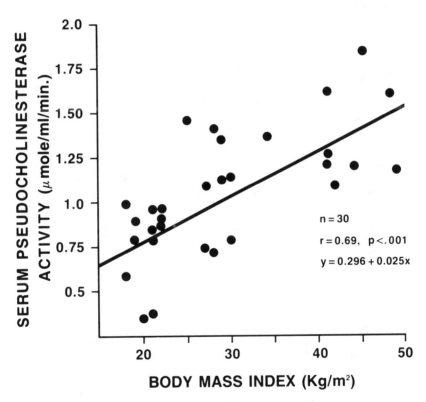

FIG 7–4.
Relationship of pseudocholinesterase activity and body mass index. (Redrawn from Bentley
JB, Bereal JD, Vaughan RW, et al: Weight, pseudocholinesterase activity and succinylcholine
requirement. *Anesthesiology* 1982; 57:48–49. Used by permission.)

PHARMACOKINETICS

The classical pharmacokinetic data have not been obtained for succinylcholine because of the lack of an appropriate assay. However, the elimination half-life can be calculated from the relationship between the log dose and duration of action.[63, 64] If the value of the rate constant of elimination, estimated from the slope of the line, is about 0.15 to 0.17 per minute, the estimated half-life is 4 to 4.6 minutes.[65, 66] Surprisingly, the elimination half-life calculated in a similar way is only 1.7 minutes for infants and 1.8 minutes for children,[66, 67] despite the increased volume of distribution and decreased PCHE in infants. Such discrepancies cannot be explained.

NEUROMUSCULAR BLOCKADE

Site of Action

It is assumed that succinylcholine acts exclusively on the post-junctional structures of the neuromuscular junction. However, several actions other than blockade of neuromuscular transmission can be observed, including inducing a repetitive response to a single stimulus, alternating post-tetanic neural repetitive activity, and initiation of motor nerve action potentials independent of an external stimulus.[68] Drugs that inhibit these presynaptic actions at the nerve terminal, such as nondepolarizing muscle relaxants and diphenylhydantoin, also prevent the occurrence of fasciculations.[69]

Characteristics of Block

The effects of succinylcholine vary markedly between species,[4] and to a lesser extent in different muscles within the same species.[70] For example, rats are much more resistant to succinylcholine than humans or cats, and in humans, respiratory muscles appear to be more resistant than hand muscles.[71] Therefore, discussion will be limited to the effect of succinylcholine on the commonly recorded adductor pollicis muscle in humans, unless some other information is relevant. It should be remembered, however, that the response of other muscles is different. For example, the effects of succinylcholine on the diaphragm are less than on the muscles of the hand.[72, 73]

Phase I and II Block

Before the onset of succinylcholine block, an acetylcholine-like effect is observed. Spontaneous fasciculations occur, and the contraction that follows indirect stimulation may be augmented by repetitive firing.[74, 75] The ensuing block is characterized by a diminished twitch response with indirect stimulation, but the response is sustained with repetitive stimulation. After administration of additional succinylcholine, this "phase I" block is followed by the appearance of "phase II" block, characterized by a fade in response to repetitive stimulation and post-tetanic potentiation. The term *phase I* is preferred to *depolarizing* and *acetylcholine-like*, and *phase II* is used instead of *dual, desensitizing, nondepolarizing*, and *curare-like*, because *phase I* and *phase II* are purely descriptive terms and do not imply a mechanism of action. When train-of-four stimulation is used, a phase II block is defined as a train-of-four ratio or T4/T1 of less than 0.5. The appearance of phase II block is a gradual process. The time and dose necessary to produce it depend on the criteria used to define it and the choice of anesthetic agent (Table 7–3).[62–64, 78, 84] In infants and children succinylcholine requirements increase and phase II block develops sooner but after a greater dose than in adults.[79, 80]

Tachyphylaxis.—As phase II block develops, succinylcholine requirements increase. This is seen either as a decreased effect with the same dose or, as during an infusion, an increase in the dose necessary to obtain the same effect.[76, 77, 81] Although this relationship between tachyphylaxis and phase II block has been disputed,[82] the phenomenon is thought to represent antagonism between phase I and phase II block.[81] Plasma cholinesterase activity does not change with time so that tachyphylaxis cannot be explained on the basis of enzyme induction.[83] During succinylcholine infusions, the rate must be increased by about 80% to keep the block constant, but there are wide variations in the published literature.[10–12]

Bradyphylaxis.—When succinylcholine is administered for more than 90 minutes, succinylcholine requirements decrease during anesthesia with an anesthetic vapor, but not with nitrous oxide and narcotic (Fig 7–5).[70, 69] Whether this is due to a decrease in the antagonistic effect of phase I block or a potentiating effect of inhalation agents on phase II block remains uncertain.

TABLE 7–3.
Onset of Phase II Block in Different Conditions

PATIENT	DEFINITION OF PHASE II BLOCK	ANESTHETIC	DOSE, MG/KG	TIME, MIN	REFERENCE
Adults	T4/T1 = 0.5 at 90% T1 block	Halothane	2.1	32	Futter et al. (1983)[86]
		Isoflurane	2.6	37	Donati and Bevan (1983)[84]
		Enflurane	2.2	31	Donati and Bevan (1983)[84]
		Narcotic	3.2	51	Donati and Bevan (1983)[84]
Adults	T4/T1 = 0.5 at 70% T1 block	Halothane	5.1		Hilgenberg and Stoelting (1981)[78]
		Enflurane	4.4		Hilgenberg and Stoelting (1981)[78]
		Narcotic	6.4		Hilgenberg and Stoelting (1981)[78]
Children >1 year old	T4/T1 = 0.5 at 90% T1 block	Halothane	4.1	29	DeCook and Goudsouzian (1980)[79]
Adults	T4/T1, <0.7 after 10 minutes of spontaneous recovery	Halothane	6	70	Futter et al. (1983)[86]
		Isoflurane	8	100	Donati and Bevan (1983)[84]
		Enflurane	6	90	Donati and Bevan (1983)[84]
		Narcotic	13	170	Donati and Bevan (1983)[84]

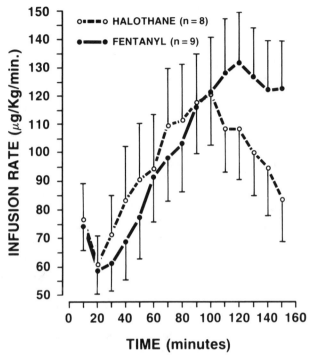

FIG 7–5.
Succinylcholine infusion rate required to maintain constant 90% block during anesthesia with narcotics or halothane. (Redrawn from Futter ME, Donati F, Bevan DR: Prolonged suxamethonium infusion during nitrous oxide anaesthesia supplemented with halothane or fentanyl. *Br J Anaesth* 1983; 55:947–953. Used by permission.)

Supramaximal Twitches.—At the termination of succinylcholine block, the force of contraction of the indirectly stimulated muscle returns to a level greater than control, both in animals[70, 74] and in man.[75] This supramaximal twitch occurs without change in the shape of the electromyographic events associated with the contraction, which suggests that succinylcholine might also act directly on the muscle. The clinical implications of this finding are unclear at this time.

Recovery From Phase II Block.—The rate of recovery from phase II block depends on the anesthetic agent and total dose of succinylcholine (see Table 7–3). Ten minutes after the infusion is stopped, in adults, the train-of-four ratio recovers to greater than 0.7 as long as the d5se of succinylcholine has not exceeded 6 mg/kg during anesthesia with anesthetic vapors or 13 mg/kg using narcotics. If T4/T1 is less than 0.7 at this time, rapid recovery follows the administration of edrophonium (10 to 20 mg)[85] or neostigmine (1.2 to 2.5 mg).[10, 11, 75, 86]

Potency

The potency of succinylcholine has not been established clearly, mainly because it is used only to produce 100% neuromuscular block. Nevertheless, the ED95 following single-bolus injections is in the order of 0.15 to 0.2 mg/kg. Such a figure is deceiving because 70% of the drug has been metabolized before maximal blockade has developed.

Onset and Duration of Action

Following injection of intravenous bolus doses of 1 mg/kg in adults, 100% neuromuscular blockade is achieved within 1 minute; recovery commences at about 4 to 6 minutes and is complete by 10 to 12 minutes[31] although there are wide individual variations.[87] Surprisingly, the duration of action of succinylcholine appears to be slightly shorter in London than in New York (90% recovery after administration of 1 mg/kg, 9.1 ± 2.9 vs. 14.6 ± 3.6 minutes).[88] Perfect intubating conditions are achieved with succinylcholine, 1 mg/kg, by about 60 to 90 seconds,[89, 90] although this may be delayed by a slow circulation time.[91]

Infants and small children require increased doses of succinylcholine on a milligram-per-kilogram basis as a result of an increase in ECF volume. Also, the pediatric requirements are modified by decreased PCHE activity and increased sensitivity of the junction to succinylcholine.

CARDIOVASCULAR EFFECTS

Succinylcholine, because of its structural resemblance to acetylcholine, may exhibit a large number of parasympathomimetic effects because nicotinic and muscarinic receptors are stimulated as it imitates acetylcholine.

Stimulation of muscarinic receptors in the sinus node leads to sinus bradycardia with nodal or ventricular escape beats.[92, 93] Bradycardia is common in nonatropinized patients, especially in children,[94] or after repeated doses of succinylcholine[92] in adults. These arrhythmias can be prevented or treated with atropine or glycopyrrolate.[95, 96] The weak nicotinic stimulation of autonomic ganglia is of little practical importance.[97]

Succinylcholine also leads to an increase in the release of catecholamines, particularly norepinephrine,[98] which may increase tenfold, and their release may be responsible for arrhythmias and tachycardia in atropinized subjects.[99–101] The arrhythmias occur frequently after

TABLE 7–4.
Complications of Initial Stimulation

Fasciculations
Muscle pain
Hyperkalemia
Increased intragastric pressure
Increased intraocular pressure
Myoglobinemia
Myoglobinuria

intubation and are more common in the presence of hypoxia and hypercapnia. Severe ventricular arrhythmias may result when succinylcholine induces hyperkalemia in the burned or injured patient (see section on complications of initial stimulation).

Normally, succinylcholine is associated with few severe cardiovascular effects because succinylcholine-induced catecholamine release is attenuated by coincident muscarinic stimulation.[102] Cardiovascular reactions are rare when succinylcholine is given by infusion even when large doses (2 to 3 gm) are given in the absence of atropine.[10–12, 84]

Anaphylaxis

The combination of bronchospasm, hypotension, and facial or periorbital edema has been described occasionally following the use of succinylcholine[103, 104] and an anaphylactic basis is suggested by skin testing and basophil degranulation.[105] Fortunately, such reactions are rare: only 36 cases were reported between 1957 and 1981.

COMPLICATIONS OF INITIAL STIMULATION

Several of the problems associated with succinylcholine are a result of its initial stimulating activity (Table 7–4).

Fasciculations

Succinylcholine gives rise to fasciculations a few seconds after its administration, especially in young, muscular adults. Fasciculations are less common in children. Many anesthetists like to observe these fasciculations as an indicator of the onset of the block. Others prefer to prevent their occurrence because of the increased intragastric pressure and the possible association between fasciculations and muscle pain. A subparalyzing dose of nondepolarizing relaxant (d-tubocurarine, 3 to 6 mg; gallamine, 10 to 20 mg; metocurine, 1 to 2 mg; pancuronium, 0.5 to 1.0 mg; atracurium, 2 to 4 mg; alcuronium, 2 mg; or vecuronium, 0.5 to 1.0 mg in the average adult) given 3 minutes before succinylcholine will prevent fasciculations in most patients and will attenuate their severity.[31, 89, 90, 106–109] A higher dose of succinylcholine (1.5 mg/kg) is required after precurarization because of the antagonism of depolarizing block by nondepolarizing muscle relaxants.[110] No increase is necessary after pancuronium because of its PCHE inhibition.[31] Complaints of heavy eyelids and blurred vision are common after precurarization and difficulty in breathing may be experienced.[111] Thus, the dose of precurarizing drug should be as small as possible, in the lower limit of the range mentioned above. Pretreatment with succinylcholine (10 mg) has been advocated as an effective way of abolishing fasciculations.[112, 113] The major disadvantage of pretreatment is that the small doses produce significant block in some patients,[114–116] and gallamine may produce tachycardia and hypertension.[117] The incidence of fasciculations is diminished by giving succinylcholine slowly (1 mg/second or less).[118] Pretreatment with diazepam,[119] lidocaine (Xylocaine),[120] fentanyl,[121] thiopental,[122] calcium gluconate,[123] vitamin C,[124] magnesium sulfate,[125] and dantrolene[126] have also been proposed. The results are no better than with nondepolarizing relaxants, and the drugs used may have some undesirable effects of their own. The optimal interval between precurarization with nondepolarizing relaxants and succinylcholine is at least 3 minutes.[127] In the prevention of fasciculations, d-tubocurarine appears to be superior to pancuronium or gallamine.[128]

Muscle Pains

Postoperatively, patients who have received succinylcholine often complain of myalgia, which is similar to the pain that follows violent exercise. A wide range of complaints has been reported regarding the incidence of the problem and the efficacy of various measures to prevent or attenuate it. These inconsistencies are a reflection of the subjective nature of the complaint, but young patients who undergo minor procedures and who are ambulatory soon after surgery appear to be more at risk. Precurarization provided a protective effect in some studies[129, 130] but not in others.[131] Many theories have been proposed to account for the muscle pains, including the formation of lactic acid as a consequence of fasciculations, the effect of hyperkalemia, and muscle damage from uncoordinated contractions, but the cause remains elusive.

Intragastric Pressure

A transient increase in intragastric pressure of up to 40 cm H_2O occurs after the administration of succinylcholine. Precurarization abolishes this increase almost completely,[120] and this has been used as an argument for precurarizing patients with full stomachs. However, lower esophageal sphincter pressure increases more than intragastric pressure during succinylcholine fasciculations, and this increase in pressure gradient might itself lessen the risk of aspiration.[132]

Intraocular Pressure

Succinylcholine increases intraocular pressure by 5 to 10 mm Hg. Precurarization does not provide protection for this effect[133-135] (Fig 7–6). Although the increase in pressure is of no clinical significance in most subjects, it may be important in patients with poorly controlled glaucoma or penetrating eye injuries. Succinylcholine is probably best avoided in these cases, but the alternative induction technique must be chosen carefully because laryngoscopy and intubation cause greater increases in intraocular pressure in lightly anesthetized, partially paralyzed patients.[136] Indeed, in some centers, succinylcholine is still used in penetrating eye injuries, despite the theoretical objections. Libonati, et al.[137] reported recently that over 10 years and 250 patients, no expulsion of global contents or gastric aspiration had occurred when an anesthetic technique was used that relied on deep anesthesia and d-tubocurarine and gallamine pretreatment before succinylcholine. However, the report was followed by vigorous debate in the correspondence columns! Most would prefer to replace succinylcholine with atracurium[135, 138] or vecuronium[139] in doses of about 2 to 3 × ED95.

Intracranial Pressure

The traditional belief is that succinylcholine is contraindicated in patients with intracranial hypertension because small yet transient increases in intracranial pressure (ICP) had been observed in cats[140] and humans.[141] Others have failed to confirm these observations,[142, 143] and Minton, et al.[144] demonstrated that any increase could be prevented by pretreatment with vecuronium. In man, the ICP response to succinylcholine is variable and is only marked during light anesthesia or in association with hypercapnia.[145]

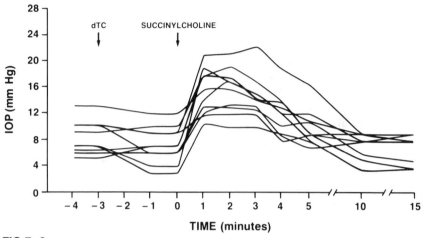

FIG 7–6.
Failure of pretreatment *d*-tubocurarine (dTC) to prevent increase in intraocular pressure
(IOP) after succinylcholine. (Redrawn from Cook JH: The effect of suxamethonium on intra-
ocular pressure. *Anaesthesia* 1981; 36:359–361. Used by permission.)

Hyperkalemia

In normal individuals, serum potassium concentration increases by
approximately 0.5 mEq/L after administration of succinylcholine.[146]
This increase is not completely abolished by precurarization.[147, 148] The
β-adrenoreceptor is important in the acute regulation of serum potassium concentration, and in dogs the increase in potassium following
administration of succinylcholine was èxaggerated after pretreatment
with propranolol (0.25 mg/kg),[149] but not after verapamil (0.15 mg/kg
bolus followed by 4 ng/kg/minute infusion),[150] which suggests succinylcholine should be used cautiously in patients receiving β-blockade.
Hyperkalemia following administration of succinylcholine has been
reported in several conditions including burns[151] and cold injury,[152]
trauma,[153, 154] infections,[155, 156] radiation injury,[157] and in association
with several neurologic conditions—peripheral neuropathies,[158] denervation,[159] stroke,[160] cerebral aneurysm,[161] head injury,[162] brachial
plexus injury,[163] and Parkinson's disease.[164]

The mechanism for the increase appears to be leakage of potassium
from the inside of the muscle cell as a result of prolonged depolarization
at the end-plate. Thus, serum potassium concentration tends to reach
high levels in patients with denervation hypersensitivity, since the
number of receptors on the muscle membrane has increased in response
to lack of stimulation by the incoming nerve.[165] Cord transection,[151]

major trauma,[153] and, to a lesser extent, central nervous system injuries[166, 167] and prolonged immobility[168] also induce receptor multiplication. Receptors take a few days to form, and succinylcholine may be contraindicated, at least until resolution of the injury or complete healing.

Nevertheless, it should not be assumed that those conditions associated with receptor multiplication will necessarily be associated with hyperkalemia. Several investigators have failed to demonstrate an exaggerated increase in serum potassium in patients with brain tumors[169] and children with myelomeningocele.[170] Nevertheless, the use of an alternative short-acting muscle relaxant with a rapid onset of action would be a considerable advantage. Preoperative hyperkalemia is also a contraindication to succinylcholine. Patients with renal failure do not exhibit larger increases in serum potassium than normal patients.[171, 172] Therefore, they can receive succinylcholine provided their preoperative level of serum potassium is within normal limits.

DRUG INTERACTIONS

Inhalation Anesthesia

The depth of the block following administration of succinylcholine given as a bolus dose has been reported to be greater with isoflurane than with other agents as a result of increased muscle blood flow.[173] However, succinylcholine requirements to maintain a constant 90% block are not affected by the presence of volatile agents, at least for the first 90 minutes of infusion.[10-12] Tachyphylaxis and phase II block develop to a similar degree when either a narcotic or a volatile agent is used, but these phenomena occur faster with a volatile agent (see Table 7–3).

Nondepolarizing Relaxants

Succinylcholine phase I block is antagonized by nondepolarizing muscle relaxants. Subparalyzing doses of d-tubocurarine, gallamine, or metocurine delay the onset of succinylcholine block and shorten its duration.[31, 89, 90] Pancuronium prolongs the duration of the block by inhibiting succinylcholine metabolism.[174] Nondepolarizing relaxants diminish the incidence and severity of fasciculations[89, 90, 106] by occupying too few receptors to cause paralysis but contributing to a reduction of free receptors available for the depolarizing effect of succinylcholine. Phase II block, on the other hand, is potentiated by nondepolarizing relaxants.[175]

The administration of an intubating dose of succinylcholine reduces the subsequent requirement for nondepolarizing relaxants,[176, 177] and this effect persists for at least 30 minutes. The reason for the interaction is not clear because it is unlikely that such doses produce any significant degree of phase II block.

Anticholinesterases

Neostigmine, edrophonium, and pyridostigmine inhibit plasma cholinesterase and thus decrease the rate of succinylcholine metabolism;[178] neostigmine given before succinylcholine therefore substantially increases the effect of the latter.[179, 180] In addition, anticholinesterases potentiate phase I and antagonize phase II block.[181, 182] Lee[85] has suggested that the reversibility of succinylcholine block by anticholinesterases can be predicted by using train-of-four monitoring. In his study, edrophonium accelerated recovery when the train-of-four ratio was 0.4 or less. Reversibility can be improved by waiting 10 minutes after the end of a succinylcholine infusion. In this situation, blocks with train-of-four ratios up to 0.7 can be antagonized with neostigmine.[12, 183] In fact, the degree of reversibility improves with increasing train-of-four ratio. This suggests that if time is allowed for most of the succinylcholine present in the plasma to be metabolized, train-of-four fade indicates a recovering phase II block, and neostigmine is readily effective.[86, 184] The only reports of failure of anticholinesterases to antagonize phase II block reflect situations in which a significant plasma concentration of succinylcholine was present in patients with atypical cholinesterases[184, 185] or when an anticholinesterase was given during an infusion of succinylcholine.[178, 186]

Other Drugs

Many other drugs, including oral contraceptives, monoamine oxidase inhibitors, cyclophosphamide, and echothiopate iodide, potentiate the effect of succinylcholine by decreasing plasma cholinesterase activity.[13] Others, such as lithium,[187] trimethaphan,[188] and magnesium[189] increase the blocking effect of succinylcholine by their direct action on the neuromuscular junction.

MODE OF ADMINISTRATION

Despite its side effects, succinylcholine offers distinct advantages over long-acting and intermediate-acting nondepolarizing muscle relaxants. When its use is not contraindicated, it can provide excellent conditions for intubation and relaxation during short and long surgical procedures.

Intubation

In a dose of 1 mg/kg, succinylcholine leads to better intubating conditions more rapidly than the available nondepolarizing muscle relaxants. Even in large doses, neither atracurium nor vecuronium leads to complete disappearance of the twitch or ideal intubating conditions in less than 2 to 2.5 minutes. Such ideal conditions are achieved within 1 to 1.5 minutes with succinylcholine (1 mg/kg). After precurarization, a higher dose should be employed (1.5 mg/kg). This rapid onset of action is of great value when the airway must be secured quickly, as in the case of a full stomach or in anesthesia for cesarean section. In the latter, succinylcholine does not cross the placenta.[189]

Maintenance Infusions

Succinylcholine infusions are well suited to short procedures requiring moderate to profound relaxation, such as laparoscopy, bronchoscopy, cesarean section, and appendectomy. A relative overdose of succinylcholine is usually without sequelae because of its rapid metabolism. However, the management of succinylcholine infusions is much easier with neuromuscular monitoring.

Reversal of Phase II Block.—Phase II block is readily reversible with anticholinesterases in patients with quantitatively and qualitatively normal plasma cholinesterase. Therefore, defining an upper limit to the duration and total dose of succinylcholine compatible with its safe administration is difficult, if not impossible. However, neostigmine or edrophonium is rarely needed if the total dose does not exceed 7 mg/kg.

OTHER USES

It is sometimes tempting to use succinylcholine in the presence of nondepolarizing relaxants. For instance, more relaxation might be requested for peritoneal closure, and it may be desirable to avoid the prolonged effect of additional nondepolarizing relaxants. A small dose of succinylcholine may either antagonize the nondepolarizing relaxant or produce a depolarizing block, and this will depend upon the degree of residual nondepolarizing block.[190] If anticholinesterase has been given to antagonize the nondepolarizing block, the effect of succinylcholine will be potentiated and prolonged because of the inhibition of succinylcholine metabolism by the anticholinesterase. Avoidance of this situation is perhaps the wiser course.

CONCLUSION

Clinicians have widely different views on the role of succinylcholine in clinical practice. Some suggest that it be relegated to the emergency cart, while others use it for most patients. Most anesthetists probably lie somewhere between these extremes. Nevertheless, succinylcholine has puzzled researchers and practicing physicians alike for more than 30 years. Whether future efforts will focus on the understanding of its complicated effects or on the search for a better substitute remains to be seen.

REFERENCES

1. Brucke H, Ginzel KH, Klupp H, et al: Bis-Cholinester von Dicarbonsäuren als Muskelrelaxantien in der Narkose. *Wien Klin Wochenschr* 1951; 63:464–466.
2. Browne JG, Collier HOJ, Somers GF: Succinylcholine (succinoxylcholine): Muscle relaxant of short duration. *Lancet* 1952; 1:1225–1228.
3. Waud DR, Waud BE: Depolarization block and phase II block at the neuromuscular junction. *Anesthesiology* 1975; 43:10–20.
4. Zaimis E, Head S: Depolarising neuromuscular blocking drugs, in Zaimis E (ed): *Neuromuscular Junction: Handbook of Experimental*

Pharmacology. Berlin, Springer-Verlag, 1976, vol 42, pp 365–419.

5. Burns BD, Paton WDM: Depolarization of the motor end-plate by decamethonium and acetylcholine. *J Physiol* 1951; 115:41–73.
6. Waud DR: The nature of "depolarization block". *Anesthesiology* 1968; 29:1014–1024.
7. Litwiller RW: Succinylcholine hydrolysis: A review. *Anesthesiology* 1969; 31:356–360.
8. Organe GSW, Paton WDM, Zaimis EJ: Preliminary trials of bis-trimethylammonium decane and pentone diiodide (C_{10} and C_5) in man. *Lancet* 1949; 1:21–23.
9. Hale Enderby GE: Twenty years experience with decamethonium, in Zaimis E (ed): *Neuromuscular Junction: Handbook of Experimental Pharmacology.* Berlin, Springer-Verlag, 1976, vol 42, pp 661–675.
10. Donati F, Bevan DR: Effect of enflurane and fentanyl on the clinical characteristics of long-term succinylcholine infusion. *Can Anaesth Soc J* 1982; 29:59–64.
11. Donati F, Bevan DR: Long-term succinylcholine infusion during isoflurane anesthesia. *Anesthesiology* 1983; 58:6–10.
12. Futter ME, Donati F, Bevan DR: Prolonged suxamethonium infusion during nitrous oxide anaesthesia supplemented with halothane or fentanyl. *Br J Anaesth* 1983; 55:947–953.
13. Whittaker M: Plasma cholinesterase variants and the anaesthetist. *Anaesthesia* 1980; 35:174–197.
14. Hall GM, Wood GJ, Patterson JL: Half-life of plasma cholinesterase. *Br J Anaesth* 1984; 56:903–904.
15. Kalow W, Lindsay HA: A comparison of optical and manometric methods for the assay of human serum cholinesterase. *Can J Biochem Physiol* 1955; 33:568–574.
16. Wakid NW, Tubbeh R, Baraka A: Assay of serum cholinesterase with succinylcholine and propionylthiocholine as substrates. *Anesthesiology* 1985; 62:509–512.
17. Stoddart JC: The suxamethonium-pseudocholinesterase relationship. *Br J Anaesth* 1960; 32:466–469.
18. Viby-Mogensen J: Correlation of succinylcholine duration of action with plasma cholinesterase activity in subjects with the genotypically normal enzyme. *Anesthesiology* 1980; 53:517–520.
19. Mirakhur RK, Elliott P, Lavery TD: Plasma cholinesterase methods for the assay of human serum cholinesterase. *Can J Biochem Physiol* 1955; 33:568–574.
20. Evans RT, Wroe JM: Plasma cholinesterase changes during pregnancy. *Anaesthesia* 1980; 35:651–654.
21. Robson N, Robertson I, Whittaker M: Plasma cholinesterase changes during the puerperium. *Anaesthesia* 1986; 41:243–249.
22. Zsigmond EK, Downs JR: Plasma cholinesterase activity in newborns and infants. *Can Anaesth Soc J* 1971; 18:278–285.

23. Blitt CD, Petty WC, Alberternst EE, et al: Correlation of plasma cholinesterase activity and duration of action of succinylcholine during pregnancy. *Anesth Analg* 1977; 56:78–83.
24. Leighton BL, Check TG, Gross JB, et al: Succinylcholine pharmacodynamics in peripartum patients. *Anesthesiology* 1986; 64:202–205.
25. Ferguson A, Whittaker M, Britten J, et al: Suxamethonium apnoea associated with pregnancy and liver dysfunction in a treated cretin. *Anaesthesia* 1983; 38:567–571.
26. Davies JM, Carmichael D, Dymond C: Plasma cholinesterase and trophoplastic disease. *Anaesthesia* 1983; 38:1071–1074.
27. Jackson SH, Bailey GWH, Stevens G: Reduced plasma cholinesterase following haemodilutional cardiopulmonary bypass. *Anaesthesia* 1982; 37:319–320.
28. Wood GJ, Hall GM: Plasmaphoresis and plasma cholinesterase. *Br J Anaesth* 1978; 50:945–947.
29. Paterson JL, Walsh EJ, Hall GM: Progressive depletion of plasma cholinesterase during daily plasma exchange. *Br Med J* 1979; 2:280.
30. Zsigmond EK, Winnie AP, Barabas E, et al: The inhibitory effect of glycopyrrolate on human plasma cholinesterase. *Can Anaesth Soc J* 1985; 32:20–22.
31. Ferguson A, Bevan DR: Mixed neuromuscular block: The effect of precurarization. *Anaesthesia* 1981; 36:661–666.
32. Whittaker M, Britten JJ, Wicks RJ: Inhibition of plasma cholinesterase variants by propranolol. *Br J Anaesth* 1981; 53:511–516.
33. Wang RI, Ross CA: Prolonged apnea following succinylcholine in cancer patients receiving AB-132. *Anesthesiology* 1963; 24:363–367.
34. Zsigmond EK, Robins G: The effect of a series of anti-cancer drugs on plasma cholinesterase activity. *Can Anaesth Soc J* 1972; 19:75–82.
35. Baraka A: Suxamethonium-neostigmine interaction in patients with normal or atypical cholinesterase. *Br J Anaesth* 1977; 49:479–484.
36. Sunew KY, Hicks RG: Effects of neostigmine and pryidostigmine on duration of succinylcholine action and pseudocholinesterase activity. *Anesthesiology* 1978; 49:188–191.
37. Baraka A, Wakid N, Mansour R, et al: Effects of neostigmine and pyridostigmine on the plasma cholinesterase activity. *Br J Anaesth* 1981; 53:849–851.
38. Mirakhur RK, Lavery TD, Briggs LP, et al: Effects of neostigmine and pyridostigmine on serum cholinesterase activity. *Can Anaesth Soc J* 1982; 29:55–58.
39. Pantuck EJ: Echothiopate iodide eye drops and prolonged response to suxamethonium. *Br J Anaesth* 1966; 38:406–407.
40. Donati F, Bevan DR: Controlled succinylcholine infusion in a patient receiving echothiophate eye drops. *Can Anaesth Soc J* 1981; 28:488–490.
41. Gesko T: Prolonged apnoea after suxamethonium injection associated with eye drops containing an anticholinesterase agent. *Br J Anaesth* 1966; 38:408–410.

42. Lanks KW, Sklar GS: Pseudocholinesterase levels and rates of chloroprocaine hydrolysis in patients receiving adequate doses of phospholene iodide. *Anesthesiology* 1980; 52:434–435.
43. Barabas E, Zsigmond EK, Kirkpatrick AF: The inhibitory effect of esmolol on human plasmacholinesterase. *Can Anaesth Soc J* 1986; 33:332–335.
44. Kalow W, Genest K: A method for the detection of atypical forms of human serum cholinesterase: Determination of dibucaine numbers. *Can J Biochem Physiol* 1957; 35:339–346.
45. King J, Griffin D: Differentiation of serum cholinesterase variants by succinylcholine inhibition. *Br J Anaesth* 1973; 45:450–454.
46. Bush GH: Prolonged apnoea due to suxamethonium. *Br J Anaesth* 1961; 33:454–462.
47. Viby-Mogensen J: Succinylcholine neuromuscular blockade in subjects homozygous for atypical plasma cholinesterase. *Anesthesiology* 1981; 55:429–434.
48. Oshita S, Sari A, Fuju, S, et al: Prolonged neuromuscular blockade following succinylcholine in a patient homozygous for the silent gene. *Anesthesiology* 1983; 59:71–73.
49. Viby-Mogensen J: Succinylcholine neuromuscular blockade in subjects heterozygous for abnormal plasma cholinesterase. *Anesthesiology* 1984; 55:231–235.
50. Owen H, Hunter AR: Heterozygotes for atypical cholinesterase. *Br J Anaesth* 1983; 55:315–318.
51. McQueen MJ, Lepinskie E, Strickland RD, et al: Abnormal enzyme phenotype ($E_1{}^a E_1{}^f$): Normal response to succinylcholine. *Can Anaesth Soc J* 1979; 26:99–103.
52. Vickers MDA: The mismanagement of suxamethonium apnoea. *Br J Anaesth* 1963; 35:260–268.
53. Savarese JJ, Ali HH, Murphy JD, et al: Train-of-four nerve stimulation in the management of prolonged neuromuscular blockade following succinylcholine. *Anesthesiology* 1975; 42:106–111.
54. Bevan DR, Donati F: Succinylcholine apnoea: Attempted reversal with anticholinesterases. *Can Anaesth Soc J* 1983; 30:536–539.
55. Dykes MH, Cheng SC, Cohen H, et al: Multiple neuromuscular blocking agents and reversal in a patient with absent plasma cholinesterase. *Can Anaesth Soc J* 1986; 33:657–661.
56. Epstein HM, Jarzemsky D, Zuckerman L, et al: Plasma cholinesterase activity in bank blood. *Anesth Analg* 1980; 49:211–214.
57. Scholler KL, Goedde HW, Benkmann HG: The use of serum cholinesterase in succinylcholine apnoea. *Can Anaesth Soc J* 1977; 24:396–400.
58. Carnie J: A pre-induction test dose for suxamethonium. *Anaesthesia* 1986; 41:358–362.
59. Azar I, Betcher AM: Response of patient with atypical pseudocholinesterase to small intermittent succinylcholine doses. *Anesthesiology* 1981; 54:519–520.

60. Cass NM, Doolan LA, Gutteridge GA: Repeated administration of suxamethonium in a patient with atypical plasma cholinesterase. *Anaesth Intensive Care* 1982; 10:25−28.
61. Bentley JB, Borel JD, Vaughan RW, et al: Weight, pseudocholinesterase activity, and succinylcholine requirement. *Anesthesiology* 1982; 57:48−49.
62. Sugmari T: Shortened action of succinylcholine in individuals with cholinesterase C_5 isoenzyme. *Can Anaesth Soc J* 1986; 33:321−327.
63. Levy G: Kinetics of pharmacologic activity of succinylcholine in man. *J Pharm Sci* 1967; 56:1687−1688.
64. Levy G: Pharmacokinetics of succinylcholine in newborns. *Anesthesiology* 1970; 32:551−2.
65. Walts LF, Dillon JB: Clinical studies on succinylcholine chloride. *Anesthesiology* 1967; 28:372−376.
66. Cook DR, Wingard LB, Taylor FH: Pharmacokinetics of succinylcholine in infants, children and adults. *Clin Pharmacol Ther* 1976; 20:493−498.
67. Cook DR, Fischer CG: Neuromuscular blocking effects of succinylcholine in infants and children. *Anesthesiology* 1975; 42:662−665.
68. Standaert FG, Adams JE: The actions of succinylcholine on the mammalian motor nerve terminal. *J Pharmacol Exp Ther* 1965; 149:113−123.
69. Hartman GS, Flamengo SA, Riker WF: Succinylcholine: Mechanism of fasciculations and their prevention by d-tubocurarine or diphenylhydantoin. *Anesthesiology* 1986; 65:405−413.
70. Sutherland GA, Squire IB, Gibb AJ, et al: Neuromuscular blocking and autonomic effects of vecuronium and atracurium in the anaesthetized cat. *Br J Anaesth* 1983; 55:1119−1126.
71. Williams JP, Bourke DL, Jones RM: Comparison of respiratory and skeletal muscle dynamics during low-dose suxamethonium infusion in man. *Br J Anaesth* 1983; 55:912P.
72. Foldes FF, Swerdlow M, Lipschitz E, et al: Comparison of the respiratory effects of suxamethonium and suxethonium in man. *Anesthesiology* 1956; 17:559−568.
73. Williams JP, Bourke DL: Effects of succinylcholine on respiratory and nonrespiratory muscle strength in humans. *Anesthesiology* 1985; 63:299−303.
74. Bowman WC: *Pharmacology of Neuromuscular Function.* Baltimore, University Park Press, 1980.
75. Donati F, Bevan DR: Muscle electromechanical correlations during succinylcholine infusion. *Anesth Analg* 1984; 63:891−894.
76. Lee C: Dose relationships of phase II, tachyphylaxis and train-of-four fade in suxamethonium-induced dual neuromuscular block in man. *Br J Anaesth* 1975; 47:841−845.
77. Lee C, Barnes A, Katz RL: Magnitude, dose requirement and mode of development of tachyphylaxis to suxamethonium in man. *Br J Anaesth* 1978; 50:189−194.

78. Hilgenberg JC, Stoelting RK: Characteristics of succinylcholine-produced phase II neuromuscular block during enflurane, halothane, and fentanyl anesthesia. *Anesth Analg* 1981; 60:192–196.
79. DeCook TH, Goudsouzian NG: Tachyphylaxis and phase II block development during infusion of succinylcholine in children. *Anesth Analg* 1980; 59:639–643.
80. Bevan JC, Donati F, Bevan DR: Prolonged infusion of suxamethonium in infants and children. *Br J Anaesth* 1986; 58:839–843.
81. Lee C: Self-antagonism: A possible mechanism of tachyphylaxis in suxamethonium-induced neuromuscular block in man. *Br J Anaesth* 1976; 48:1097–1102.
82. Ramsey FM, Lebowitz PW, Savarese JJ, et al: Clinical characteristics of long-term succinylcholine neuromuscular blockade during balanced anesthesia. *Anesth Analg* 1980; 59:110–116.
83. Delisle S, Lebrun M, Bevan DR: Plasma cholinesterase activity and tachyphylaxis during prolonged succinylcholine infusion. *Anesth Analg* 1982; 61:941–944.
84. Donati F, Bevan DR: Potentiation of succinylcholine phase II block with isoflurane. *Anesthesiology* 1983; 58:552–555.
85. Lee C: Train-of-four fade and edrophonium antagonism of neuromuscular block by succinylcholine in man. *Anesth Analg* 1976; 55:663–667.
86. Futter ME, Donati F, Sadikot AS, et al: Neostigmine antagonism of succinylcholine phase II block: A comparison with pancuronium. *Can Anaesth Soc J* 1983; 30:575–580.
87. Katz RL, Ryan JF: The neuromuscular effects of suxamethonium in man. *Br J Anaesth* 1969; 41:381–390.
88. Katz RL, Norman J, Seed RF, et al: A comparison of the effects of suxamethonium and tubocurarine in patients in London and New York. *Br J Anaesth* 1969; 41:1041–1047.
89. Cullen DJ: The effect of pretreatment with nondepolarizing muscle relaxants on the neuromuscular blocking action of succinylcholine. *Anesthesiology* 1971; 35:572–578.
90. Blitt CD, Carlson GL, Rolling GD, et al: A comparative evaluation of pretreatment with nondepolarizing blockers prior to the administration of succinylcholine. *Anesthesiology* 1981; 55:687–689.
91. Harrison GA, Junius F: The effect of circulation time on the neuromuscular action of suxamethonium. *Anaesth Intensive Care* 1972; 1:33–40.
92. Williams CH, Deutsch S, Linde HW, et al: Effects of intravenously administered succinylcholine on cardiac rate, rhythm, and arterial blood pressure in anesthetized man. *Anesthesiology* 1961; 22:947–954.
93. Schoenstadt DA, Witcher CE: Observations on the mechanism of succinyldicholine-induced cardiac arrhythmias. *Anesthesiology* 1963; 24:358–362.
94. Lerman J, Chinyanga HM: The heart rate response to succinylcholine in children: A comparison of atropine and glycopyrrolate. *Can Anaesth Soc J* 1983; 30:377–381.

95. Sorensen O, Eriksen S, Hommelgaard P, et al: Thiopental-nitrous oxide-halothane anesthesia and repeated succinylcholine: Comparison of preoperative glycopyrrolate and atropine administration. *Anesth Analg* 1980; 59:686–689.

96. Viby-Mogensen J, Wisberg K, Sorensen O: Cardiac effects of atropine and gallamine in patients receiving suxamethonium. *Br J Anaesth* 1980; 52:1137–1142.

97. Paton WDM: The effects of muscle relaxants other than muscle relaxation. *Anesthesiology* 1959; 20:453–460.

98. McCulloch LS, Nigrovic C, Wajskol A, et al: Release of catecholamines by succinylcholine in man. *Anesth Analg* 1982; 61:203.

99. Lupprian KG, Churchill-Davidson HC: Effect of suxamethonium on cardiac rhythm. *Br Med J* 1960; 2:1174–1177.

100. Barreto RS: Effect of intravenously administered succinylcholine upon cardiac rate and rhythm. *Anesthesiology* 1960; 21:401–403.

101. Perez HR: Cardiac arrhythmias after succinylcholine. *Anesth Analg* 1970; 49:33–36.

102. Nigrovic V: Succinylcholine, cholinoceptors and catecholamines: Proposed mechanism of early adverse haemodynamic reactions. *Can Anaesth Soc J* 1984; 31:382–394.

103. Cohen S, Liu KH, Marx GL: Upper airway edema: An anaphylactoid reaction to succinylcholine? *Anesthesiology* 1982; 56:467–468.

104. Smith NL: Histamine release by suxamethonium. *Anaesthesia* 1957; 12:293–298.

105. Laxenaire MC, Maneret-Vautrin DA, Boileau S: Choc anaphylactique au suxamethonium. *Ann Fr Anesth Reanim* 1982; 1:29–36.

106. Erkola O, Salmenpera A, Kuoppamaki R: Five nondepolarizing muscle relaxants in precurarization. *Acta Anaesthesiol Scand* 1983; 27:427–432.

107. Laurence AS: Biochemical changes following suxamethonium. *Anaesthesia* 1985; 40:854–859.

108. Manchikanti L, Grow JB, Colliver JA, et al: Atracurium pretreatment for succinylcholine induced fasciculations and postoperative myalgia. *Anesth Analg* 1985; 64:1010–1014.

109. Ferres CJ, Mirakhur RK, Craig HJC, et al: Pretreatment with vecuronium as a prophylactic against post-suxamethonium muscle pain. *Br J Anaesth* 1983; 55:735–741.

110. Freund FG, Rubin AP: The need for additional succinylcholine after d-tubocurarine. *Anesthesiology* 1972; 36:185–187.

111. Howardy-Hansen P, Chraemmer Jorgensen B, Orgind H, et al: Pre-treatment with non-depolarizing muscle relaxants: The influence on neuromuscular transmission and pulmonary function. *Acta Anaesthesiol Scand* 1980; 24:419–422.

112. Baraka A: Self-taming of succinylcholine-induced fasciculations. *Anesthesiology* 1977; 46:292.

113. Brodsky JB, Brock-Utne JG: Does "self-taming" with succinylcholine

prevent post-operative myalgia? *Anesthesiology* 1979; 50:265–267.
114. Massey SA, Glazebrook CW, Goat VA: Suxamethonium: A new look at pretreatment. *Br J Anaesth* 1983; 55:729–733.
115. Bruce DL, Downs JB, Kulkarni PS, et al: Precurarization inhibits maximal ventilatory effort. *Anesthesiology* 1984; 61:618–621.
116. Rao TLK, Jacobs HK: Pulmonary function following "pretreatment" dose of pancuronium in volunteers. *Anesth Analg* 1980; 59:659–661.
117. Kingsley BP, Vaughan MS, Vaughan RW: Cardiovascular effects of nondepolarizing relaxants employed for pretreatment prior to succinylcholine. *Can Anaesth Soc J* 1984; 31:13–19.
118. Feingold A, Velasquez JL: Suxamethonium infusion rate and observed fasciculations: A dose-response study. *Br J Anaesth* 1979; 51:241–245.
119. Fahmy NR, Malek NS, Lappas DG: Diazepam prevents some adverse effects of succinylcholine. *Clin Pharmacol Ther* 1979; 26:395–398.
120. Miller RD, Way WL: Inhibition of succinylcholine-induced increased intragastric pressure by nondepolarizing muscle relaxants and lidocaine. *Anesthesiology* 1971; 34:185–188.
121. Lindgren L, Saarnivaara L: Effect of competitive myoneural blockade and fentanyl on muscle fasciculations caused by suxamethonium in children. *Br J Anaesth* 1983; 55:747–751.
122. Manani G, Valenti S, Segatto A, et al: The influence of thiopentone and alfathesin on succinylcholine-induced fasciculations and myalgias. *Can Anaesth Soc J* 1981;28:253–258.
123. Shrivastava OP, Chatterji S, Kachhawa S, et al: Calcium gluconate pretreatment for prevention of succinylcholine-induced myalgia. *Anesth Analg* 1983; 62:59–62.
124. Gupta SR, Savant NS: Post suxamethonium pains and vitamin C. *Anaesthesia* 1971; 26:436–440.
125. James MFM, Cork RC, Dennett JE: Succinylcholine pretreatment with magnesium sulfate. *Anesth Analg* 1986; 65:373–376.
126. Collier DB: Dantrolene and suxamethonium: The effect of pre-operative dantrolene on the action of suxamethonium. *Anesthesiology* 1979; 34:152–158.
127. Horrow JC, Lambert DH: The search for an optimal interval between pretreatment dose of d-tubocurarine and succinylcholine. *Can Anaesth Soc J* 1984; 31:528–533.
128. Erkola O, Salmenpera A, Kuoppamaki R: Five nondepolarizing muscle relaxants in precurarization. *Acta Anaesthesiol Scand* 1983; 27:427–432.
129. Lamoreaux LF, Urbach KF: Incidence and prevention of muscle pain following the administration of succinylcholine. *Anesthesiology* 1960; 21:394–396.
130. Bennetts FE, Khalil KI: Reduction of post-suxamethonium pain by pretreatment with four nondepolarizing agents. *Br J Anaesth* 1981; 53:531–536.
131. Brodsky JB, Ehrenwerth J: Post-operative muscle pains and suxamethonium. *Br J Anaesth* 1980; 52:215–217.

132. Smith G, Dalling R, Williams TIR: Gastro-oesophageal pressure gradient changes produced by induction of anaesthesia and suxamethonium. *Br J Anaesth* 1978; 50:1137–1143.

133. Meyers EF, Krupin T, Johnson M, et al: Failure of nondepolarizing neuromuscular blockers to inhibit succinylcholine-induced increased intraocular pressure, a controlled study. *Anesthesiology* 1978; 48:149–151.

134. Cook JH: The effect of suxamethonium on intraocular pressure. *Anaesthesia* 1981; 36:359–365.

135. Lavery GG, McGalliard JN, Mirakhur RK, et al: The effects of atracurium on intraocular pressure during steady state anaesthesia and rapid sequence induction: A comparison with succinylcholine. *Can Anaesth Soc J* 1986; 33:437–442.

136. Wynands JE, Crowell DE: Intraocular tension in association with succinylcholine and endotracheal intubation: A preliminary report. *Can Anaesth Soc J* 1960; 7:39–43.

137. Libonati MM, Leahy JJ, Ellison N: The use of succinylcholine in open eye surgery. *Anesthesiology* 1985; 62:637–640.

138. Badrinath SK, Vazecry A, McCarthy RJ, et al: The effect of different methods of inducing anesthesia on intraocular pressure. *Anesthesiology* 1986; 65:431–435.

139. Schneider MJ, Stirt JA, Finholt DA: Atracurium, vecuronium, and intraocular pressure in humans. *Anesth Analg* 1986; 65:877–882.

140. Cottrell JE, Hartung J, Giffin JP, et al: Intracranial and hemodynamic changes after succinylcholine administration in cats. *Anesth Analg* 1983; 62:1006–1009.

141. Marsh ML, Dunlop BJ, Shapiro HM, et al: Succinylcholine-intracranial pressure effects in neurosurgical patients. *Anesth Analg* 1980; 59:550–551.

142. Bormann BE, Smith RB, Bunegin L, et al: Does succinylcholine raise intracranial pressure? *Anesthesiology* 1980; 53:S262.

143. Stullken EH Jr, Sokoll MD: Anesthesia and subarachnoid intracranial pressure. *Anesth Analg* 1975; 54:494–498.

144. Minton MD, Grosslight K, Stirt JA, et al: Increases in intracranial pressure from succinylcholine: Prevention by prior non-depolarizing blockade. *Anesthesiology* 1986; 65:165–169.

145. Lam AM, Gelb AW: Succinylcholine and intracranial pressure—A cause for 'pause,' letter. *Anesth Analg* 1984; 63:620.

146. Weintraub HD, Heisterkamp DV, Cooperman LH: Changes in plasma potassium concentration after depolarizing blockers in anaesthetized man. *Br J Anaesth* 1969; 41:1048–1052.

147. Bali IM, Dundee JW, Doggart JR: The source of increased plasma potassium following succinylcholine. *Anesth Analg* 1975; 54:680–686.

148. Bourke DL, Rosenberg M: Changes in total serum Ca^{2+}, Na^+, and K^+ with administration of succinylcholine. *Anesthesiology* 1978; 49:361–363.

149. McCammon RL, Stoelting RK: Exaggerated increase in serum potassium

following succinylcholine in dogs with beta blockade. *Anesthesiology* 1984; 61:723–725.

150. Roth JL, Nugent M, Gronert GA: Verapamil does not alter succinylcholine induced increases in serum potassium during halothane anesthesia in normal dogs. *Anesth Analg* 1985; 64:1202–1204.
151. Tolmie JD, Joyce TH, Mitchell GD: Succinylcholine danger in the burned patient. *Anesthesiology* 1967; 28:467–470.
152. Laycock JRD, Loughman E: Suxamethonium-induced hyperkalaemia following cold injury. *Anaesthesia* 1986; 41:739–741.
153. Birch AA, Mitchell GD, Playford GA, et al: Changes in serum potassium response to succinylcholine following trauma. *JAMA* 1969; 210:490–493.
154. Mazze RI, Escue HM, Houston JB: Hyperkalemia and cardiovascular collapse following administration of succinylcholine to the traumatized patient. *Anesthesiology* 1969; 31:540–544.
155. Khan TZ, Khan RM: Changes in serum potassium following succinylcholine in patients with infections. *Anesth Analg* 1983; 62:327–331.
156. Kohlschutter B, Baur H, Roth F: Suxamethonium-induced hyperkalaemia in patients with severe intra-abdominal infections. *Br J Anaesth* 1976; 48:557–561.
157. Cairdi VJ, Ivankovich AD, Vucicevic D, et al: Succinylcholine-induced hyperkalemia in the rat following radiation injury to muscle. *Anesth Analg* 1982; 61:83–86.
158. Fergusson RJ, Wright DJ, Willey RF, et al: Suxamethonium is dangerous in polyneuropathy. *Br Med J* 1981; 282:298–299.
159. John DA, Tobey RE, Homer LD, et al: Onset of succinylcholine induced hyperkalemia following denervation. *Anesthesiology* 1976; 45:294–298.
160. Cooperman LH, Strobel GE Jr, Kennell EM: Massive hyperkalemia after administration of succinylcholine. *Anesthesiology* 1970; 32:161–164.
161. Iwatsuki N, Kuroda N, Amaha K, et al: Succinylcholine-induced hyperkalemia in patients with ruptured cerebral aneurysms. *Anesthesiology* 1980; 53:64–67.
162. Stevenson PH, Birch AA: Succinylcholine-induced hyperkalemia in a patient with closed head injury. *Anesthesiology* 1979; 51:89–90.
163. Kelly EP: A rise in serum potassium after suxamethonium following brachial plexus injury. *Anaesthesia* 1982; 37:694–702.
164. Gravlee GP: Succinylcholine-induced hyperkalemia in a patient with Parkinson's disease. *Anesth Analg* 1980; 59:444–446.
165. Gronert GA, Theye RA: Effect of succinylcholine on skeletal muscle with immobilization atrophy. *Anesthesiology* 1974; 40:268–271.
166. Smith RB, Grenvik A: Cardiac arrest following succinylcholine in patients with central nervous system injuries. *Anesthesiology* 1970; 33:558–560.
167. Cowgill DB, Mostello LA, Shapiro HM: Encephalitis and a hyperkalemic response to succinylcholine. *Anesthesiology* 1974; 40:409–411.

168. Gronert GA, Theye RA: Pathophysiology of hyperkalemia induced by succinylcholine. *Anesthesiology* 1975; 43:89–99.
169. Minton MD, Stirt JA, Bedford RF: Serum potassium following succinylcholine in patients with brain tumours. *Can Anaesth Soc J* 1986; 33:328–331.
170. Dierdorf SF, McNiece WL, Rao CC, et al: Failure of succinylcholine to alter plasma potassium in children with myelomeningocoele. *Anesthesiology* 1986; 64:272–273.
171. Miller RD, Way WL, Hamilton WK, et al: Succinylcholine-induced hyperkalemia in patients with renal failure? *Anesthesiology* 1972; 36:138–141.
172. Koide M, Waud BE: Serum potassium concentrations after succinylcholine in patients with renal failure. *Anesthesiology* 1972; 36:142–145.
173. Miller RD, Way WL, Dolan WM, et al: Comparative neuromuscular effects of pancuronium, gallamine and succinylcholine during forane and halothane anesthesia in man. *Anesthesiology* 1971; 35:509–514.
174. Stovner J, Oftedal N, Holmboe J: The inhibition of cholinesterases by pancuronium. *Br J Anaesth* 1975; 47:949–954.
175. Foldes FF, Wnuck A, Hamer-Hodges RJ, et al: The mode of action of depolarizing relaxants. *Anesth Analg* 1957; 36:23–37.
176. Katz RL: Modification of the action of pancuronium by succinylcholine and halothane. *Anesthesiology* 1971; 35:602–606.
177. d'Hollander AA, Agoston S, DeVille A, et al: Clinical and pharmacological actions of a bolus injection of suxamethonium: Two phenomena of distinct duration. *Br J Anaesth* 1983; 55:131–134.
178. Barrow MEH, Johnson JK: A study of the anticholinesterase and anticurare effects of some cholinesterase inhibitors. *Br J Anaesth* 1966; 38:420–431.
179. Baraka A: Suxamethonium-neostigmine interaction in patients with normal or atypical cholinesterase. *Br J Anaesth* 1977; 49:479–484.
180. Baraka A, Wakid N, Mansour R, et al: Effect of neostigmine and pyridostigmine on plasma cholinesterase activity. *Br J Anaesth* 1981; 53:849–851.
181. Brennan HJ: Dual action of suxamethonium chloride. *Br J Anaesth* 1956; 28:159–168.
182. Crul JF, Long GJ, Brunner EA, et al: The changing pattern of neuromuscular blockade caused by succinylcholine in man. *Anesthesiology* 1966; 27:729–741.
183. Donati F, Bevan DR: Intensity of phase II succinylcholine block and its antagonism with neostigmine. *Can Anaesth Soc J* 1984; 31:S88–S89.
184. Bevan DR, Donati F: Anticholinesterase antagonism of succinylcholine phase II block, editorial. *Can Anaesth Soc J* 1983; 30:569–572.
185. Viby-Mogensen J: Succinylcholine neuromuscular blockade in subjects homozygous for atypical plasma cholinesterase. *Anesthesiology* 1981; 42:106–111.
186. Gissen AJ, Katz RL, Karis JH, et al: Neuromuscular block in man during

prolonged arterial infusion of succinylcholine. *Anesthesiology* 1966; 27:242–249.

187. Hill GE, Wong KC, Hodges MR: Potentiation of succinylcholine neuromuscular blockade by lithium carbonate. *Anesthesiology* 1976; 44:439–442.

188. Poulton TJ, James FM, Lockridge O: Prolonged apnea following trimethaphan and succinylcholine. *Anesthesiology* 1979; 50:54–56.

189. Ghoneim MM, Long JP: The interaction between magnesium and other neuromuscular blocking agents. *Anesthesiology* 1970; 32:23–27.

190. Rouse JM, Bevan DR: Mixed neuromuscular block. *Anaesthesia* 1979; 34:608–617.

8

Malignant Hyperthermia

Malignant hyperthermia (MH) is the most dangerous complication of succinylcholine administration. It manifests, in skeletal muscles of susceptible individuals, as an acute hypermetabolic response to the triggering effects of some drugs or stress.

EPIDEMIOLOGY, INCIDENCE, AND MORTALITY

Fatal pyrexial reactions to general anesthesia were unexplained until the syndrome of malignant hyperthermia was described by Denborough[1] in Australia in 1963. Fulminant MH crises during general anesthesia are rare, with reported incidences of 1 in 11–250,000 in Denmark,[2] 1 in 7–110,000 in Japan,[3] and 1 in 15–150,000 in North America.[4] In some areas, such as Wisconsin and Canada, there is a concentration of cases with a high incidence of 1 in 1,500[5] because of the familial nature of the disorder. Inheritance is primarily autosomal dominant, but the variable severity in different families suggests a multifactorial genetic basis.[6] It is most common between the ages of 3 and 30 years. Males are more often affected than females due to their larger muscle mass and increased risk of sports injury.[7] Mortality from an untreated MH crisis used to be greater than 70%, but earlier recognition and symptomatic treatment reduced this to 28%. Specific treatment with dantrolene, available since 1979, has dramatically altered the outcome so that the current survival rate exceeds 90%.[8]

TRIGGERING AGENTS

The onset of MH can occur acutely during the induction of anesthesia or be delayed several hours after surgery. Succinylcholine and halothane are the most potent triggering agents,[9] but the response has been described after administration of a variety of anesthetic agents including most volatile agents.[10-12] Amide local anesthetics, nitrous oxide,[13] ketamine,[14] and d-tubocurarine[15] have all been blamed but with unconvincing evidence.[16] No reservations are now placed on their use, and mepivacaine[17] and lidocaine are recommended for muscle biopsy in suspected individuals. The MH reaction may be aggravated by epinephrine, cardiac glycosides, calcium salts, and theophylline derivatives. However, Flewellen and Nelson,[18] from contractile responses in positive biopsy specimens, allow the cautious use of aminophylline in therapeutic doses and a moderate caffeine intake in MH-susceptible individuals.

The neuroleptic malignant syndrome is associated with the chronic administration of psychotropic drugs including butyrophenones, phenothiazines, monoamine oxidase inhibitors, or lithium. Although exhibiting some of the features of MH, this syndrome has a slow onset of days or weeks, and recovery extends over a prolonged period after discontinuance of the drugs.[19] Sudden infant death syndrome[20] and heat stroke[21] may involve a similar response but are infrequently related to MH susceptibility. True MH reactions can be initiated by stress such as muscular exercise or emotional reactions in the absence of any pharmacologic trigger, possibly in response to endogenous norepinephrine.[22]

PATHOPHYSIOLOGY

Malignant hyperthermia is a functional disorder of calcium metabolism with abnormalities in skeletal muscle physiology. However, the site of these changes within the cell remains speculative. Similarities have been found between MH and the porcine stress syndrome[23-26] that have allowed further investigation of the etiology of the syndrome and the metabolic and physiologic changes that occur.

The most plausible theory to explain the MH reaction is loss of calcium control. Exposure to a triggering agent causes a sudden increase in myoplasmic calcium concentration,[27-29] which is followed by a rise from 10^{-7} to 10^{-5} moles/L. in the intracellular free ionized calcium concentration in skeletal muscle during contraction. The site of the primary defect has not been identified but concerns calcium uptake, binding, or release in the sarcoplasmic reticulum (SR).[28, 30, 31] The normal calcium flux that occurs during muscular relaxation is distorted, and results in persistent contraction of the muscle.

The variable severity of MH reactions may depend on the amount of trigger calcium released. If this is insufficient to excite contraction, it may still promote metabolic activity with increased oxygen consumption and production of heat, carbon dioxide, and lactic acid.[27, 28] Energy-dependent enzyme systems in the cell fail, and cellular metabolism is inactivated.[4, 28, 32, 33]

The earliest abnormality is respiratory acidosis with hypercapnia and hypoxemia within two minutes of succinylcholine injection.[34, 35] Tachycardia and cardiac arrhythmias are also early manifestations. After 5 to 10 minutes, muscle temperature may increase, and by 20 minutes, body temperature is elevated.[36] Serum concentrations of potassium, magnesium, calcium, sodium, and chloride then increase and are associated with sympathetic overactivity, hyperglycemia, and increased circulatory catecholamines. The sympathetic responses of the reaction can be blocked by spinal anesthesia[37] and adrenergic blockade[38] without altering the clinical course, while infusions of phenylephrine or noradrenaline with propranolol can induce an MH reaction.[39] Sympathetic dysfunction is, therefore, a secondary rather than primary response in MH but may account for many of the features of the fulminating reaction. The acute episode may be followed by pulmonary edema and electrolyte disturbances. Late complications include hemolysis, myoglobinemia, and myoglobinuria with disseminated intravascular coagulation causing multiple organ failure and death from cerebral or renal failure.

Calcium control is important throughout the body so that skeletal muscle may not be the only tissue altered in MH. Abnormalities may also exist in cardiac muscle, smooth muscle, nerves, platelets, lymphocytes, and pancreatic islet cells.[40]

IDENTIFICATION OF MALIGNANT HYPERTHERMIA SUSCEPTIBILITY

A fulminating MH crisis is incontrovertible evidence of MH susceptibility. However, the diagnosis of a mild or atypical response may be less clear but have important implications for future management. The avoidance of MH crises during anesthesia ultimately relies on preoperative detection of susceptibility.

CLINICAL FEATURES

Susceptible individuals may have a family history of unexplained deaths or complications during general anesthesia. Usually they appear healthy, but common localized muscle abnormalities such as strabismus, ptosis, hernia, and kyphoscoliosis may have an association with MH. However, the King-Denborough syndrome, characterized by musculoskeletal abnormalities, short stature, and mental retardation is constantly linked with MH.[41] Other conditions in which a relationship is suspected include Duchenne muscular dystrophy,[42] nonspecific myopathies,[43] central core disease,[44] heat stroke,[21] sudden infant death syndrome,[20] and neuroleptic malignant syndrome.[19]

Clinical diagnosis of a fulminating reaction (Table 8–1) is based on the acute metabolic changes and muscular rigidity. Otherwise, the earliest detectable signs of increased metabolism are hypoxia and hypercapnia. Thus, continuous end-tidal carbon dioxide monitoring is invaluable in suggesting the possibility of MH.[34, 35] Tachypnea and tachycardia with cardiac arrhythmias, cyanosis, sweating, rigidity, and unstable blood pressure follow. Arterial blood gas analysis will confirm

TABLE 8–1.
Recognition of Malignant Hyperthermia
During General Anesthesia

Clinical
  Tachycardia
  Tachypnea
  Blood pressure instability
  Cardiac arrhythmias
  Cyanosis
  Sweating
  Fever (2°C/hr rise or >42.2°C)
  Fasciculations
  Generalized rigidity
  Localized masseter spasm
  Discolored urine
  Dark blood in wound

Pathophysiological
  Central venous desaturation
  Central venous hypercapnia
  Arterial hypercapnia
  Metabolic acidosis
  Respiratory acidosis
  Hyperkalemia
  Myoglobinemia
  Myoglobinuria
  Elevated CPK

the respiratory and metabolic acidosis. Body temperature is not inevitably elevated. Differential diagnosis in the early stages can be difficult as similar signs may be seen in hyperthyroidism and pheochromocytoma or may be due to technical complications of anesthesia. Masseter muscle rigidity following halothane anesthesia and succinylcholine can precede fulminating MH.[45]

PATHOPHYSIOLOGIC TESTS

Pathophysiologic tests have been applied to the identification of MH susceptibility with limited success. Creatinine phosphokinase (CPK) levels of over 20,000 IU in the perioperative period may be indicative of MH,[46] but there is considerable normal variation, and raised levels are found in muscle disorders[47] and unrelated causes of muscle breakdown. Phosphorylase ratios are sometimes raised,[48] but false positive results are often seen in nonsusceptible patients.[49] Measurement of platelet adenosine triphosphate (ATP) depletion, a test based on the similarity of platelets to skeletal muscle,[50, 51] is a poorly reproducible test.[52] Determination of calcium uptake by the sarcoplasmic reticulum has dubious reliability,[53] while attempts to differentiate MH-susceptible patients on the basis of electrophoresis of muscle proteins give inconsistent results.[54] The tourniquet test depends on enhancement of the postischemic evoked twitch response of the thumb by ulnar nerve stimulation in MH-susceptibe patients, but it is difficult to evaluate.[55, 56]

Histologic examination of muscle biopsy specimens from affected individuals may yield normal results or show nonspecific abnormalities, particularly variation in fiber diameter.[57] The most reliable screening tests developed for MH susceptibility in patients and family members are based on in vitro contracture responses of excised muscle to halothane and caffeine.[58–60] Three diagnostic contracture phenotypes were described by Nelson et al.[61] to relate the contracture responses to the severity of clinical MH. Phenotype H is an unequivocal MH response to 3% halothane; phenotype K shows an equivocal response, requiring a combination of halothane and caffeine to induce contracture; and phenotype N is unequivocally negative.

The interpretation of contracture responses has been inconsistent because of the variability of test procedures in different laboratories and the absence of comparative normal data. A consensus on standardization of testing techniques and reporting has been reached by the European Malignant Hyperpyrexia Group.[62] It recommends static and dynamic contracture testing with halothane and the static cumulative caffeine test. Diagnoses are categorized as MHS, showing a definite susceptibility to MH; MHN, indicating that the individual is not susceptible to MH (but reserved to describe a person from a family known to have MH members); and MHE, an equivocal diagnosis resulting in treating the person clinically as MH susceptible. The MHE category allows for constant review of those cases (1% to 2% of all patients investigated) in which the clinical circumstances are suspicious but unconfirmed by laboratory findings.

Therefore, definitive diagnosis of MH susceptibility is based on clinical reactions and specific muscle contracture tests. The latter have been criticized because they require a substantial amount of muscle, and in the child, these tests leave a disfiguring scar. In view of the excellent prognosis of an unexpected MH crisis, MH-susceptible patients can be managed more confidently by treatment with dantrolene and the comparatively safe nontriggering anesthesia. An expectant policy might, therefore, be appropriate for children exhibiting possible MH reactions under anesthesia, and muscle biopsy might be delayed for some years. It is important that patients who fall into the gray area of uncertain diagnosis are not labeled as MH susceptible without being subjected to careful periodic review.

MASSETER SPASM

Masseter spasm following succinylcholine administration is presumptive evidence of MH susceptibility until excluded by further investigation. Although it must be distinguished from inadequate anesthesia and insufficient relaxation, the masseter rigidity is characterized by a tight trismus without involvement of other muscles.[63] It takes 10 to 20 minutes to resolve but may precede an acute MH episode.[4, 64] Relatively common, it occurs in 1 in 800 children to whom general anesthetics have been administered.[65] However, masseter spasm is limited to children given succinylcholine intravenously during inhalation of halothane, and in this group the incidence may be as high as 1 in 100. No cases have been reported in children below age 1 or over age 11 years.

The significance of masseter spasm in relationship to MH susceptibility has been evaluated by in vitro contracture testing.[27, 66–68] In patients who proved to be MH susceptible, by halothane-induced contractures, masseter spasm was twice as common as in nonsusceptible patients. However, if the muscles are exposed to succinylcholine after halothane administration, then a significant contracture response was obtained in all specimens from patients who exhibited masseter spasm. These studies recognized that half the patients who develop masseter spasm cannot be shown to be MH susceptible. Of these, electromyographic abnormalities consistent with myotonia congenita or myotonic dystrophy could account for the abnormal reaction to succinylcholine in some of the patients tested.[27, 66] These conditions are not constantly associated with MH, and muscle rigidity follows succinylcholine but not halothane administration, but without any hypermetabolic reaction. Other conditions such as polymyositis[69] and rhabdomyolysis after succinylcholine administration may be involved, but a number of cases of masseter spasm remain unexplained.

The association of masseter spasm with MH in 50% of cases warrants a conservative approach to the management of patients exhibiting trismus during halothane and succinylcholine anesthesia.[45, 66, 67] In elective cases, anesthesia should be terminated and MH susceptibility determined according to CPK values (>20,000 IU is suggestive), muscle biopsy, and electromyographic investigation. In emergency situations, it is advisable to discontinue all agents that might trigger MH. At present, it is uncertain whether this will ensure a safe continuation of anesthesia. Moreover, the need for dantrolene treatment is not clear, and an expectant approach is advised.

MANAGEMENT OF AN ACUTE MALIGNANT HYPERTHERMIC REACTION

Recognition of an MH reaction during general anesthesia requires immediate and vigorous treatment. Prompt intervention with withdrawal of volatile agents and institution of intravenous (IV) dantrolene therapy is the essence of a successful treatment regimen (Table 8–2). Supportive measures should be instituted including hyperventilation with 100% oxygen, administration of sodium bicarbonate to correct metabolic acidosis, and active cooling. Cardiac arrhythmias are usually abolished by these measures, but if drug therapy is indicated, the use of procainamide is recommended. Hyperkalemia can be controlled with dextrose and insulin infusions and urine output maintained with diuretics. These immediate and aggressive measures should be followed by control of biochemical factors based on results of serial monitoring of blood gases and electrolytes. Late complications, such as disseminated intravascular coagulopathy and renal failure, require appropriate supportive therapy.

Until dantrolene became available in 1979, the most commonly

TABLE 8–2.
Treatment of Malignant Hyperthermia Crisis*

1. Stop anesthesia and surgery.
2. Change to vapor-free anesthetic machine.
3. Hyperventilate with 100% oxygen.
4. Administer dantrolene sodium (2.5 mg/kg IV initially followed by infusion to a cumulative dose of 10 mg/kg).
5. Monitor ECG, temperature, urine, arterial pressure, central venous pressure, end-tidal CO_2, O_2 saturation.
6. Cool patient.
   Administer iced saline IV, 15 ml/kg; repeat three times.
   Apply ice to body surface.
   Place patient on hypothermia blanket.
   Lavage stomach and body cavities with iced saline.
   Establish extracorporeal circulation or femoral-femoral heat exchange.
   Stop when temperature is less than 38.3°C.
7. Treat arrhythmias (procainamide, IV, 15 mg/kg over 10 min).
8. Correct acidosis (sodium bicarbonate, 1–2 mEq/kg initially, then according to blood gas analysis).
9. Maintain urine output greater than 2 ml/kg/hr (mannitol, 0.125 gm/kg, and/or furosemide, 1 mg/kg; repeat four times if necessary).
10. Treat hyperkalemia (insulin, 0.2 ug/kg, in 50% dextrose 1 ml/kg IV).
11. Treat postoperatively.
    Continue dantrolene orally/IV for 1–3 days.
    Continue monitoring for 48 hr.
    Follow-up family investigations.

*The emergency MH hotline number of the Malignant Hyperthermia Association (USA) is (209) 634–4917. Ask for "Index Zero."

recommended treatment for MH was procaine or procainamide.[70, 71] These drugs had limited therapeutic benefit, which may have been expected from their membrane stabilizing properties. The skeletal muscle relaxant dantrolene was effective in preventing or terminating halothane-induced porcine MH.[72–74] Comparative studies of dantrolene and procainamide[75] demonstrated that dantrolene, 2 mg/kg, blocked the twitch response of muscle in susceptible pigs. Doses equivalent to 0.8 mg/kg in vivo prevented or reversed the halothane-induced contracture responses in MH susceptible human muscle biopsy specimens, while therapeutic doses of procainamide had no effect. Thus, the effectiveness of dantrolene in MH was confirmed for treatment and prophylaxis of MH.

DANTROLENE

Dantrolene (Fig 8–1) is available in bottles of a lyophilized mixture of 20 mg of dantrolene sodium with 3000 mg mannitol and sodium hydroxide to adjust the pH to 9.5. It is reconstituted with 60 ml sterile water to provide a solution of 0.33 mg/ml. Crystals will dissolve more quickly if the bottle is warmed under tap water, but mixing takes several minutes. As the initial dose will require 2 to 3 bottles for a 10-kg child and 7 to 10 bottles for an adult, reconstitution can entail some delay in administration.

Britt[76] has reviewed the contradictory evidence available and concluded that dantrolene, in both normal and MH-susceptible muscle, probably acts to prevent the release of calcium ions from the SR to the myoplasm.

The recommended therapeutic and prophylactic dose of dantrolene of 2.4 mg/kg IV was suggested by studies in pigs[77] and humans.[78] This efficacy of this dose was confirmed by the finding of a multicenter study of the use of intravenous therapy in the acute MH crisis.[79] This study found that the mean dose of dantrolene needed to reverse a clinical MH crisis was 2.5 mg/kg. With prompt administration, all patients survived. However, it is possible that the criteria for recognition of MH were such that a number of patients were misdiagnosed, but others, with clearly hypermetabolic episodes, survived without any adverse effects.

Oral dantrolene has been recommended for preoperative prophylaxis in doses of 1 to 2 mg/kg four times daily for 24 to 48 hours. However, absorption and metabolism of orally administered dantrolene are uncertain, and therapeutic levels are difficult to achieve. Gastrointestinal side effects can be severe, and physical activity is limited by sedation and muscular weakness.

Rather than accept the limitations and risk of side effects of oral therapy, it is preferable to administer dantrolene intravenously immediately before the induction of anesthesia in a dose of 2.5 mg/kg infused over 10 to 15 minutes.[78] Reports of failures of both oral[80, 81] and intravenous dantrolene prophylaxis in the prevention of MH reactions emphasize the importance of adequate dosage, because therapeutic levels may not have been achieved by the dose regimens followed in these cases.

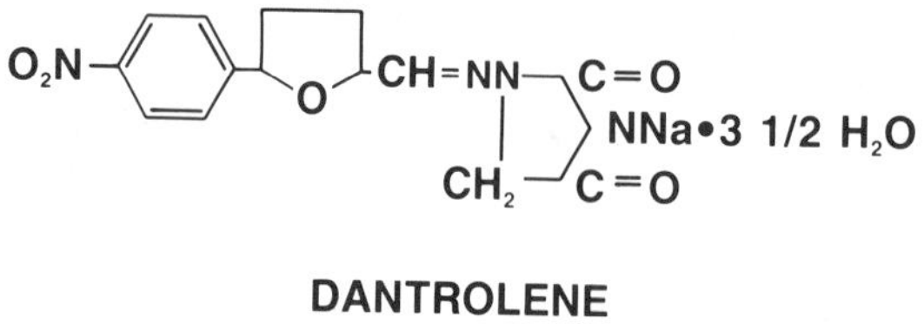

DANTROLENE

FIG 8–1.
Structure of dantrolene.

Treatment of an MH crisis during anesthesia requires prompt and adequate intravenous administration of dantrolene to normalize the clinical signs and symptoms. As soon as MH is diagnosed, dantrolene therapy should be instituted with an initial bolus of 2.5 mg/kg IV followed by repeated doses or an infusion up to a total dose of 10 mg/kg over 5 to 10 minutes. Resolution of the acute MH episode should be followed by an infusion of 0.25 to 0.50 mg/kg or oral dantrolene, 1 to 2 mg four times a day, until there is no likelihood of a further MH reaction. At these dosages, side effects are unusual, but a report of fatal cardiovascular collapse in two pigs during dantrolene administration cautions against the rapid administration of large doses of 10 mg/kg IV,[82] although doses of 1 to 7 mg/kg have been used to treat human MH without complications.[81] Calcium-channel blocking drugs are contraindicated with dantrolene therapy.[83, 84] To avoid myocardial depression due to the accumulation of dantrolene and verapamil, the combination of the two drugs is not recommended for treatment of human MH,[84, 85] and no support exists for the use of verapamil alone. If an antiarrhythmic agent is indicated in combination with dantrolene, procainamide is preferable.[84]

Side effects of dantrolene include venous thrombophlebitis, gastrointestinal upset, muscular weakness, elevation of serum potassium, and hepatic dysfunction.

SUBSEQUENT MANAGEMENT OF MALIGNANT HYPERTHERMIA–SUSCEPTIBLE PATIENTS

Survival of an MH episode should be followed by investigation of the patient and, if necessary, the family to confirm MH susceptibility. Investigations should include a family history to determine any complications relatives may have experienced during anesthesia and careful physical examination to exclude a predisposing condition. If laboratory investigations are inconclusive or unavailable, future management will be based on clinical evidence that the patient is MH susceptible.

Management of MH susceptible patients for elective anesthesia now follows accepted principles to avoid known triggering factors. Recommendations include the use of any of the common local anesthetic agents, including the amide group. General anesthesia should be approached with the minimum of stress and adequate premedication with barbiturates, narcotics, or diazepam. Volatile anesthetic agents should be avoided, and a technique using oxygen and nitrous oxide supplemented with a narcotic is satisfactory. Nondepolarizing muscle relaxants may be used. Pancuronium is established as being satisfactory, but atracurium[86] and vecuronium[87] appear to be safe, although dantrolene may delay recovery from vecuronium neuromuscular blockade.[88] Reversal with atropine and neostigmine at the end of surgery is not contraindicated. Dantrolene prophylaxis should be given intravenously at induction of anesthesia and continued postoperatively by slow intravenous infusion or orally for at least 48 hours.

REFERENCES

1. Denborough MA, Forster JE, Lovell RRH, et al: Anaesthetic deaths in a family. *Br J Anaesth* 1962; 34:395–396.
2. Ording H: Incidence of malignant hyperthermia in Denmark. *Anesth Analg* 1985; 64:700–704.
3. Kinoshita H, Kikuchi H, Yuge O, et al: Statistical review of malignant hyperthermia in Japan. *Hiroshima J Anesth* 1981; 17:53–58.
4. Britt BA, Kalow W: Malignant hyperthermia: A statistical review. *Can Anaesth Soc J* 1970; 17:293–315.
5. Henschel EO, Locher WG: The Wausau study—Malignant hyperthermia in Wisconsin, in Henschel EO (ed): *Malignant Hyperthermia: Current Concepts.* New York, Appleton-Century-Crofts, 1977, pp 3–7.
6. Kalow W, Britt BA, Chan FY: Epidemiology and inheritance of malignant hyperthermia. *Int Anesthesiol Clin* 1979; 17:119–140.
7. Britt BA, Kwong, FHF, Endrenyi L: The clinical and laboratory features of malignant hyperthermia management—A review, in Henschel EO (ed): *Malignant Hyperthermia: Current Concepts.* New York, Appleton-Century-Crofts, 1977.
8. Gronert GA: Malignant hyperthermia. *Semin Anesth* 1983; 2:197–204.
9. New causes of malignant hyperpyrexia, editorial. *Br Med J* 1974; 2:488.
10. Denborough MA, Hird FJR, King JO: Malignant hyperpyrexia. *Br Med J* 1971; 2:636–637.
11. Pan TH, Wollak AR, DeMarco JA: Malignant hyperthermia associated with enflurane anesthesia. *Anesth Analg* 1975; 54:47–49.
12. Boheler J, Hamrick JC Jr, McKnight RL, et al: Isoflurane and malignant hyperthermia, letter. *Anesth Analg* 1982; 61:712–713.
13. Ellis FR, Clarke IMC, Appleyard TN, et al: Malignant hyperpyrexia induced by nitrous oxide and treated with dexamethasone. *Br Med J* 1974; 4:270–271.
14. Roervik S, Stovner J: Ketamine-induced acidosis, fever, and creatinine-kinase rise. *Br Med J* 1974; 2:1384–1385.
15. Britt BA, Webb GE, LeDuc C: Malignant hyperthermia induced by curare. *Can Anaesth Soc J* 1974; 21:371–375.
16. Adragna MG: Medical protocol by habit—The avoidance of amide local

anesthetics in malignant hyperthermia susceptible patients. *Anesthesiology* 1985; 62:99–100.

17. Berkowitz A, Rosenberg H: Femoral block with mepivacaine for muscle biopsy in malignant hyperthermia patients. *Anesthesiology* 1985; 62:651–652.
18. Flewellen EH, Nelson TE: Is theophylline, aminophylline, or caffeine (methylxanthines) contraindicated in malignant hyperthermia susceptible patients? *Anesth Analg* 1983; 52:115–118.
19. Weinberg S, Twersky RS: Neuroleptic malignant syndrome. *Anesth Analg* 1983; 62:845–880.
20. Denborough MA, Galloway GJ, Hopkinson KC: Malignant hyperpyrexia and sudden infant death. *Lancet* 1982; 2:1068–1069.
21. Jardon OM: Physiologic stress, heat stroke, malignant hyperthermia—A perspective. *Milit Med* 1982; 147:8–14.
22. Gronert GA, Thompson RL, Onofrio BM: Human malignant hyperthermia: Awake episodes and correction by dantrolene. *Anesth Analg* 1980; 59:377–378.
23. Hall LW, Trim CM, Woolf N: Further studies of porcine malignant hyperthermia. *Br Med J* 1972; 1:145–148.
24. Harrison GG, Biebuyck JF, Terblanche J, et al: Hyperpyrexia during anaesthesia. *Br Med J* 1968; 3:594.
25. Hall LW, Woolf N, Bradley JWP, et al: Unusual reaction to suxamethonium chloride. *Br Med J* 1966; 4:1305.
26. Harrison GG, Saunders SJ, Biebuyck JF, et al: Anaesthetic-induced malignant hyperpyrexia and a method for its prediction. *Br J Anaesth* 1969; 41:844–855.
27. Flewellen EH, Nelson TE: Masseter spasm induced by succinylcholine in children: Contracture testing for malignant hyperthermia: Report of six cases. *Can Anaesth Soc J* 1982; 29:42–49.
28. Aldrete JA, Britt BA: *Second International Symposium on Malignant Hyperthermia.* New York, Grune & Stratton, 1978.
29. Lopez JR, Alamo L, Caputo C, et al: Intracellular ionized calcium concentration in muscles from humans with malignant hyperthermia. *Muscle Nerve* 1985; 3:355–358.
30. Nelson TE: Abnormality in calcium release from skeletal sarcoplasmic reticulum of pigs susceptible to malignant hyperthermia. *J Clin Invest* 1983; 72:862–870.
31. Rosenberg H, Merrill H: The importance of T tubular function in the pathophysiology of malignant hyperthermia (abstract). *Anesthesiology* 1983; 59:229.
32. Britt BA: Etiology and pathophysiology of malignant hyperthermia. *Fed Proc* 1979; 38:44–48.
33. Lucke JN, Hall GM, Lister D: Porcine malignant hyperthermia. I: Metabolic and physiological changes. *Br J Anaesth* 1976; 48:297–304.
34. Baudendistel L, Goudsouzian NG, Cote CJ, et al: End-tidal CO_2 monitoring: Its use in the diagnosis and management of malignant hyperthermia. *Anaesthesia* 1984; 39:1000–1003.

35. Neubauer KR, Kaufman RD: Another use for mass spectrometry: Detection and monitoring of malignant hyperthermia. *Anesth Analg* 1985; 64:837–839.

36. Hall GM, Bendall JR, Lucke JN, et al: Porcine malignant hyperthermia. II: Heat production. *Br J Anaesth* 1976; 48:305–308.

37. Gronert GA, Milde JH, Theye RA: Role of sympathetic activity in porcine malignant hyperthermia. *Anesthesiology* 1977; 47:411–415.

38. Lister D, Hall GM, Lucke JN: Porcine malignant hyperthermia. III: Adrenergic blockade. *Br J Anaesth* 1976; 48:831–837.

39. Hall GM, Lucke JN, Lister D: Porcine malignant hyperthermia. V: Fatal hyperthermia in the Pietrian pig, associated with the infusion of α-adrenergic agonists. *Br J Anaesth* 1976; 48:855–863.

40. Denborough MA, Warne GL, Moulds RFW, et al: Insulin secretion in malignant hyperpyrexia. *Br Med J* 1974; 3:493–495.

41. Kaplan AM, Bergeson PS, Gregg SA: Malignant hyperthermia associated with myopathy and normal muscle enzymes. *J Pediatr* 1977; 91:431.

42. Brownell AKW, Passuke RT, Elash A, et al: Malignant hyperthermia in Duchenne muscular dystrophy. *Anesthesiology* 1983; 58:180–182.

43. Gronert GA: Malignant hyperthermia. *Anesthesiology* 1980; 53:395–423.

44. Denborough MA, Dennett X, Anderson R, et al: Central-core disease and malignant hyperpyrexia. *Br Med J* 1973; 1:272–273.

45. Rosenberg H, Fletcher JE: Masseter muscle rigidity and malignant hyperthermia susceptibility. *Anesth Analg* 1986; 65:161–164.

46. Ellis FR, Clarke IMC, Modgill M, et al: Evaluation of creatinine phosphokinase in screening patients for malignant hyperpyrexia. *Br Med J* 1975; 3:511–513.

47. Isaacs H, Barlow MB: Malignant hyperpyrexia during anaesthesia: Possible correlation with subclinical myopathy. *Br Med J* 1970; 1:275.

48. Willner JH, Woods DS, Cerri C, et al: Increased myophosphorylase A in malignant hyperthermia. *N Engl J Med* 1980; 303:138–140.

49. Traynor CA, Van Dyke RA, Gronert GA: Phosphorylase ratio and susceptibility to malignant hyperthermia. *Anesth Analg* 1983; 62:324–326.

50. Rosenberg H, Fisher CA, Reed SB, et al: Platelet aggregation in patients susceptible to malignant hyperthermia. *Anesthesiology* 1981; 55:621–624.

51. Giger U, Kaplan RF: Halothane-induced ATP depletion in platelets from patients susceptible to malignant hyperthermia and from controls. *Anesthesiology* 1983; 58:347–352.

52. Solomons CC, McDermott N, Mahowald M: Screening for malignant hyperthermia with platelet bioassay, correspondence. *N Engl J Med* 1980; 303:642.

53. Schwartz L, Rockoff MA, Koka BV: Masseter spasm with anesthesia: Incidence and implications. *Anesthesiology* 1984; 61:772–775.

54. Walsh MP, Brownell AKW, Littman V, et al: Electrophoresis of muscle proteins is not a method for diagnosis of malignant hyperthermia susceptibility. *Anesthesiology* 1986; 64:473–479.

55. Jones PIE, Britt BA, Steward DJ, et al: Tourniquet test as a predictor of malignant hyperthermia susceptibility. *Anesth Analg* 1981; 60:256.
56. Roberts JF, Ryan JF, Ali HH, et al: Abnormally high regional oxygen consumption in malignant hyperthermia patients induced by a non-anesthetic stress (ten minutes ischemia to the upper extremity). *Anesthesiology* 1982; 57:A229.
57. Nelson TE, Schochet SS: Malignant hyperthermia: A disease of specific myofibrotype. *Can Anaesth Soc J* 1982; 29:163–167.
58. Ellis RF, Keaney NP, Harrim DGF, et al: Screening for malignant hyperpyrexia. *Br Med J* 1972; 3:559–561.
59. Moulds RFW, Denborough MA: Identification of susceptibility to malignant hyperpyrexia. *Br Med J* 1974; 2:245–247.
60. Ranklev E, Fletcher R, Blomquist S: Static v. dynamic tests in the in vitro diagnosis of malignant hyperthermia susceptibility. *Br J Anaesth* 1986; 58:646–648.
61. Nelson TE, Flewellen EH, Gloyna DF: Spectrum of susceptibility to malignant hyperthermia—Diagnostic dilemma. *Anesth Analg* 1983; 62:545–552.
62. The European Malignant Hyperthermia Group: A protocol for the investigation of malignant hyperpyrexia (MH) susceptibility. *Br J Anaesth* 1984; 56:1267–1269.
63. Ryan JF: Malignant hyperthermia, in Ryan JF, Todres ID, Cote CJ, et al (eds): *A Practice of Anesthesia for Infants and Children.* New York. Grune & Stratton, 1986, p 245.
64. Donlon JV, Newfield P, Streter FA, et al: Implications of masseter spasm after succinylcholine. *Anesthesiology* 1978; 49:298–301.
65. Schwartz L, Rockoff MA, Koka BV: Masseter spasm with anesthesia: Incidence and implications. *Anesthesiology* 1984; 61:772–775.
66. Ellis FR, Halsall PJ: Suxamethonium spasm: A differential diagnostic conundrum. *Br J Anaesth* 1984; 56:381–384.
67. Flewellen EH, Nelson TE: Halothane-succinylcholine induced masseter spasm: Indicative of malignant hyperthermia susceptibility? *Anesth Analg* 1984; 63:693–697.
68. Fletcher FE, Rosenberg H: In vitro interaction between halothane and succinylcholine in human skeletal muscle: Implications for malignant hyperthermia and masseter muscle rigidity. *Anesthesiology* 1985; 63:190–194.
69. Davies DD: Hypertonic syndrome associated with suxamethonium administration. *Br J Anaesth* 1970; 42:656.
70. Harrison GG: Anaesthetic-induced malignant hyperpyrexia: A suggested method of treatment. *Br Med J* 1971; 3:454–456.
71. Moulds RFW, Denborough MA: Procaine in malignant hyperpyrexia. *Br Med J* 1972; 4:526–528.
72. Lister D: Correction of adverse response to suxamethonium of susceptible pigs. *Br Med J* 1973; 1:208–210.
73. Hall GM, Lucke JN, Lister D: Treatment of porcine malignant hyperther-

mia: A review based on experimental studies. *Anaesthesia* 1975; 30:308–317.

74. Harrison GG: Control of the malignant hyperpyrexic syndrome in MHS swine by dantrolene sodium. *Br J Anaesth* 1975; 47:62–65.
75. Nelson TE, Flewellen EH: Rationale for dantrolene vs procainamide for treatment of malignant hyperthermia. *Anesthesiology* 1979; 50:118–122.
76. Britt BA: Dantrolene. *Can Anaesth Soc J* 1984; 31:61–75.
77. Flewellen EH, Nelson TE: Dantrolene dose response in malignant hyperthermia-susceptible (MHS) swine: Method to obtain prophylaxis and therapeusis. *Anesthesiology* 1980; 52:303–308.
78. Flewellen EH, Nelson TE, Jones WP, et al: Dantrolene dose response in awake man: Implications for management of malignant hyperthermia. *Anesthesiology* 1983; 59:275–280.
79. Kolb ME, Horne ML, Martz R: Dantrolene in human malignant hyperthermia. *Anesthesiology* 1982; 56:254–262.
80. Fitzgibbons DC: Malignant hyperthermia following preoperative oral administration of dantrolene. *Anesthesiology* 1981; 54:73–75.
81. Ruhland G, Hurkle AJ: Malignant hyperthermia after oral and intravenous pretreatment with dantrolene in a patient susceptible to malignant hyperthermia. *Anesthesiology* 1984; 60:159–160.
82. Chapin JW: Asystole after intravenous dantrolene sodium in pigs, correspondence. *Anesthesiology* 1981; 54:527–528.
83. Gallant EM, Foldes FF, Rempel WE, et al: Verapamil is not a therapeutic adjunct to dantrolene in porcine malignant hyperthermia. *Anesth Analg* 1985; 64:601–606.
84. Carter JC, Gergis SD, Carter A, et al: The caffeine-halothane challenge test and calcium blockers. *Anesthesiology* 1983; 59:A226.
85. Durbin CG, Fisher NA, Lynch C III: Cardiovascular effects in dogs of intravenous dantrolene alone and in the presence of verapamil. *Anesthesiology* 1983; 59:A227.
86. Morrell DG, Harrison GG: The screening of atracurium in MHS swine. *Br J Anaesth* 1986; 58:444–446.
87. Buzello W, Williams CH, Chandra P, et al: Vecuronium and porcine malignant hyperthermia. *Anesth Analg* 1985; 64:515–519.
88. Driessen JJ, Wuis EW, Gieden JM: Prolonged vecuronium neuromuscular blockade in a patient receiving oral dantrolene. *Anesthesiology* 1985; 62:523–524.

9

Pharmacology: Antagonists

The use of curare in 19th century Europe was limited to restricting movement in experimental animals. Until 1900, resuscitation of the animals was only possible using artificial ventilation. However, during the course of investigating the action of anticholinesterases on the gut, Pal[1] noticed that spontaneous breathing was restored after injecting physostigmine. When curare was introduced into clinical practice, reversal was seldom required because of the small doses administered,[2] but this practice was associated with an increase in surgical mortality.[3] Antagonism with neostigmine became necessary with the use of large doses of curare, and routine reversal of nondepolarizing relaxants was accepted. Recently, with the introduction of the intermediate-acting relaxants atracurium and vecuronium and the increased use of neuromuscular monitoring, the need for routine reversal has been questioned again.[4]

The pharmacologic principle involved in the reversal of muscle relaxants is the reduction of the effect of competitive blocking drugs by increasing the concentration of the neurotransmitter acetylcholine at the neuromuscular junction. This is usually achieved with anticholinesterases that inhibit acetylcholinesterase.

ANTICHOLINESTERASES

Pharmacology

Physostigmine (eserine), an alkaloid isolated from the calabar bean (esere nut) and used as an "ordeal" poison by West African tribes, was

293

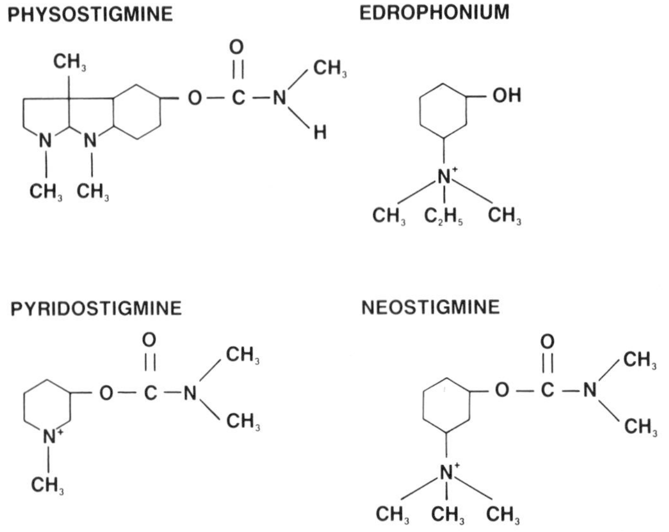

PHYSOSTIGMINE

EDROPHONIUM

PYRIDOSTIGMINE

NEOSTIGMINE

FIG 9–1.
Structure of physostigmine, edrophonium, pyridostigmine, and neostigmine.

the model for the development of many anticholinesterase compounds including edrophonium, neostigmine, and pyridostigmine. Physostigmine (Fig 9–1), a tertiary amine, crosses the blood-brain barrier and thus is not used in the clinical reversal of relaxants. Although it may be effective in counteracting overdosage with diazepam,[5] ketamine,[6] or monoamine oxidase inhibitors,[7] it will not be discussed further as doses up to 4 mg do not antagonize the relaxants in man.[8] Galanthamine, another tertiary amine, is an anticholinesterase that has been used to reverse the respiratory depression of opioids. It has a prolonged duration of action because of a long terminal half-life.[9] Its central effects limit its use in the reversal of muscle relaxants.

The structures of edrophonium, neostigmine, and pyridostigmine are shown in Figure 9–1. All are quaternary ammonium compounds, ionized, water soluble, and, therefore, excreted via the kidney.

Mechanism of Action

The active surface of the acetylcholinesterase molecule, where acetylcholine is hydrolyzed, consists of an anionic and an esteratic site.[10] Edrophonium combines by an electrostatic bond at the anionic site and by a hydrogen bond at the esteratic site (Fig 9–2), and these bonds are rapidly broken. Neostigmine and pyridostigmine are also attached at the anionic and esteratic sites but produce a longer-lasting inhibition.

Eventually, they are hydrolyzed by cholinesterase in a manner similar to acetylcholine but more slowly (half-life of 30 minutes vs. 42 microseconds for acetylcholine).[11, 12] The interaction of neostigmine and pyridostigmine with acetylcholinesterase inactivates them whereas edrophonium is unaffected during the inhibition.

Irreversible anticholinesterases have been developed that make permanent bonds with acetylcholinesterase. Activity can then only be restored by regeneration of the enzyme. They are used as insecticides (parathion, naphthyl carbamates) and for chemical warfare (sarin, soman, tabun).[11]

There is considerable controversy whether the reversal of nondepolarizing relaxants is achieved only by inhibition of acetylcholinesterase or by other actions at the neuromuscular junction. In the presence of neostigmine, a single nerve impulse results in a brief tetanus instead of a twitch. This is most likely a presynaptic event. Neostigmine-induced nerve terminal depolarization often reaches threshold after a single nerve impulse. This may pass antidromically to involve other nerve terminals of the motor unit and cause repetitive firing.[13–16]

Because the anticholinesterases also produce direct depolarization

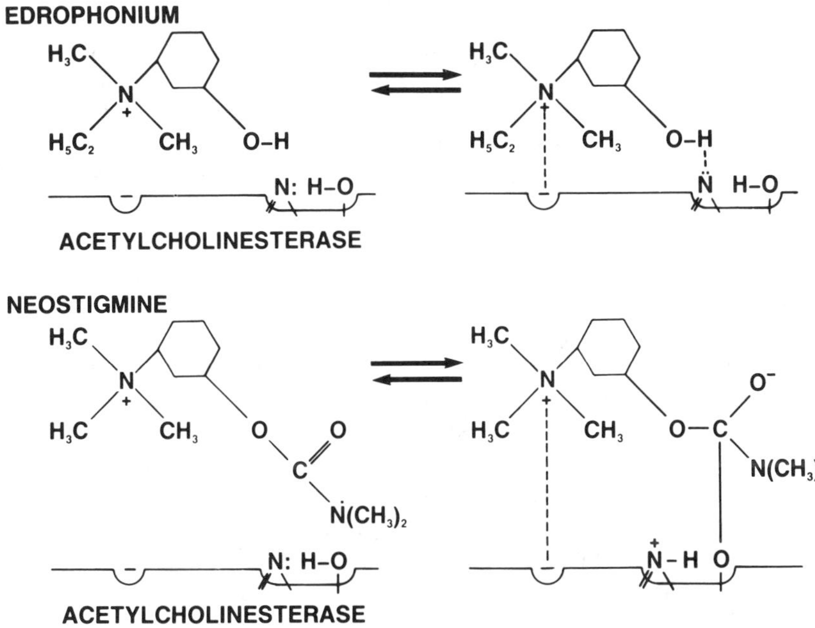

FIG 9–2.
Binding of edrophonium and neostigmine to acetylcholinesterase.

of motor nerve terminals and of postsynaptic receptors, they are in direct competition with the muscle relaxants. When muscle relaxants are absent or when their action has almost ceased, a brief reduction in neuromuscular transmission may occur.[17] Finally, anticholinesterases may increase the mobilization and the release of acetylcholine.[15, 16] Thus, the antagnosim of curare-like relaxants may result from a combination of actions at the nerve terminal and postjunctional receptor as well as from inhibition of acetylcholinesterase.

Pharmacokinetics

Assays for the anticholinesterases that enable the determination of distribution, metabolism, and excretion are now available. Despite individual variation of response to anticholinesterases, assay insensitivity, and the small numbers of persons so far studied, prediction of activity can be made in normal and diseased states. The results of several studies from one laboratory are shown in Table 9–1.

The volumes of distribution, central (V_1) and steady state (V_{dss}), are larger than the plasma and extracellular fluid volumes, respectively, and more than twice the values found for nondepolarizing muscle relaxants (see Chapter 5). The anticholinesterases are polar compounds, and this would be expected to limit diffusion across cell membranes. These larger volumes represent tissue localization such as binding to various proteins. Plasma clearances (Cp) are more rapid than for the long-acting relaxants and result in shorter elimination half-lives in spite of larger volumes of distribution. Surprisingly, the pharmacokinetic behavior of edrophonium is similar to that of neostigmine and pyridostigmine. Indeed, any variations in clinical activity among the reversal agents cannot be based upon pharmacokinetic differences. In renal failure, plasma clearances are decreased and elimination half-lives increased for all anticholinesterases. Thus, plasma concentrations decrease more slowly (Fig 9–3), which suggests that reparalysis as a result of proportionately greater prolongation of action of the relaxants compared with the antagonists[18] cannot be supported by pharmacokinetic alterations.

Neostigmine and pyridostigmine are metabolized to 3–hydroxy phenyl trimethyl ammonium (PTMA) and 3–hydroxy-N-methyl pyridinium (MP) during inhibition of cholinesterase. The latter has no effect as a relaxant antagonist, and PTMA has only weak reversal activity.[19]

TABLE 9–1.
Mean Pharmacokinetic Variables (±SD) of Neostigmine, Edrophonium, and Pyridostigmine in Normal and Renal Failure Patients*

ANTAGONIST	PATIENT	$t_{1/2\alpha}$, MIN	$t_{1/2\beta}$, MIN	V_1, L/KG	V_{dss}, L/KG	C_p, ML/KG/ MIN
Neostigmine	Normal	3.4 ± 1.1	77 ± 47	0.2 ± 0.07	0.7 ± 0.2	9.2 ± 2.6
	Renal failure	2.5 ± 0.4	181 ± 54	0.42 ± 0.2	1.6 ± 0.2	7.8 ± 2.6
Edrophonium	Normal	7.2 ± 3.9	110 ± 34	0.32 ± 0.09	1.1 ± 0.2	9.6 ± 2.7
	Renal failure	—	206 ± 62	—	0.7 ± 0.1	2.7 ± 1.4
Pyridostigmine	Normal	6.8 ± 1.1	112 ± 12	0.3 ± 0.1	1.1 ± 0.3	8.6 ± 1.7
	Renal failure	3.9 ± 3.1	379 ± 162	0.2 ± 0.1	1.0 ± 0.1	2.1 ± 0.6

*Adapted from references 117–120.

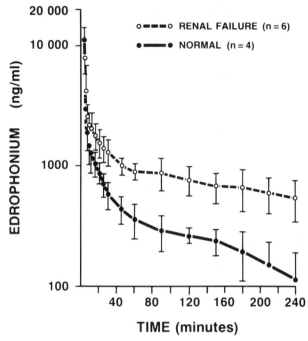

FIG 9–3.
Plasma clearance of edrophonium in patients with renal failure. (From Morris RB, Cronnelly R, Miller RD, et al: Pharmacokinetics of edrophonium in anephric and renal transplant patients. *Br J Anaesth* 1981; 53:1311–1314. Used by permission.)

Potency

The potency of the anticholinesterase agents in antagonizing neuromuscular blocking drugs depends on the circumstances of the paralysis. Potency varies with different relaxants and their modes of administration, the extent of spontaneous recovery, and age of recipient. The method of measurement of neuromuscular activity used may also influence the assessment of reversal.

Recently, dose-response curves have been constructed from data obtained during reversal of a block[20, 21] produced by a bolus dose of pancuronium. One of three doses of either edrophonium or neostigmine was given at 10% recovery of twitch activity (Fig 9–4). The log dose-response curves were parallel, and neostigmine was found to be 16 times more potent than edrophonium. Previously, dose-response curves had been produced after giving edrophonium, neostigmine, or pyridostigmine during the course of the administration of d-tubocurarine infused continuously at a rate to maintain 90% neuromuscular blockade.[22] Dose-response curves for edrophonium were flatter than those for neostigmine or pyridostigmine. Eighty percent antagonism was achieved with doses of edrophonium (0.5 μg/kg) that were about 12 times larger than for neostigmine (0.043 mg/kg), and the duration of antagonism achieved with edrophonium was only slightly shorter than after neostigmine or pyridostigmine (Fig 9–5). Neostigmine was found to be approximately five times as potent as pyridostigmine.

Actions at Other Sites

Cardiovascular Activity

The most important cardiovascular effect seen in man during reversal of the neuromuscular relaxants is bradycardia that results from muscarinic stimulation of the heart. At higher doses in animals, a variety of effects may follow direct and indirect actions on the muscarinic receptors and ganglia.

Traditionally, atropine has been used as the anticholinergic agent to prevent bradycardia. When equipotent doses of antagonist are used, the atropine requirement for pyridostigmine is similar to that of neostigmine,[23] but the requirement is reduced by half when edrophonium is used[22] (Fig 9–6).

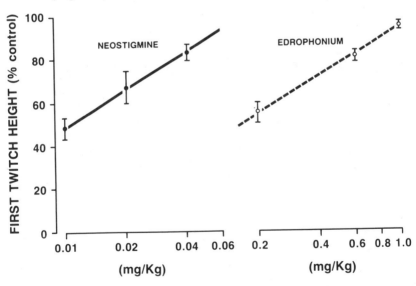

FIG 9–4.
Dose-response curves for neostigmine *(left)* and edrophonium *(right)* in the reversal of pancuronium. (From Breen PJ, Doherty WG, Donati F, et al: The potencies of edrophonium and neostigmine as antagonists of pancuronium. *Anesthesia* 1985; 40:844–847. Used by permission.)

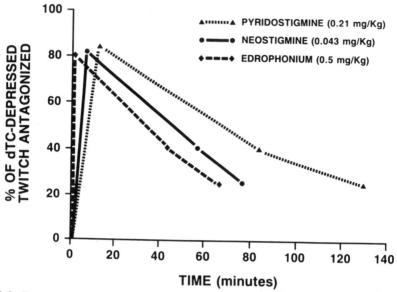

FIG 9–5.
Duration of antagonism of approximately equipotent doses of edrophonium, neostigmine or pyridostigmine during the course of an infusion of *d*-tubocurarine (dTC). (From Cronnelly R, Morris RB, Miller RD: Edrophonium: Duration of action and atropine requirement in humans during halothane anesthesia. *Anesthesiology* 1982; 57:261–266. Used by permission.)

Atropine vs. Glycopyrrolate.—A number of anesthetic deaths[24, 25] followed the bradycardic action of neostigmine so it became common practice to administer atropine 2 to 3 minutes before the anticholinesterase to "protect" the heart.[26] Some practitioners persist with this practice, although it has been demonstrated that when given together, a moderate increase in heart rate precedes a moderate bradycardia.[27] Clearly, the atropine acts on the heart before neostigmine.

Several methods have been tried to avoid acute alterations of heart rate during reversal. When atropine is given together with neostigmine, heart rate changes are reduced if the mixture is given slowly (over 3 minutes)[28] and in the presence of enflurane rather than halothane both in adults[29] and children.[30]

The introduction of the slower-acting glycopyrrolate has made it possible to match the time scale of action of the anticholinergic with the anticholinesterase agent. Glycopyrrolate is a good choice when combined with neostigmine[31, 32] (Fig 9–7) or pyridostigmine.[33] Similarly, the rapid onset of action of atropine is better suited to edrophonium.[22, 34] The use of glycopyrrolate with neostigmine is particularly appropriate in the elderly[35] or those with cardiac disease.[36] It seems that the problems described following administration of the mixtures of anticholinergic and anticholinesterase were caused either by using too little atropine[24, 25] or by their administration during respiratory acidosis.[8] Most anesthetists now administer these drugs in a combination.[37]

Gastrointestinal Activity

Anticholinesterases produce an increase in bowel activity when given either together with or after anticholinergics.[38, 39] It has been suggested that such activity may, in part, be responsible for anastamotic leakage, particularly of ileorectal anastamoses.[40] The definitive experiment has yet to be performed. Although it was found that the incidence of anastomotic dehiscence following colon resection was 23% with relaxants and their reversal compared with 7.4% with spinal analgesia, the difference was not statistically significant.[41] Also, the risk of res-

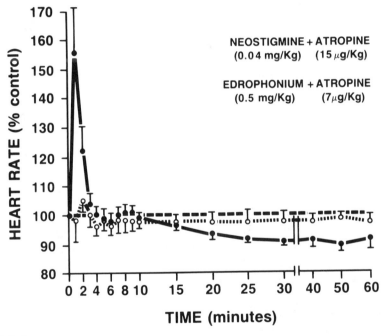

FIG 9–6.
Heart rate changes following equipotent doses of neostigmine (solid line) and edrophonium (small dashed line) with atropine. (From Cronnelly R, Morris RB, Miller RD: Edrophonium: Duration of action and atropine requirement in humans during halothane anesthesia. *Anesthesiology* 1982; 57:261–266. Used by permission.)

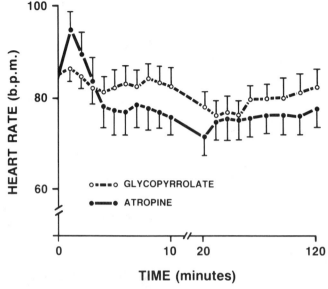

FIG 9–7.
Heart rate changes following reversal with neostigmine (50 µg/kg) with either atropine (20 µg/kg) or glycopyrrolate (10 µg/kg). (From Mirakhur RK, Jones CJ, Dundee JW: Heart rate changes following reversal of neuromuscular block with glycopyrrolate or atropine given before or with neostigmine. *Indian J Anaesth* 1981; 29:83–87. Used by permission.)

piratory insufficiency when the action of long-acting competitive relaxants was not reversed was too great to recommend the avoidance of antagonism in this situation; atracurium and vecuronium may have changed the situation.

Neuromuscular Disorders

Anticholinesterases increase the concentration of acetylcholine at the neuromuscular junction so that problems similar to those associated with succinylcholine might be anticipated.[42, 43] It follows that anticholinesterases should be avoided in patients who have conditions for which succinylcholine is contraindicated. This suspicion has not been supported. Most reports describe the uneventful use of nondepolarizing relaxants and their antagonists in myotonia, although Buzello, et al.[44] observed intensification of paralysis after administration of neostigmine in one patient. They also showed that tonic muscular contraction was induced by a small dose of neostigmine (0.5 mg) in a patient with progressive muscular dystrophy. Clearly, patients with neurologic or neuromuscular disease may demonstrate abnormal reactions to neuromuscular blocking drugs and their antagonists. Generally, problems are more severe after succinylcholine administration so it should be avoided. At present there is insufficient evidence to incriminate the competitive relaxants or their antagonists, particularly if their effects are titrated using neuromuscular stimulation. The introduction of the new relaxant drugs atracurium and vecuronium, which are associated with rapid recovery, may allow anticholinesterases to be omitted.

Anticholinesterase agents remain the first line of treatment for patients with myasthenia gravis[45] (see Chapter 12). Dosage remains empirical so that the operative management requires careful assessment of neuromuscular activity to avoid the Scylla of myasthenic weakness and the Charybdis of cholinergic crisis. Although several authors have described the "safe" use of small doses of muscle relaxants,[46-50] most anesthetists have avoided them to prevent potential problems with the relaxants and their antagonists. Muscle relaxation in these patients is usually easy to achieve with inhalational anesthetic agents.

Clinical Use

Nondepolarizing neuromuscular blocking drugs can be antagonized with edrophonium, neostigmine, or pyridostigmine. Understanding the pharmacology of these anticholinesterases, particularly with regard to potency, metabolism, and clearance, has encouraged more logical use. When given in equipotent doses at a time when spontaneous recovery of neuromuscular activity is well established, the most important difference among them is in the onset of action. Edrophonium is the quickest and pyridostigmine the slowest[51-56] (Fig 9-8). When train-of-four stimulation is used for the same degree of antagonism of first-twitch depression, the train-of-four fade is reversed more with edrophonium than neostigmine, which is superior to pyridostigmine[57] (Fig 9-9). It has been suggested that these differences represent presynaptic activity for edrophonium and postsynaptic predominance for pyridostigmine.[58] It might be expected that a combination of antagonists having different sites of action would be synergistic. They are not. Combinations of edrophonium and neostigmine or pyridostigmine have only additive effects.[20, 59] Recently, it has been suggested that neostigmine is more effective when given in divided doses[60], i.e., "priming," but this report awaits confirmation.

Satisfactory reversal of the effect of muscle relaxants in children is particularly important because of the severe consequences of respiratory inadequacy. Fortunately, when given on a weight-for-weight basis, the reversal of nondepolarizing neuromuscular blocking drugs is more rapid than in adults and is achieved more rapidly with edrophonium than neostigmine.[61] These differences are not the result of pharmaco-kinetic changes[62, 63] but may reflect altered responses of the neuro-muscular junction or a more rapid circulation time in infants with diversion of a greater portion of the cardiac output to the muscles. Alternatively, the differences in children may simply represent more rapid spontaneous recovery from the effect of the relaxant in the young.

Thus, for a recovering neuromuscular block, any of the three anti-cholinesterases is effective in restoring neuromuscular activity. Differences in onset time and cardiovascular activity can be observed, but when used in equipotent dosage (neostigmine, 2.5 mg; pyridostigmine, 12.5 mg; and edrophonium, 40 mg are equipotent), all are effective when spontaneous recovery is well established. The greater the degree of neuromuscular block, the more difficult it is to antagonize. Neostig-

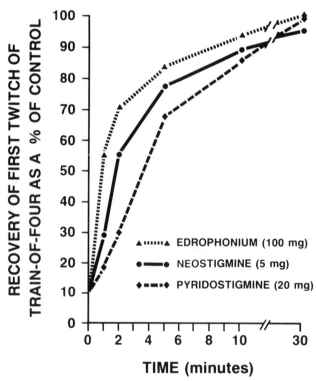

FIG 9–8.
Onset of action of edrophonium, neostigmine, and pyridostigmine in the reversal of pan-curonium-induced neuromuscular blockade. (From Cronnelly R: Muscle relaxant antagonists. *Semin Anaesth* 1985; 4:31–40. Used by permission.)

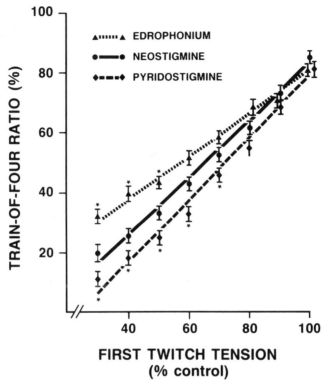

FIG 9–9.
Train-of-four ratio vs. first twitch tension after reversal of pancuronium with edrophonium, neostigmine, or pyridostigmine. (From Donati F, Ferguson A, Bevan DR: Twitch depression and train-of-four ratio after antagonism of pancuronium with edrophonium, neostigmine, or pyridostigmine. *Anesth Analg* 1983; 62:314–316. Used by permission.)

mine is more effective in antagonizing intense neuromuscular block (>90%) whether recovery is assessed by single twitch or train-of-four. This has now been confirmed using roughly equipotent doses of edrophonium and neostigmine in antagonizing atracurium,[64–69] vecuronium,[66, 69, 70] and pancuronium.[71]

Factors Affecting Reversal of Blockade
Extent of Spontaneous Recovery.—Trial and error have shown that neostigmine in doses of 2 to 3 mg (or its equivalent for edrophonium and pyridostigmine) will reverse most neuromuscular blocks.[72, 73] However, the more intense the block, the longer will recovery take.[68] When single-twitch tension has recovered to more than 20% of control or when train-of-four stimulation demonstrates four visible twitches, the

block is easily reversed. More intense blocks may still be reversible with larger doses of anticholinesterase, but total, 100%, blocks may be irreversible.[74] There is seldom any advantage in giving doses in excess of the equivalent of neostigmine, 5 mg/70 kg. Complete blocks induced with atracurium or vecuronium cannot be reversed rapidly. Thus, their activity cannot be made to mimic the time course of succinylcholine by giving anticholinesterases shortly after their administration.

Choice of Relaxant.—Gallamine is reversed by neostigmine more slowly than is *d*-tubocurarine or pancuronium whether the reversal agent is administered in a single bolus (0.05 mg/kg)[75] or by small doses (0.25 mg) repeated every 3 minutes.[73] Dose-response curves for edrophonium, neostigmine, or pyridostigmine have been obtained during reversal of 90% neuromuscular blockade by pancuronium or d-tubocurarine. The ED50 values required for all these antagonists to reverse d-tubocurarine, were similar but slightly greater than those obtained to reverse pancuronium (Table 9–2).

Atracurium and vecuronium have more rapid rates of spontaneous recovery so that the recovery after neostigmine appears to be enhanced.[76–78] However, antagonism with neostigmine of neuromuscular block during the course of a vecuronium infusion is no more rapid than with pancuronium,[79] which suggests that enhanced recovery after a bolus injection simply represents more rapid spontaneous recovery. Recovery after these intermediate agents may be so rapid that the need for reversal is obviated.

Pharmacokinetic Factors.—Anticholinesterases reverse neuromuscular blocking drugs (NMBDs) by accelerating spontaneous recovery. Decreased plasma clearance of relaxants in renal or hepatic failure increases the elimination half-life and delays spontaneous recovery. Thus, reversal appears to be delayed in these situations. However, the block, when antagonized, produces complete recovery that is sustained.[80] Recurarization[81] does not occur. Similarly, decreased clear-

TABLE 9–2.
ED50 Values Obtained From Dose-Response Curves in
Antagonizing Pancuronium and *d*-Tubocurarine

ANTAGONIST	PANCURONIUM	*d*-TUBOCURARINE	*p*
	ED50, mg/kg		
Neostigmine	0.013 ± 0.0015	0.017 ± 0.0012	NS
Pyridostigmine	0.085 ± 0.0054	0.11 ± 0.005	<.001
Edrophonium	0.17 ± 0.024	0.27 ± 0.027	<.006

ance of relaxants in the elderly[82] may produce an apparent delay in reversal, whereas antagonism of atracurium and vecuronium is rapid.

Drug Interactions.—The action of neuromuscular relaxants may be potentiated by many drugs including antibiotics, anesthetic vapors, local anesthetic agents, and calcium-channel blocking drugs (see Chapter 13). Administration of anticholinesterase agents will only antagonize the block produced by the relaxants so that overall recovery may be impaired, and this has been confirmed, at least for enflurane.[83] However, neuromuscular blockades produced by combinations of pancuronium and lidocaine or verapamil appear to be reversed with edrophonium as completely as similar blocks obtained by pancuronium alone.[84, 85]

Neuromuscular blockade induced by a sequence of depolarizing and nondepolarizing relaxants is complicated but predictable. Succinylcholine antagonizes a nondepolarizing block before its own depolarizing block develops. This can be observed when succinylcholine is administered after "precurarization"[86] or at the end of surgery when used to assist peritoneal closure. The action of succinylcholine is prolonged considerably if it is administered after neostigmine and pyridostigmine because they[87, 88] but not edrophonium[89] also inhibit plasma cholinesterase. Usually phase II succinylcholine block can be antagonized with anticholinesterases.[90, 91] However, the prolonged paralysis associated with abnormal plasma cholinesterase cannot be antagonized despite a train-of-four appearance typical of nondepolarizing relaxants[92, 93] (see Chapter 7).

Acid-Base and Electrolyte Imbalance.—"Neostigmine-resistant curarization" was a description given to the state of prolonged cardio-respiratory insufficiency that occurred in ill, cachectic patients after major surgery[94] but that appeared to respond to sodium bicarbonate.[95] Subsequently, controlled animal studies demonstrated incomplete antagonism by neostigmine of blocks produced by d-tubocurarine and pancuronium during respiratory acidosis or metabolic alkalosis.[96, 97] This has been confirmed in man during hypercapnia[98] and may have considerable importance in the postoperative period in patients with residual anesthesia, narcotic analgesia, and respiratory insufficiency.

Hypokalemia, hypermagnesemia, and hypocalcemia may be associated with prolonged relaxant action and, thus, an apparent delay in recovery after reversal.[99, 100] Cats made hypokalemic by chlorothiazide administration had increased sensitivity to pancuronium, and the amount of neostigmine required to antagonize the block was also increased.[101]

4–AMINOPYRIDINE

4–Aminopyridine antagonizes nondepolarizing NMBDs by increasing transmitter release. This occurs as a result of a decrease in potassium conductance that prolongs the duration of the nerve action potential leading to greater calcium influx and increased acetylcholine release.[102] Given alone, in man, it has a weak, slow, anticurare effect, and its use is limited by restlessness, excitation, and confusion due to its crossing of the blood-brain barrier. However, in smaller doses, it has been shown to potentiate neostigmine and to antagonize the neuromuscular blockade produced by antibiotics[103] as well as by muscle relaxants.[104] Clinical use is limited because of the narrow therapeutic index.[105]

GERMINE MONOACETATE

Germine monoacetate (GMA), a *Veratrum* alkaloid, has been shown to antagonize depolarizing and nondepolarizing neuromuscular blockade.[106, 107] Its mode of action is uncertain. In vitro experiments of nerve-muscle preparations in the presence of succinylcholine or *d*-tubocurarine demonstrate repetitive end-plate potentials followed by a repetitive action potential in response to a single indirect stimulus. The effects it produces are not the result of alteration in transmitter release or activity. Although it has been suggested that GMA may be useful in restoring neuromuscular activity in myasthenia gravis and the Eaton-Lambert syndrome and in antagonizing neuromuscular blocking drugs, it has not been introduced into clinical practice.

THE ADEQUACY OF REVERSAL

The purpose of antagonizing neuromuscular blockade is to restore neuromuscular activity. Thus, it is disturbing to realize the high incidence of residual curarization of patients on arrival in the recovery room. Viby-Mogensen et al. found in Scandinavia that 24% of patients could not sustain head lift for 5 seconds, and 42% had a train-of-four ratio (TOFR) of less than 0.7.[108] Similarly, 21 of 100 patients in Australia had a TOFR of less than 0.7 on arrival in the recovery room after surgery.[109]

The goals of reversal are the reestablishment of spontaneous respiration and the ability to protect the airway. In the conscious, co-operative patient, many crude tests have been recommended including

TABLE 9–3.
Correlation Between Tests of Neuromuscular Activity and Respiratory Function*

RESPIRATORY FUNCTION	NEUROMUSCULAR FUNCTION
Normal tidal volume	Reduced twitch height and sustained tetanus at 30 Hz
Normal expiratory flow and vital capacity	Normal train-of-four
Normal inspiratory force	Sustained tetanus at 100 Hz
Normal head lift and hand grip	Sustained tetanus at 200 Hz

*Adapted from Miller RD: Antagonism of neuromuscular blockade. *Anesthesiology* 1976; 44:318–329.

sustained head lift for 5 seconds, tongue protrusion, sustained arm lift for 45 seconds,[110] and in children an ability to lift the leg off the bed.[111] Difficulties occur in the assessment of patients who are not awake. However, several studies have correlated clinical tests, respiratory measurement, and neuromuscular stimulation[112–115] (Table 9–3). Most indices obtained during spontaneous recovery from curare blockade have returned to normal when the TOFR exceeds 0.7, and this end point is used for the adequacy of reversal. However, without appropriate transducers, such a small decrement is difficult to detect clinically so that residual weakness should be anticipated until the response to TOF stimulation is fully restored.

The safe use of neuromuscular relaxants is dependent on the accurate titration of the relaxants and their antagonists with the help of neuromuscular monitoring. Too often monitoring stops at the end of surgery, and patients are at greatest risk in the recovery room in an environment where monitoring and personnel may be in short supply.

REFERENCES

1. Pal J: Physostigmin ein gegengift des curare. *Zentralbl Physiol* 1900; 14:255–258.
2. Griffith HR, Johnson GE: The use of curare in general anesthesia. *Anesthesiology* 1942; 3:418–420.
3. Beecher HK, Todd DP: A study of the deaths associated with anesthesia and surgery. *Ann Surg* 1954; 140:2–34.
4. Payne JP, Hughes R: Atracurium in anaesthetized man. *Br J Anaesth* 1981; 53:1366.
5. Larson GF, Hurlbert BJ, Wingard DW: Physostigmine reversal of diazepam-induced depression. *Anesth Analg* 1977; 56:348–351.
6. Toro-Matos A, Rendon-Platas AM, Avila-Valdez E, et al: Physostigmine antagonizes ketamine. *Anesth Analg* 1980; 59:764–767.
7. Johnson PB: Physostigmine in tricyclic antidepressant overdose. *J Am Coll Emerg Physicians* 1976; 5:443–445.

8. Riding JE, Robinson JS: The safety of neostigmine. *Anaesthesia* 1961; 16:346–354.

9. Westra P, van Thiel MSJ, Vermeer GA, et al: Pharmacokinetics of galanthamine (a long-acting anticholinesterase drug) in anaesthetized patients. *Br J Anaesth* 1986; 58:1303–1307.

10. Kitz RJ: The chemistry of anticholinesterase activity. *Acta Anaesthesiol Scand* 1964; 8:197–218.

11. Wilson IB, Harrison MA: Turnover number of acetylcholinesterase. *J Biol Chem* 1961; 236:2292–2295.

12. Koelle GB: Anticholinesterase agents, in Goodman LS, Gilman A (eds): *The Pharmacological Basis of Therapeutics.* New York, Macmillan Publishing Co, 1975, pp 445–466.

13. Blaber LC, Bowman WC: Studies on the repetitive discharges evoked in ulnar nerve and skeletal muscle after injection of anticholinesterase drugs. *Br J Pharmacol* 1963; 20:326–344.

14. Riker WF, Standaert FG: The action of facilitatory drugs and acetylcholine on neuromuscular transmission. *Ann NY Acad Sci* 1966; 135:163–176.

15. Riker WF, Okamoto MO: Pharmacology of motor nerve terminals. *Ann Rev Pharmacol* 1969; 9:173–208.

16. Blaber LC: The mechanism of the facilitatory action of edrophonium in cat skeletal muscle. *Br J Pharmacol* 1972; 46:498–507.

17. Payne JP, Hughes R, Al Azari S: Neuromuscular blockade by neostigmine in anaesthetized man. *Br J Anaesth* 1980; 52:69–76.

18. Miller RD, Cullen DJ: Renal failure and postoperative respiratory failure: Recurarization. *Br J Anaesth* 1976; 48:253–256.

19. Hennis PJ, Cronnelly R, Sharma M, et al: Metabolites of neostigmine and pyridostigmine do not contribute to antagonism of neuromuscular blockade in the dog. *Anesthesiology* 1984; 61:534–539.

20. Breen PJ, Doherty WG, Donati F, et al: The potencies of edrophonium and neostigmine as antagonists of pancuronium. *Anaesthesia* 1985; 40:844–847.

21. Donati F, McCarroll SM, Antzaka C, et al: Dose-response relationships for edrophonium and d-tubocurarine. *Can Anaesth Soc J* 1986; 33:S87–S88.

22. Cronnelly R, Morris RB, Miller RD: Edrophonium: Duration of action and atropine requirement in humans during halothane anesthesia. *Anesthesiology* 1982; 57:261–266.

23. Fogdall RP, Miller RD: Antagonism of d-tubocurarine and pancuronium-induced blockade by pyridostigmine in man. *Anesthesiology* 1973; 39:504–509.

24. Clutton Brock J: Death following neostigmine. *Br Med J* 1949; 1:1007.

25. MacIntosh RR: Death following injection of neostigmine. *Br Med J* 1949; 1:1852.

26. Bain WA, Broadbent JL: Death following neostigmine. *Br J Med* 1949; 1:1137.

27. Rosner V, Kepes ER, Foldes FF: The effects of atropine and neostigmine on heart rate and rhythm. *Br J Anaesth* 1971; 43:1066–1074.
28. Harper KW, Bali IM, Gibson FM, et al: Reversal of neuromuscular block: Heart rate changes with slow injection of neostigmine and atropine mixtures. *Anaesthesia* 1984; 39:772–775.
29. Samra SK, Pandit UA, Pandit SK, et al: Modification by halogenated anaesthetics of chronotropic response during reversal of neuromuscular blockade. *Can Anaesth Soc J* 1983; 30:48–52.
30. Satwant KS, Cohen PJ: Modifications of chronotropic response to anticholinergics by halogenated anaesthetics in children. *Can Anaesth Soc J* 1980; 27:540–545.
31. Mirakhur RK, Dundee JW, Jones CJ, et al: Reversal of neuromuscular blockade: Dose determination studies with atropine and glycopyrrolate given before or in a mixture with neostigmine. *Anesth Analg* 1981; 60:557–562.
32. Mirakhur RK, Jones CJ, Dundee JW: Heart rate changes following reversal of neuromuscular block with glycopyrrolate or atropine given before or with neostigmine. *Indian J Anaesth* 1981; 29:83–87.
33. Mirakhur RK, Briggs LP, Clarke RSJ, et al: Comparison of atropine and glycopyrrolate in a mixture with pyridostigmine for the antagonism of neuromuscular block. *Br J Anaesth* 1981; 53:1315–1320.
34. Mirakhur RK: Antagonism of the muscarinic effects of edrophonium with atropine or glycopyrrolate. *Br J Anaesth* 1985; 57:1216–1220.
35. Mirakhur RK: Antagonism of neuromuscular block in the elderly: A comparison of atropine and glycopyrrolate in a mixture with neostigmine. *Anaesthesia* 1985; 40:254–258.
36. Muravchick S, Owens LD, Felts JA: Glycopyrrolate and cardiac dysrhythmias in geriatric patients after reversal of neuromuscular block. *Can Anaesth Soc J* 1979; 26:22–25.
37. Mirakhur RK, Clarke RSJ, Dundee JW, et al: Anticholinergic drugs in anaesthesia: A survey of the present position. *Anaesthesia* 1978; 33:133–138.
38. Hannington-Kiff JG: Timing of atropine and neostigmine in the reversal of muscle relaxants. *Br Med J* 1969; 1:418–420.
39. Wilkins JL, Hardcastle JD, Mann CV, et al: Effects of neostigmine and atropine on motor activity of ileum, colon and rectum of anaesthetized subjects. *Br Med J* 1970; 1:793–794.
40. Bell CMA, Lewis CB: Effect of neostigmine on integrity of ileorectal anastamoses. *Br Med J* 1968; 2:587–588.
41. Aitkenhead AR, Wishart HY, Brown DA: High spinal block for large bowel anastomosis: A retrospective study. *Br J Anaesth* 1978; 50:177–183.
42. Ellis FR: Inherited muscle disease. *Br J Anaesth* 1980; 52:153–164.
43. Mitchell MM, Ali HH, Savarese JJ: Myotonia and neuromuscular blocking agents. *Anesthesiology* 1978; 49:44–48.

44. Buzello W, Krieg H, Schlickewei A: Hazards of neostigmine in patients with neuromuscular disorders. *Br J Anaesth* 1982; 54:529–534.

45. Drachman DB: Myasthenia gravis. *N Engl J Med* 1978; 298:186–193.

46. Baraka A, Afifi A, Musallem M, et al: Neuromuscular effects of halothane, suxamethonium, and tubocurarine in a myasthenic undergoing thymectomy. *Br J Anaesth* 1971; 43:91–95.

47. Blitt CD, Wright LA, Peat J: Pancuronium and the patient with myasthenia gravis. *Anesthesiology* 1975; 42:624–626.

48. Azar I: The response of patients with neuromuscular disorders to muscle relaxants: A review. *Anesthesiology* 1984; 61:173–187.

49. Bell CF, Florence AM, Hunter JM, et al: Atracurium in the myasthenic patient. *Anaesthesia* 1984; 39:961–968.

50. Vacanti CA, Ali HH, Schweiss JF, et al: The response of myasthenia gravis to atracurium. *Anesthesiology* 1985; 62:692–694.

51. Kopman AF: Edrophonium antagonism of pancuronium-induced neuromuscular blockade in man: A reappraisal. *Anesthesiology* 1979; 51:139–142.

52. Bevan DR: Reversal of pancuronium with edrophonium. *Anaesthesia* 1979; 34:614–619.

53. Ferguson A, Egerszegi P, Bevan DR: Neostigmine, pyridostigmine, and edrophonium as antagonists of pancuronium. *Anesthesiology* 1980; 53:390–394.

54. Jones RM, Pearce AC, Williams JP: Recovery characteristics following antagonism of atracurium with neostigmine or edrophonium. *Br J Anaesth* 1984; 56:453–457.

55. Harper NJW, Bradshaw EG, Healey TEJ: Antagonism of alcuronium with edrophonium or neostigmine. *Br J Anaesth* 1984; 56:1089–1094.

56. Baird WLM, Bowman WC, Kerr WJ: Some actions or ORG NC 45 and of edrophonium in the anaesthetized cat and in man. *Br J Anaesth* 1982; 54:375–385.

57. Donati F, Ferguson A, Bevan DR: Twitch depression and train-of-four ratio after antagonism of pancuronium with edrophonium, neostigmine, or pyridostigmine. *Anesth Analg* 1983; 62:314–316.

58. Cronnelly R: Muscle relaxant antagonists. *Semin Anesthesia* 1985; 4:31–40.

59. Cronnelly R, Miller RD: Onset and duration of edrophonium pyridostigmine mixtures. *Anesthesiology* 1984; 61:A301.

60. Abdulatif M, Naguib M: Accelerated reversal of atracurium blockade with divided doses of neostigmine. *Can Anaesth Soc J* 1986; 33:723–728.

61. Meakins G, Sweet PT, Bevan JC, et al: Neostigmine and edrophonium as antagonists of pancuronium in infants and children. *Anesthesiology* 1983; 59:316–321.

62. Fisher DM, Cronnelly R, Miller RD, et al: The neuromuscular pharmacology of neostigmine in infants and children. *Anesthesiology* 1983; 59:220–225.

63. Fisher DM, Cronnelly R, Sharma M, et al: Clinical pharmacology of edrophonium in infants and children. Anesthesiology 1984; 61:428–433.
64. Hughes R, Astley BA, Payne PJ: Reversal of atracurium blockade by neostigmine and edrophonium. Br J Anaesth 1984; 56:796P–797P.
65. Hunter JM, Bell CF, Jones RS: Reversal of block from atracurium with edrophonium in anephric patients. Br J Anaesth 1984; 56:1285P–1286P.
66. Rupp SM, McChristian JW, Miller RD: Neostigmine antagonizes a profound neuromuscular blockade more rapidly than edrophonium. Anesthesiology 1984, 61:A297.
67. Lavery GG, Mirakhur RK, Gibson FM: A comparison of edrophonium and neostigmine for the antagonism of atracurium-induced neuromuscular block. Anesth Analg 1985; 64:867–870.
68. Hennart D, d'Hollander A, Plasman C, et al: Importance of the level of paralysis recovery for a rapid antagonism of atracurium neuromuscular blockade with moderate doses of edrophonium. Anesthesiology 1986; 64:384–387.
69. Caldwell JE, Robertson EW, Baird WLM: Antagonism of profound neuromuscular blockade induced by vecuronium or atracurium. Br J Anaesth 1986; 58:1285–1289.
70. Engbaek J, Ording H, Ostergaard D, et al: Edrophonium and neostigmine for reversal of the neuromuscular blocking effect of vecuronium. Acta Anaesthesiol Scand 1985; 29:544–546.
71. Lahoud J, Donati F, Bevan DR, et al: Neostigmine, edrophonium and pyridostigmine as antagonists of deep pancuronium block. Can Anaesth Soc J 1986; 33:S88–S89.
72. Katz RL: Clinical neuromuscular pharmacology of pancuronium. Anesthesiology 1971; 34:550–556.
73. Miller RD, Larson CP, Way WL: Comparative antagonism of d-tubocurarine, gallamine, and pancuronium-induced neuromuscular blockade by neostigmine. Anesthesiology 1972; 37:503–509.
74. Lee C, Katz RL: Neuromuscular pharmacology: A clinical update and commentary. Br J Anaesth 1980; 52:173–188.
75. Monks PS: The reversal of non-depolarizing relaxants: A comparison of tubocurarine, gallamine and pancuronium. Anaesthesia 1972; 27:313–318.
76. Fahey MR, Morris RB, Miller RD, et al: Clinical pharmacology of ORG NC 45 (Norcuron™). Anesthesiology 1981; 55:6–11.
77. Williams A, Gyasi H, Melloni C, et al: Clinical experience with ORG NC 45 (Norcuron) as the sole muscle relaxant. Can Anaesth Soc J 1982; 29:567–572.
78. Stirt JA, Murray AL, Katz RL, et al: Atracurium during halothane anesthesia in humans. Anesth Analg 1983; 62:207–210.
79. Gencarelli PJ, Miller RD: Antagonism of ORG NC 45 (vecuronium) and pancuronium neuromuscular blockade by neostigmine. Br J Anaesth 1982; 54:53–56.

80. Bevan DR, Archer D, Donati F, et al: Antagonism of pancuronium in renal failure: No recurarization. *Br J Anaesth* 1982; 54:63–68.
81. Miller RD, Cullen DJ: Renal failure and postoperative respiratory failure: Recurarization? *Br J Anaesth* 1976; 48:253–256.
82. Marsh RHK, Chimielewski AT, Goat VA: Recovery from pancuronium: A comparison between old and young patients. *Anaesthesia* 1980; 35:1193–1196.
83. Delisle S, Bevan DR: Impaired neostigmine antagonism of pancuronium during enflurane anaesthesia in man. *Br J Anaesth* 1982; 54:441–445.
84. van Poorten JF, Dhasmana KM, Kuypers RSM, et al: Verapamil and reversal of vecuronium neuromuscular blockade. *Anesth Analg* 1984; 63:155–157.
85. Carpenter RL, Mulroy MF: Edrophonium antagonizes combined lidocaine-pancuronium and verapamil-pancuronium neuromuscular blockade in cats. *Anesthesiology* 1986; 65:506–510.
86. Ferguson A, Bevan DR: Mixed neuromuscular block: The effect of precurarization. *Anaesthesia* 1981; 36:661–666.
87. Sunew KY, Hicks RG: Effects of neostigmine and pyridostigmine on duration of succinylcholine action and pseudocholinesterase activity. *Anesthesiology* 1978; 49:188–191.
88. Baraka A, Walord A, Mansour R, et al: Effect of neostigmine and pyridostigmine on the plasma cholinesterase activity. *Br J Anaesth* 1985; 53:849–851.
89. Mirakhur RK: Edrophonium and plasma cholinesterase activity. *Can Anaesth Soc J* 1986; 33:588–590.
90. Donati F, Bevan DR: Antagonism of phase II succinylcholine block by neostigmine. *Anesth Analg* 1985; 64:773–776.
91. Futter ME, Donati D, Bevan DR: Neostigmine antagonism of succinylcholine phase II block: A comparison with pancuronium. *Can Anaesth Soc J* 1983; 30:575–580.
92. Savarese JJ, Ali HH, Murphy JD, et al: Train-of-four stimulation in the management of prolonged neuromuscular block following succinylcholine. *Anesthesiology* 1975; 42:106–111.
93. Bevan DR, Donati F: Succinylcholine apnoea: Attempted reversal with anticholinesterases. *Can Anaesth Soc J* 1983; 30:536–539.
94. Hunter AR: Neostigmine resistant curarization. *Br Med J* 1950; 2:919–921.
95. Brooks DK, Feldman SA: Metabolic acidosis: A new approach to "neostigmine resistant curarization." *Anaesthesia* 1962; 17:161–169.
96. Miller RD, Van Nyhuis LS, Eger EI, et al: The effect of acid-base balance on neostigmine antagonism of *d*-tubocurarine-induced neuromuscular blockade. *Anesthesiology* 1975; 42:377–383.
97. Miller RD, Roderick LL: Acid-base balance and neostigmine antagonism of pancuronium neuromuscular blockade. *Br J Anaesth* 1978; 50:317–324.

98. Wirtavouri K, Salmenpera M, Tauristo T: Effect of hypocarbia and hypercarbia on the antagonism of pancuronium induced neuromuscular blockade with neostigmine in man. *Br J Anaesth* 1982; 54:57–61.

99. Feldman SA: Effect of changes in electrolytes, hydration and pH upon the reactions to muscle relaxants. *Br J Anaesth* 1963; 35:546–550.

100. Ghoneim MM, Long JP: The interaction between magnesium and other neuromuscular blocking agents. *Anesthesiology* 1970; 33:23–29.

101. Miller RD, Roderick LL: Diuretic-induced hypokalaemia, pancuronium neuromuscular blockade and its antagonism by neostigmine. *Br J Anaesth* 1978; 50:541–544.

102. Bowman WC, Savage AD: Pharmacological actions of aminopyridines and related compounds. *Rev Pure Appl Pharmacol Sci* 1981; 2:317–371.

103. Booij LHD, Miller RD, Crul JF: Neostigmine and 4-aminopyridine antagonism of neomycin-pancuronium neuromuscular blockade in man. *Anesth Analg* 1978; 57:316–321.

104. Miller RD, Booij LHD, Agoston S, et al: 4–Aminopyridine potentiates neostigmine in man. *Anesthesiology* 1979; 50:416–420.

105. Agoston S, Langreter D, Newton DEF: Pharmacology and possible clinical applications of 4-aminopyridine. *Semin Anesthesia* 1985; 4:81–86.

106. Detwiler PB: The effects of germine-3-acetate on neuromuscular transmission. *J Pharmacol Exp Ther* 1972; 180:244–254.

107. Higashi H, Yonemura K, Slimoji K: Antagonism of neuromuscular blocks by germine monoacetate. *Anesthesiology* 1973; 38:145–152.

108. Viby-Mogensen J, Chraemmer Jorgensen B, Ording H: Residual curarization in the recovery room. *Anesthesiology* 1979; 50:539–541.

109. Beamer GH, Rozental P: Postoperative neuromuscular function. *Anaesth Intensive Care* 1986; 14:41–45.

110. Bar ZG: The armlift test: An alternative to the headlift test for assessing recovery from neuromuscular blockade. *Anaesthesia* 1985; 40:630–633.

111. Mason LJ, Betts EK: Leg lift and maximum inspiratory force, clinical signs of neuromuscular blockade reversal in neonates and infants. *Anesthesiology* 1980; 52:441–442.

112. Brand JB, Cullen DJ, Wilson NE, et al: Spontaneous recovery from nondepolarizing neuromuscular blockade: Correlation between clinical and evoked responses. *Anesth Analg* 1977; 56:55–58.

113. Ali HH, Savarese JJ, Lebowitz PW, et al: Twitch, tetanus and train-of-four as indices of recovery from nondepolarizing neuromuscular blockade. *Anesthesiology* 1981; 54:294–297.

114. Viby-Mogensen J: Clinical assessment of neuromuscular transmission. *Br J Anaesth* 1982; 54:209–223.

115. Miller RD: Antagonism of neuromuscular blockade. *Anesthesiology* 1976; 44:318–329.

116. Morris RB, Cronnelly R, Miller RD, et al: Pharmacokinetics of edrophonium in anephric and renal transplant patients. *Br J Anaesth* 1981; 53:1311–1314.

117. Cronnelly R, Stanski DR, Miller RD, et al: Renal function and the pharmacokinetics of neostigmine in anesthetized man. *Anesthesiology* 1979; 51:222–226.

118. Cronnelly R, Stanski DR, Miller RD, et al: Pyridostigmine kinetics with and without renal function. *Clin Pharmacol Ther* 1980; 28:78–81.

119. Morris RB, Cronnelly R, Miller RD, et al: Pharmacokinetics of edrophonium and neostigmine when antagonizing d-tubocurarine neuromuscular block in man. *Anesthesiology* 1981; 54:399–402.

120. Morris RB, Cronnelly R, Miller RD, et al: Pharmacokinetics of edrophonium in anephric and renal transplant patients. *Br J Anaesth* 1981; 53:1311–1314.

10

Renal and Hepatic Disease

Muscle relaxant drugs are eliminated via the kidneys and liver. Thus, when renal or hepatic function is impaired, the behavior of the neuromuscular blocking drugs (NMBDs) is also disturbed. The relationship is complicated because the relative importance of each organ differs among the relaxants.

RENAL FAILURE

Muscle relaxant drugs and their antagonists are ionized, water-soluble compounds. Consequently, after filtration at the glomerulus, their water solubility prevents them from being reabsorbed as they pass along the nephron, and they are excreted in the urine. Thus, their clearance from the plasma is dependent on glomerular filtration, and when this decreases in the elderly or in renal failure, excretion is diminished. This will be associated with an increased duration of action unless alternative routes of excretion, metabolism, or redistribution exist. The clearance of the acetylcholinesterase inhibitors is also decreased in renal failure so that it is unlikely that prolonged duration of action of the relaxants exceeds that of the reversal agent to induce "recurarization."[1]

A large proportion of the muscle relaxants in plasma is bound to plasma.[2-6] Only the free portion is filtered at the glomerulus, but the bound to unbound fraction is restored rapidly so that the extent of the protein binding probably has little effect on renal excretion.

There are several reports of persistent paralysis or failure to reverse the action of muscle relaxants in patients with renal failure,[7-10] although

317

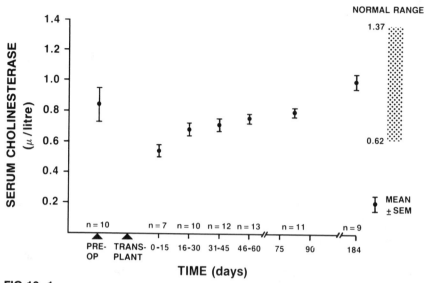

FIG 10–1.
Mean serum cholinesterase concentrations before and after renal transplantation. (Redrawn with permission from Ryan DW: Postoperative serum cholinesterase activity following successful renal transplantation. *Br J Anaesth* 1979; 51:881–884.)

often other contributing factors, such as gentamicin treatment[11] and the presence of myasthenia,[12] exist. Almost every review of the anesthetic management of the renal failure patient includes examples of prolonged paralysis,[13–16] which usually results from a relative or absolute overdose of NMBD together with inadequate monitoring of the neuromuscular junction. Often neuromuscular activity can be restored by hemodialysis.[17] Problems are more frequent with gallamine, which has no alternative route of excretion.[18] Conversely, the newer intermediate relaxants atracurium and vecuronium have normal or near-normal activity in patients with renal failure.

Succinylcholine

Renal excretion plays little part in the duration of action of succinylcholine because it is metabolized by plasma cholinesterase. Following renal transplantation, serum cholinesterase concentration may be decreased for up to 2 weeks (Fig 10–1).[19] The cause is uncertain but may reflect extracellular fluid compartment changes and not decreased enzyme production by the liver. The small decrease in concentration, 25% to 30%, is unlikely to be associated with clinical effects. However, prolonged duration of action of succinylcholine has been reported in two patients with renal failure who received succinylcholine for a second operation several hours after renal transplantation.[20] The cause was assumed to be inhibition of plasma cholinesterase by retention of neostigmine that had been used to reverse d-tubocurarine after the first operation.

Theoretically, administration of the immunosuppressive agent azathioprine to the renal transplant recipient may potentiate succinylcholine by increasing transmitter release,[21] but this has not been observed in man.

The increase in serum potassium concentration after single (1 mg/kg) or repeated doses of succinylcholine in patients with renal failure is no different from normal. Average increases of about 0.5 mEq/L are seen,[22, 23] although increases up to 1.2 mEq/L have been reported.[24] The increase is not prevented by "precurarization" will small doses of d-tubocurarine.[25] Hyperkalemic cardiac arrest during renal transplantation is more likely a consequence of failing to flush the donor kidney of preservative fluids such as Collins' or Saks' solutions that contain high concentrations of potassium.[26] Cardiac arrest has also accompanied acidosis and hyperglycemia in a diabetic patient.[27]

Thus, succinylcholine is not contraindicated in the patient with renal failure. It is useful to facilitate endotracheal intubation in the emergency renal transplant recipient and has been used in intermittent doses or by continuous infusion throughout the transplantation procedure.[28]

Nondepolarizing Relaxants

Pharmacokinetics

There is a wide spectrum of disturbance of plasma clearance of relaxants in patients with renal failure. For example, in some patients atracurium and vecuronium clearance is affected little, while gallamine clearance is decreased by more than 80% (Table 10–1). The pharmacokinetics variables reported for individual drugs are shown in Table 10–2.

TABLE 10–1.
Decrease in Relaxant Clearance in Renal Failure

DECREASE IN CLEARANCE	RELAXANT
None or little	Atracurium, Vecuroniun
1.5–5 times	Alcuronium, Fazadinium, Metocurine, Pancuronium, d-Tubocurarine
More than 5 times	Gallamine

TABLE 10-2.
Pharmacokinetic Variables of Nondepolarizing Relaxants in Renal Failure (Mean ± SEM)

	NORMAL VS. RENAL FAILURE	N	V_{dss}, L/KG	$t_{1/2\beta}$, MIN	C_p, ML/MIN/KG	REFERENCE
Atracurium	N	10	0.18 ± 0.01	20.6 ± 1.2	6.1 ± 0.3	30
	RF	9	0.22 ± 0.02	23.7 ± 0.9	6.7 ± 0.6	30
	N	6	0.14 ± 0.02	17.0 ± 0.8	5.8 ± 0.8	31
	RF	5	0.17 ± 0.02	18.0 ± 1.3	6.3 ± 0.9	31
Fazadinium	N		0.29 ± 0.04	85.0 ± 5	2.2 ± 0.29	32
	RF		0.31 ± 0.08	140.0 ± 17	1.6 ± 0.25	32
	N		0.23 ± 0.08	50.1 ± 6.4	3.7 ± 1.1	33
	RF		0.34 ± 0.1	80.2 ± 29.5	2.8 ± 0.7	33
Gallamine	N	17	0.21 ± 0.01	131.0	1.2 ± 0.1	34
	RF	8	0.28 ± 0.03	752.4	0.2 ± 0.1	34
Pancuronium	N	6	0.15 ± 0.01	100.4 ± 3.4	1.0 ± 0.1	35
	RF	7	0.24 ± 0.03	489.2 ± 74.8	0.3 ± 0.03	35
	N	7	0.34 ± 0.02	132.5 ± 10.0	1.9 ± 0.24	36
	RF	10	0.33 ± 0.07	257.3 ± 44	0.9 ± 0.08	36
Metocurine	N	5	0.15 ± 0.01	360.0 ± 57	1.3 ± 0.1	37
	RF	5	0.24 ± 0.03	684.0 ± 90	0.4 ± 0.1	37
d-Tubocurarine	N		0.39	239.0	1.9	38
	RF			330.0		39
Vecuronium	N	7	0.51 ± 0.11	117.0	3.2 ± 0.2	40
	RF	8	0.47 ± 0.17	149.0	2.6 ± 0.3	40
	N	4	0.19 ± 21.2	79.5 ± 6.8	3.0 ± 0.2	41
	RF	4	0.24 ± 31.3	97.1 ± 18.9	2.5 ± 0.3	41

TABLE 10–3.
Pharmacodynamics of Atracurium in Renal Failure*

	DOSE, MG/KG	N	TIME TO MAXIMUM BLOCK, MIN	TIME TO 90% RECOVERY, MIN	25%–75% RECOVERY, MIN
Normal	0.5	10	1.8 ± 0.1	69.5 ± 5.2	10.5 ± 1.1
Renal failure	0.5	10	2.0 ± 0.4	77.4 ± 3.2	13.5 ± 3.2

*From Fahey MR, Rupp SM, Fisher DM, et al: The pharmacokinetics and pharmacodynamics of atracurium in patients with and without renal failure. *Anesthesiology* 1984; 61:699–702. Used by permission.

Protein binding of d-tubocurarine, and probably all relaxants, is not affected in renal failure.[42] Although one study[37] reported that the serum concentration of metocurine to produce a given level of neuromuscular blockade in renal failure was higher than normal, this has not been confirmed in other studies. An increased volume of distribution of pancuronium in renal failure was reported in one center,[5] which suggests that differences might exist in hemodialysis control among institutions.

Pharmacodynamics

In general, the duration of action and rate of recovery is affected little or not at all for atracurium or vecuronium. Computer predictions for those agents for which plasma clearance is affected in renal failure suggest that the duration of action of large, single doses and multiple doses is affected more than when small single doses are used[38, 43] in clinical studies.

Alcuronium.—Controlled clinical studies of the use of alcuronium have not been carried out in patients with renal failure, although it has been used without apparent problems to provide muscle relaxation during renal transplantation.[29]

Atracurium.—Single doses of atracurium, 0.5 mg/kg, are associated with no significant differences in onset or duration of action, or recovery (Table 10–3).[30] Similarly, the duration of action of repeated doses is unaffected, and cumulation does not occur.[44] Although increased concentrations of the atracurium metabolite laudanosine[31] have been reported in renal failure, their significance is unknown. Atracurium is the only nondepolarizing NMBD the actions of which are not altered in renal failure. The use of alternative NMBDs is not contraindicated, but their use should be controlled carefully using neuromuscular monitoring.

Fazadinium.—When small and repeated doses of fazadinium were given, the differences in duration of action and rate of recovery of neuromuscular activity were not significantly altered in patients with renal failure.[32, 33] Also, the relationship between plasma concentration and neuromuscular blockade is unaffected in renal failure (Fig 10–2).

Gallamine.—Small doses of gallamine are not associated with prolonged neuromuscular blockade; this finding led to the suggestion, fortunately ignored, that "gallamine is an appropriate relaxant in patients with absent renal function because it may undergo an extrarenal pathway of excretion."[45] More careful pharmacokinetic studies demonstrated that after administration of small doses, the rapid redistribution of gallamine allows plasma concentration to decrease below that required for 95% block in much the same time in patients with renal failure as in normal patients. However, larger doses produce a marked prolongation of action (Fig 10–3). Thus, use of gallamine should be avoided in renal failure.

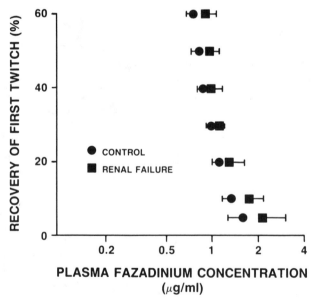

FIG 10–2.
Relationship between plasma concentrations of fazadinium and neuromuscular blockade in normal patients and those with renal failure. (Redrawn with permission from Bevan DR, d'Souza J, Rouse JM, et al: Clinical pharmacokinetics and pharmacodynamics of fazadinium in renal failure. *Eur J Clin Pharmacol* 1981; 20:293–298.)

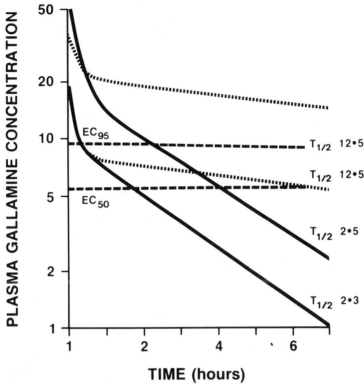

FIG 10–3.
Plasma concentration vs. time plot for gallamine from data collected in normal patients and in renal failure. (Redrawn with permission from Ramzan MI, Shanks CA, Triggs EJ: Gallamine disposition in surgical patients with chronic renal failure. *Br J Clin Pharmacol* 1981; 12:141–147.)

Metocurine.—Following administration of a single dose of metocurine, 0.3 mg/kg, the plasma concentration at 10% recovery of EMG was found to be higher in renal failure (1.05 ± 0.26 µg/ml) than normal (0.46 ± 0.11 µg/ml).[37] The decreased plasma clearance would be expected to prolong the duration of action, although that was not demonstrated in the study.

Pancuronium.—The duration of action of single doses of pancuronium is prolonged in renal failure[46] (Fig 10–4), although the degree of prolongation of small doses, 0.04 mg/kg, is much less than after 0.08 mg/kg.[47] Following reversal of blockade of pancuronium with neostigmine, recovery of neuromuscular activity proceeds steadily,[48] and no evidence of "recurarization" exists.[1]

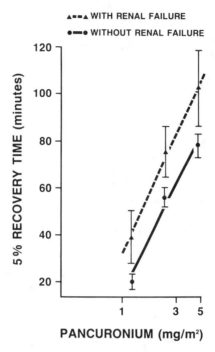

WITH RENAL FAILURE

WITHOUT RENAL FAILURE

FIG 10–4.
Duration of action of pancuronium in patients with renal failure. (Redrawn with permission from Miller RD, Stevens WC, Way WL: The effect of renal failure and hyperkalemia on the duration of pancuronium neuromuscular blockade in man. *Anesth Analg* 1973; 52:661–666.)

d-**Tubocurarine.**—The duration of action of single doses of *d*-tubo-curarine (0.16 mg/kg) is prolonged significantly, and the response seems to be more variable than after equipotent doses of atracurium or vecuronium.[49]

If use of a long-acting neuromuscular blocking drug is required in a patient with impaired renal function, metocurine, pancuronium, and d-tubocurarine are all possible alternatives. Any pharmacokinetic or pharmacodynamic differences between them are small and unimportant.

Vecuronium.—Administration of single doses of vecuronium, 0.05 mg/kg, results in a slight but significant increase in the duration of action and a slight increase in recovery index (Table 10–4) in renal failure.[50] After repeated doses, 0.01 mg/kg, a gradual increase in du-ration of action (Fig 10–5), and cumulation[51] due to gradual saturation of peripheral stores occurs. The dose-response curve for vecuronium is not different in renal failure.[51] Nevertheless, the modifications in

TABLE 10–4.
Pharmacodynamics of Vecuronium in Renal Failure*

	DOSE, MG/KG	N	TIME TO MAXIMUM BLOCK, MIN	TIME TO 90% RECOVERY, MIN	25%–75% RECOVERY, MIN
Normal	0.05	10	5.2 ± 2.0	25 ± 10	7.2 ± 3.0
Renal failure	0.05	10	5.9 ± 1.9	33 ± 10	10.5 ± 3.7

*From Meistelman C, Lienhart D, Leveque C, et al: Pharmacology of vecuronium in patients with end stage renal failure. *Anesthesiology* 1983; 59:A293. Used by permission.

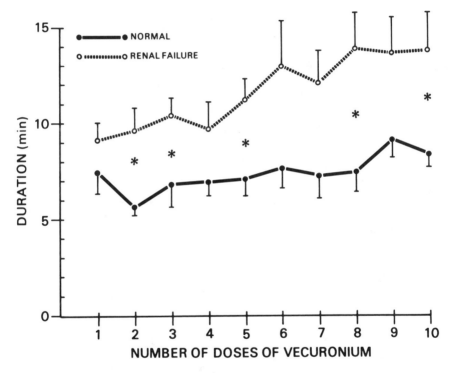

FIG 10–5.
Duration of action of repeated small doses of vecuronium (0.01 mg/kg) in renal failure. (Redrawn with permission from Bevan DR, Donati F, Gyasi H, et al: Vecuronium in renal failure. *Can Anaesth Soc J* 1984; 31:491–496.)

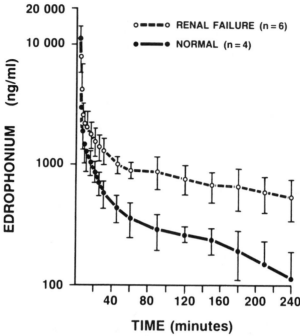

FIG 10–6.
Plasma concentration vs. time plot for edrophonium in normal patients and patients with renal failure. (Redrawn with permission from Morris RB, Cronnelly R, Miller RD, et al: Pharmacokinetics of edrophonium in anephric and renal transplant patients. *Br J Anaesth* 1981; 53:1311–1314.)

TABLE 10–5.
Pharmacokinetics of Anticholinesterases in Renal Failure (Mean ± SEM)

	NORMAL VS. RENAL FAILURE	N	V_{dss}, L/KG	$t_{1/2\beta}$ MIN	C_p, ML/MIN/KG
Neostigmine	N	8	1.4 ± 0.5	79.8 ± 16.6	16.7 ± 1.8
	RF	4	1.6 ± 0.1	181.1 ± 27.2	7.8 ± 1.3
Pyridostigmine	N	5	1.1 ± 0.1	112.0 ± 5.0	8.6 ± 0.8
	RF	4	1.0 ± 0.05	379.0 ± 82.0	2.1 ± 0.3
Edrophonium	N	4	0.9 ± 0.1	114.0 ± 24.0	8.2 ± 1.4
	RF	6	0.7 ± 0.05	206.0 ± 28.0	2.7 ± 0.6

activity of vecuronium in renal failure are small[49, 52, 93] so its use offers considerable advantage over the older agents metocurine, pancuronium, and d-tubocurarine.

Reversal of Paralysis

Pharmacokinetic analysis of the anticholinesterases neostigmine, pyridostigmine, and edrophonium demonstrated that their clearance is reduced in anephric patients[53, 54] (Fig 10–6, Table 10–5), and the extent of the decrease in clearance suggests that they are excreted by tubular secretion as well as by glomerular filtration. In addition, their volumes of distribution are approximately three to four times greater than the nondepolarizing relaxants. As quaternary amines, they do not cross lipid membranes so that rapid equilibration in the central and peripheral compartments must occur. The recently transplanted kidney restores renal clearance of the reversal agents to normal.

Clinical Recommendations

In planning a strategy for the use of muscle relaxant drugs in patients with renal failure, abnormal reactions to all agents should be anticipated. Thus, the neuromuscular junction should be monitored throughout surgery so that the smallest doses of agent necessary to achieve adequate relaxation are used. In this regard, potent inhalational anesthetic vapors potentiate the nondepolarizing relaxants, and their effect can be reversed easily at the end of surgery. The patient with renal failure may demonstrate greater variation in response to the relaxants because of fluid status, metabolic (acid-base and electrolyte) imbalance, and the influence of other drugs, e.g., antibiotics and azathioprine. Also the effects of the variation are greater than normal so that a moderate overdose will produce greater prolongation of effect.

The smallest disturbance in function is seen with succinylcholine and atracurium, and many recommend that atracurium is the drug of choice in renal failure. This may be inconvenient in lengthy surgery or in the presence of cardiovascular instability when pancuronium, metocurine, or d-tubocurarine may be substituted with appropriate monitoring and after facilitating endotracheal intubation with succinylcholine. Reversal of the block should not be difficult with the usual doses of any of the anticholinesterases.

Thus, the absence of renal function in man is likely to interfere with the clearance of the anticholinesterases more than it interferes with the excretion of pancuronium, metocurine, or d-tubocurarine so that recurarization is unlikely.

HEPATIC DISEASE

The liver plays an accessory role in the excretion of most nonde-polarizing relaxants. It has been estimated that normally it accounts for about 10% of the elimination of alcuronium,[55] fazadinium,[56] pancu-ronium,[57] and d-tubocurarine.[58] These proportions may be increased in renal failure. The liver plays a less important role for metocurine[58] and is not involved at all with the excretion of atracurium[59] or gallamine.[60] Vecuronium is different: the liver accounts for at least 35% of its elim-ination.[61, 62] Plasma cholinesterase is synthesized in the liver[63] so that impaired hepatic function, if sufficiently severe, may be associated with succinylcholine apnea.[64]

Abnormal reactions to the nondepolarizing relaxants in hepatic or biliary disease are one of two types. First, patients with hepatic disease exhibit resistance, on a mg/kg basis, to d-tubocurarine,[65, 66] pancuron-ium,[67, 68] and atracurium[69] as a result of an increased volume of distri-bution. Secondly, cholestasis is associated with prolonged duration of action of d-tubocurarine,[66] pancuronium,[70] fazadinium,[56] and vecuronium[71] because biliary excretion is impaired. However, several reasons exist for abnormal behavior of NMBDs in hepatic disease (Table 10–6).

TABLE 10–6.
Causes of Abnormal Reaction to Neuromuscular Blocking Drugs in Liver Disease and Cholestasis

Decreased hepatic uptake
Decreased metabolism
Abnormal protein binding
Secondary renal disease
Increased volume of distribution
Decreased biliary excretion

Bile Salts and Hepatic Uptake

Recent studies have demonstrated that an increase in plasma con-centration of bile salts reduces the hepatic uptake of pancuronium and particularly of vecuronium.[72–74] In addition, taurocholate, a bile salt, potentiates the action of pancuronium and gallamine but not vecuron-ium in the phrenic nerve-diaphragm preparation.

Hepatic Metabolism

Pancuronium and vecuronium undergo biotransformation to hydroxy derivatives in the liver, but there is no evidence that the decreased metabolism is responsible for the prolonged duration of action of these relaxants in cirrhosis.[75]

Protein Binding

Muscle relaxants are bound to plasma proteins in a reversible manner that obeys the law of mass action:

$$[\text{unbound drug}] + [\text{protein}] \underset{k_2}{\overset{k_1}{\rightleftharpoons}} [\text{drug-protein complex}]$$

It is the unbound fraction that is responsible for the pharmacologic results. However, the interaction of relaxants with plasma protein is dynamic, and dissociation of the drug-pattern complex occurs rapidly.[76] Muscle relaxants are also bound to other tissues including red cells and cartilage.

The neuromuscular blocking drugs are bound to protein, globulin, and albumin in varying degrees (Table 10–7). In hepatic disease, plasma albumin concentrations may be decreased, while the globulin fraction is increased so that attempts have been made to correlate alterations in the behavior of the NMBDs with changes in plasma protein concentration.[77]

However, no systematic studies have compared the pharmacokinetic and pharmacodynamic activities of the muscle relaxants with varying plasma protein concentrations. The free fraction of d-tubocurarine, fazadinium, pancuronium, and vecuronium is not altered in cirrhotic patients.[78, 82, 83]

TABLE 10–7.
Protein Binding of Neuromuscular Blocking Drugs

DRUG	% BOUND	REFERENCE
Alcuronium	40	55
Fazadinium	51	78
Gallamine	low	79
Metocurine	32–35	58, 80
Pancuronium	11–29	78, 81
d-Tubocurarine	43–51	58, 80, 82, 83
Vecuronium	30	78

TABLE 10–8.
Pharmacokinetic Variables Associated with Liver Disease and Cholestasis (Mean ± SEM)

		N	V_{dss}, L/KG	$t_{1/2\beta}$, MIN	C_p, ML/MIN/KG	REFERENCE
Atracurium	N	6	0.16 ± 0.01	21.0 ± 0.8	5.3 ± 0.3	59
	R & HF	7	0.21 ± 0.02	22.0 ± 0.8	6.5 ± 0.6	59
Fazadinium	N	11	0.29 ± 0.03	82.0 ± 5.1	2.7 ± 1.1	56
	C	8	0.45 ± 0.05	153.0 ± 19.4	2.1 ± 0.5	56
	CH	8	0.35 ± 0.03	103.0 ± 8.8	2.2 ± 0.7	56
Gallamine	N	17	0.23 ± 0.01	134.6 ± 8.0	1.2 ± 0.1	90
	CH	7	0.27 ± 0.01	160.1 ± 15.0	1.2 ± 0.1	90
	N	5	0.24 ± 0.04	162.0 ± 18.0	1.2 ± 0.2	84
	CH	4	0.25 ± 0.04	220.0 ± 41.0	0.9 ± 0.1	84
Pancuronium	N	7	0.26 ± 0.02	132.5 ± 9.4	1.9 ± 0.2	70
	CH	9	0.31 ± 0.04	269.8 ± 33.7	0.97 ± 0.1	70
	N	12	0.28 ± 0.02	114.3 ± 9.6	1.9 ± 0.1	75
	C	14	0.42 ± 0.06	208.2 ± 24.8	1.5 ± 0.1	75
	N	12	0.28 ± 0.02	141.0 ± 16.0	1.8 ± 0.2	84
	CH	7	0.43 ± 0.06	224.0 ± 21.0	1.5 ± 0.1	84
	N	5	0.20 ± 0.04	93.9 ± 16.0	1.4 ± 0.1	85
	HF	5	0.20 ± 0.03	303.0 ± 87.7	0.6 ± 0.1	85
Vecuronium	N	14	0.35 ± 0.02	58.0 ± 5.1	4.3 ± 0.4	71
	C	12	0.30 ± 0.03	84.0 ± 6.6	2.7 ± 0.3	71
	CH	9	0.29 ± 0.04	98.0 ± 19.0	2.4 ± 0.3	71

*N = normal; R = renal; HF = hepatic failure; C = cirrhosis; CH = cholestasis.

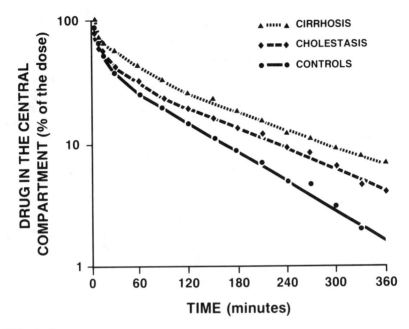

FIG 10–7.
Calculated decrease in fazadinium in the central compartment in patients with cholestasis or cirrhosis. (From Duvaldestin P, Saada J, Henzel D, et al: Fazadinium pharmacokinetics in patients with liver disease. *Br J Anaesth* 1980; 52:789–793. Used by permission.)

Secondary Renal Failure

Although renal failure is a common accompaniment of severe hepatic impairment or cholestasis, there is no evidence that decreased renal clearance of the relaxants is responsible for their modified behavior in hepatic-biliary disease.

Pharmacokinetics

Although the pharmacokinetic behavior of the relaxants in patients with hepatic disease or cholestasis shows some variation, some general patterns emerge (Table 10–8). *Cirrhosis* is associated with an increased volume of distribution due to the accumulation of extracellular fluid (ECF) and ascites. This results in increased dilution of relaxant and is the probable cause of "curare resistance." In addition, the increased volume of distribution causes an increase in terminal half-life. Conversely, *cholestasis* is associated with an increase in terminal half-life as a result of decreased biliary excretion, but the volume of distribution is normal. This pattern is well characterized for fazadinium[56] (Fig 10–7). The pattern for pancuronium is similar, except that some reports of cholestasis also showed some increase in the volume of distribution.[72, 84] In acute hepatic failure, the predominant effect is an increase in elimination half-life with a decrease in clearance.[85]

That no statistically significant pharmacokinetic changes occur in cholestatic patients after administration of gallamine[84, 90] confirms that gallamine is excreted predominantly via the renal route.[86] Similarly, the liver appears to play no part in the elimination of atracurium. Although its volume of distribution was found to be increased slightly in patients with hepatic failure, there was no change in elimination half-life.[59]

Vecuronium behaves differently. As a result of its greater lipophilicity, it is dependent on the liver for distribution and elimination.[87-89] Its normal, brief duration of action results from rapid hepatic uptake[91] so that when biliary clearance of vecuronium is reduced by cholestasis, the duration of action is prolonged considerably. Surprisingly, its volume of distribution was not increased in cirrhosis,[71] but this probably reflects the decrease in hepatic uptake allowing a larger quantity of the administered dose to be diluted elsewhere. The decrease in hepatic uptake results in delayed excretion and a prolonged duration of action.

Succinylcholine

The duration of action of succinylcholine is determined by the activity of plasma cholinesterase (PCHE), which is synthesized in the liver.[92, 93] The plasma concentrations of this stable enzyme, half-life 8 to 12 days, parallel albumin concentration in patients with chronic liver disease, although the synthesis of PCHE is independent of albumin synthesis. Consequently, hypoalbuminemia may be associated with prolonged neuromuscular blockade after succinylcholine. In practice, the PCHE concentration had to be decreased by more than 50% so that prolonged apnea occurred only once when succinylcholine was given to 69 patients with hepatic cirrhosis.[64]

Clinical Sequelae

A prolonged duration of action of most muscle relaxants can be expected in patients with either cirrhosis or cholestasis. In addition, cirrhosis will encourage the phenomenon of curare resistance. In cholestasis the lack of biliary excretion of gallamine suggested that it was the drug of choice despite its cardiovascular effects.[90] However, this selection has been altered by the introduction of atracurium. Atracurium can be used with or without succinylcholine to facilitate intubation in normal doses in patients with cirrhosis or cholestasis and a near normal reaction will ensue. Although slightly greater doses may be necessary in cirrhosis, the rate of recovery will not be affected.

ELECTROLYTES AND ACID-BASE DISTURBANCES

There are several reports of prolonged paralysis[94] and "neostigmine-resistant curarization"[95] in the severely ill. As several of these patients have associated abnormalities of fluid status, attempts to achieve electrolyte homeostasis and acid-base balance have been made to incriminate the latter as the cause of abnormal responses to curare.[96] But in vivo it is often difficult to separate the actions of individual ions from systemic disease in the ill patient.

Potassium

It has been demonstrated in vitro that potassium has presynaptic and postsynaptic actions at the neuromuscular junction. Membrane potential depends, to a large extent, on the environmental potassium concentration,[97] and at high concentrations, muscle contraction may be induced. In addition, potassium increases the frequency of miniature end-plate potentials and the amount of acetylcholine release.[98]

Studies to determine dose-response curves of the guinea pig nerve-lumbrical muscle preparation showed that an acute increase in potassium concentration (2, 4, or 6 mEq/L) decreased the sensitivity to *d*-tubocurarine and pancuronium.[99] The authors predicted that within the clinical range, the requirement for relaxant might increase by about one third as potassium increased from 3.5 to 5 mEq/L. The administration of diuretics to produce chronic hypokalemia gave conflicting results. Following administration of furosemide, the response to *d*-tubocurarine and pancuronium was unaffected, while after chlorothiazide it was enhanced.[100] However, chronic hypokalemia, induced by dietary restriction, was associated with a decrease in the ED50 of *d*-tubocurarine. Thus, acute and chronic potassium depletion might be expected to result in a decrease in requirement of nondepolarizing relaxants. If severe, the requirement of *d*-tubocurarine may decrease to one third of normal.[101]

Since serum potassium concentrations may fluctuate widely in the syndrome of hypokalemic familial periodic paralysis, and sensitivity to NMBDs is increased considerably when patients with the syndrome develop hypokalemia, some researchers have suggested the avoidance of NMBDs.[102] However, if serum potassium concentration is controlled carefully and dosage of relaxant controlled with neuromuscular monitoring, the nondepolarizing relaxants can be used safely.[103]

Calcium and Magnesium

Calcium has two opposing actions in the process of neuromuscular transmission. Presynaptically it increases acetylcholine release:[104] an increase in calcium concentration increases spontaneous quantal endplate potential (EPP) content,[98, 105] and this is augmented by evoked nerve impulses.[106] Conversely, calcium decreases postsynaptic chemosensitivity.[99] However, dose-response curves of the isolated guinea pig nerve-lumbrical preparation demonstrated that an increase in calcium concentration from 1 to 3 mmole/L decreases the sensitivity of the preparation to d-tubocurarine and pancuronium.[99] This suggests that, applied to the clinical situation, an increase in total calcium concentration from 2.1 to 2.6 mmole/L (the normal range) corresponds to a decrease in sensitivity of about 25%.[107, 108] A recent report of anesthesia in a patient with hyperparathyroidism (calcium concentration 15 mg/dl) demonstrated prolongation of action of succinylcholine but a decrease in the duration of action of atracurium.[109]

Magnesium antagonizes the action of calcium by simple competition. Thus, neuromuscular blocking drugs, both depolarizing and nondepolarizing, are potentiated in patients who have received large doses of magnesium sulfate for the control of preeclamptic toxemia.[110] Studies in cats demonstrated that the effects of magnesium and succinylcholine or d-tubocurarine were additive (Fig 10–8), and d-tubocurarine was 1000 times as potent as magnesium sulfate.[111]

If general anesthesia is required in the toxemic patient, endotracheal intubation is facilitated with succinylcholine. Usually the normal dose, 1 mg/kg, is given to ensure good intubating conditions, although a prolonged action can be anticipated. Further relaxation may be achieved with small doses of nondepolarizing relaxants with careful monitoring of the neuromuscular junction.[112]

Acid-Base Disturbances

Postoperative respiratory depression in the patient with generalized disease has been attributed to potentiation of the muscle relaxants in acidosis.[89, 113] However, supportive experimental evidence is difficult to find. Most,[114–119] but not all,[120] studies have demonstrated that the action of d-tubocurarine is potentiated by acidosis, whether metabolic

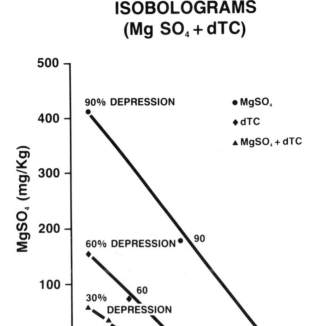

FIG 10–8.
Individual and mixed doses of *d*-tubocurarine (dTC) and magnesium sulfate required to produce neuromuscular blockade of 30%, 60%, and 90%. (Redrawn with permission from Giesecke AH, Morris RE, Dalton MD, et al: Of magnesium, muscle relaxants, toxemic parturients, and cats. *Anaesth Analg* 1968; 47:689–695.)

or respiratory, and slightly antagonized by alkalosis. Less information is available for other relaxants. Acid-base changes appear to have small but appreciable effects on the action of gallamine and metocurine,[113, 120] and respiratory acidosis reduces the blockade associated with succinylcholine. Several studies failed to make clear distinctions between effects of pH and CO_2 and ignored the often considerable circulatory disturbances induced by the method used to alter pH.

The influence of acid-base changes on the action of d-tubocurarine appears to be greater than for other relaxants, and this may result from the presence of two ionizable groups with pK values near the biologic

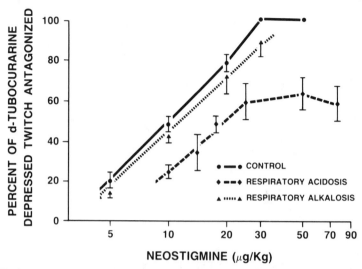

FIG 10–9.

Impaired antagonism of *d*-tubocurarine by neostigmine in respiratory acidosis and respiratory alkalosis. (Redrawn with permission from Miller RD, Van Nyhuis LS, Eger EI, et al: The effect of acid-base balance on neostigmine antagonism of *d*-tubocurarine-induced neuromuscular blockade. *Anesthesiology* 1975; 42:377–383.)

range.[121] When pancuronium or vecuronium is given to patients with varying degrees of respiratory acidosis or alkalosis, the change in pH makes no difference to the potency, duration of action, or rate of recovery.[121–123] Apparent differences that occur when the Pco_2 is changed after administration of relaxant produce a change in control twitch height[122] and account for the apparent potentiation of pancuronium and vecuronium when pH is increased.[124] The metabolism of atracurium, by the Hofmann elimination, is pH dependent. A decrease in pH caused by breathing 20% CO_2 causes only slight increase in blockade, and recovery is only marginally more rapid during alkalosis, at least in animals.[125]

The antagonism of pancuronium[126, 127] and d-tubocurarine[128] (Fig 10–9) by neostigmine is impaired by respiratory acidosis and metabolic alkalosis. Surprisingly, the altered acid-base status did not modify the infusion rate of either relaxant required to produce constant 90% twitch depression. The authors suggested that as the impaired reversal was not a direct effect of pH, it might be secondary to changes in electrolyte concentration or might reflect an effect on muscle contractility.

REFERENCES

1. Miller RD, Cullen DJ: Renal failure and postoperative respiratory failure: Recurarization? *Br J Anaesth* 1976; 48:253–256.
2. Walker JS, Shanks CA, Brown KF: Determinants of d-tubocurarine plasma protein binding in health and disease. *Anesth Analg* 1983; 62:870–874.
3. Wood M, Stone WJ, Wood AJJ: Plasma binding of pancuronium: Effects of age, sex, and disease. *Anesth Analg* 1983; 62:29–32.
4. Duvaldestin P, Henzel D: Binding of tubocurarine, fazadinium, pancuronium and ORG NC 45 to serum proteins in normal man and in patients with cirrhosis. *Br J Anaesth* 1982; 54:513–516.
5. Olsen GD, Chan EM, Riker WW: Binding of d-tubocurarine and di(methyl-^{14}C) ether iodide and other amines to cartilage, chondroitin sulfate, and human plasma proteins. *J Pharmacol Exp Ther* 1975; 195:242–250.
6. Liebel WS, Martyn JAJ, Szyfelbein SK, et al: Elevated plasma binding cannot account for the burn-related d-tubocurarine hyposensitivity. *Anesthesiology* 1981; 54:378–382.
7. Feldman SA, Levi JA: Prolonged paresis following gallamine. *Br J Anaesth* 1963; 35:804–806.
8. Singer MM, Dutton R, Way WL: Untoward results of gallamine administration during bilateral nephrectomy: Treatment with haemodialysis. *Br J Anaesth* 1971; 43:404–405.
9. Riordan DD, Gilbertson AA: Prolonged curarization in a patient with renal failure. *Br J Anaesth* 1971; 43:506–508.
10. Abrams RE, Hornbein TF: Inability to reverse pancuronium blockade in a patient with renal failure and hepatic disease. *Anesthesiology* 1975; 42:362–364.
11. Geha DG, Blitt CD, Moon BJ: Prolonged neuromuscular blockade with pancuronium in the presence of acute renal failure: A case report. *Anesth Analg* 1976; 55:343–345.
12. Bradley JP, Maisland AR, O'Connor JP: Prolonged neuromuscular blockade after renal transplantation. *Anaesth Intensive Care* 1985; 13:196–198.
13. Popescu DT: The use of muscle relaxants in anephric patients, in Spierdijk J, Feldman S (eds): *Anaesthesia and Pharmaceutics.* Leiden, Holland, Leiden University Press, 1972, pp 74–88.
14. Samuel JR, Powell D: Renal transplantation: Anaesthetic experience of 100 cases. *Anaesthesia* 1970; 25:165–170.
15. Rouse JM, Galley RLA, Bevan DR: Prolonged curarisation following renal transplantation. *Anaesthesia* 1977; 32:247–251.
16. Morgan M, Lumley J: Anaesthetic considerations in chronic renal failure. *Anaesth Intensive Care* 1975; 3:218–225.

17. Cozantis D, Haapanen E: Studies on muscle relaxants during haemodialysis. *Acta Anaesthesiol Scand* 1979; 23:225–234.
18. Churchill-Davidson HC, Way WL, de Jong RH: The muscle relaxants and renal excretion. *Anesthesiology* 1967; 28:540–546.
19. Ryan DW: Postoperative serum cholinesterase activity following successful renal transplantation. *Br J Anaesth* 1979; 51:881–884.
20. Bishop MJ, Hornbein TF: Prolonged effect of succinylcholine after neostigmine and pyridostigmine administration in patients with renal failure. *Anesthesiology* 1983; 58:384–386.
21. Dretchen KL, Morgenroth VH, Standaert FG, et al: Azathioprine: Effects on neuromuscular transmission. *Anesthesiology* 1976; 45:604–609.
22. Miller RD, Way WL, Hamilton WK, et al: Succinylcholine-induced hyperkalemia in patients with renal failure? *Anesth Analg* 1975; 54:746–748.
23. Powell DR, Miller RD: The effect of repeated doses of succinylcholine on serum potassium in patients with renal failure. *Anesth Analg* 1975; 54:746–748.
24. Walton JD, Farman JV: Suxamethonium, potassium and renal failure. *Anaesthesia* 1973; 28:628–630.
25. Koide M, Waud BE: Serum potassium concentrations after succinylcholine in patients with renal failure. *Anesthesiology* 1972; 36:142–145.
26. Hirshman CA, Leon C, Edelstein G, et al: Risk of hyperkalemia in recipients of kidneys preserved with an intracellular electrolyte solution. *Anesth Analg* 1980; 59:283–286.
27. Hirshman CA, Edelstein G: Intraoperative hyperkalemia and cardiac arrests during renal transplantation in an insulin-dependent diabetic patient. *Anesthesiology* 1979; 51:161–162.
28. Strunin L: Some aspects of anaesthesia for renal homotransplantation. *Br J Anaesth* 1966; 38:812–817.
29. Kaushik S, Grover VK, Singh H, et al: Use of alcuronium in patients undergoing renal transplantation. *Br J Anaesth* 1984; 56:1229–1233.
30. Fahey MR, Rupp SM, Fisher DM, et al: The pharmacokinetics and pharmacodynamics of atracurium in patients with and without renal failure. *Anesthesiology* 1984; 61:699–702.
31. de Bros F, Lai A, Scott R, et al: Pharmacokinetics and pharmacodynamics of atracurium under isoflurane anesthesia in normal and anephric patients. *Anesth Analg* 1985; 64:207.
32. Duvaldestin P, Bertrand JC, Concina D, et al: Pharmacokinetics of fazadinium in patients with renal failure. *Br J Anaesth* 1979; 51:943–947.
33. Bevan DR, d'Souza J, Rouse JM, et al: Clinical pharmacokinetics and pharmacodynamics of fazadinium in renal failure. *Eur J Clin Pharmacol* 1981; 20:293–298.
34. Ramzan MI, Shanks CA, Triggs EJ: Gallamine disposition in surgical patients with chronic renal failure. *Br J Clin Pharmacol* 1981; 12:141–147.

35. McLeod K, Watson MJ, Rawlins MD: Pharmacokinetics of pancuronium in patients with normal and impaired renal function. *Br J Anaesth* 1976; 48:341–345.
36. Somogyi AA, Shanks CA, Triggs EJ: The effect of renal function on the disposition and neuromuscular blocking action of pancuronium bromide. *Eur J Clin Pharmacol* 1977; 12:23–29.
37. Brotherton WP, Matteo RS: Pharmacokinetics and pharmacodynamics of metocurine in humans with and without renal failure. *Anesthesiology* 1981; 55:272–276.
38. Shanks CA: Pharmacokinetics of the nondepolarizing neuromuscular relaxants applied to calculation of bolus and infusion dosage regimens. *Anesthesiology* 1986; 64:72–86.
39. Miller RD, Matteo RS, Benet LZ, et al: The pharmacokinetics of d-tubocurarine in man with and without renal failure. *J Pharmacol Exp Ther* 1977; 202:1–7.
40. Bencini AF, Scaf AHJ, Sohn YJ, et al: Disposition and urinary excretion of vecuronium bromide in anesthetized patients with normal renal function or renal failure. *Anesth Analg* 1986; 65:245–251.
41. Fahey MR, Morris RB, Miller RD, et al: Pharmacokinetics of ORG NC45 (Norcuron) in patients with and without renal failure. *Br J Anaesth* 1981; 53:1049–1053.
42. Ghoneim MM, Kramer SE, Bannow R, et al: Binding of d-tubocurarine to plasma proteins in normal man and in patients with hepatic or renal disease. *Anesthesiology* 1973; 39:410–415.
43. Gibaldi M, Levy G, Hayton WL: Tubocurarine and renal failure. *Br J Anaesth* 1972; 44:163–165.
44. Hunter JM, Jones RS, Utting HJE: Use of atracurium in patients with no renal function. *Br J Anaesth* 1982; 54:1251–1258.
45. White RD, De Weerd JH, Dawson B: Gallamine in anesthesia for patients with chronic renal failure undergoing bilateral nephrectomy. *Anesth Analg* 1971; 50:11–16.
46. Miller RD, Stevens WC, Way WL: The effect of renal failure and hyperkalemia on the duration of pancuronium neuromuscular blockade in man. *Anesth Analg* 1973; 52:661–666.
47. d'Hollander AA, Camu F, Sanders F: Comparative evaluation of neuromuscular blockade after pancuronium administration in patients with and without renal failure. *Acta Anaesthesiol Scand* 1978; 22:21–26.
48. Bevan DR, Archer D, Donati F, et al: Antagonism of pancuronium in renal failure: No recurarization. *Br J Anaesth* 1982; 54:63–68.
49. Hunter JM, Jones RS, Utting JE: Comparison of vecuronium, atracurium and tubocurarine in normal patients and in patients with no renal function. *Br J Anaesth* 1984; 56:941–951.
50. Meistelman C, Lienhart D, Leveque C, et al: Pharmacology of vecuronium in patients with end stage renal failure. *Anesthesiology* 1983; 59:A293.

51. Bevan DR, Donati F, Gyasi H, et al: Vecuronium in renal failure. *Can Anaesth Soc J* 1984; 31:491–496.
52. Orko R, Heino A, Rosenberg PH: Vecuronium in patients with and without renal failure. *Acta Anaesthesiol Scand* 1985; 29:326–329.
53. Cronnelly R, Stanski DR, Miller RD, et al: Pyridostigmine kinetics with and without renal function. *Clin Pharmacol Ther* 1980; 28:78–81.
54. Morris RB, Cronnelly R, Miller RD, et al: Pharmacokinetics of edrophonium in anephric and renal transplant patients. *Br J Anaesth* 1981; 53:1311–1314.
55. Raaflaub J, Frey P: Zur pharmakokinetik von Diallylnortoxiferin beim menschen. *Arzneimittel-forschung* (Aylendorf) 1972; 22:72–81.
56. Duvaldestin P, Saada J, Henzel D, et al: Fazadinium pharmacokinetics in patients with liver disease. *Br J Anaesth* 1980; 52:789–793.
57. Agoston S, Vermeer GA, Kersten UW, et al: The fate of pancuronium bromide in man. *Acta Anaesthesiol Scand* 1973; 17:267–272.
58. Meijer DKF, Weitering JG, Vermeer GA, et al: Comparative pharmacokinetics of *d*-tubocurarine and metocurine in man. *Anesthesiology* 1979; 51:402–405.
59. Ward S, Neill EAM: Pharmacokinetics of atracurium in acute hepatic failure (with acute renal failure). *Br J Anaesth* 1983; 55:1169–1172.
60. Agoston S, Vermeer GA, Kersten UW, et al: A preliminary investigation of the renal and hepatic excretion of gallamine triethiodide in man. *Br J Anaesth* 1978; 50:345–351.
61. Sohn YJ, Bencini A, Scaf AHJ, et al: Pharmacokinetics of vecuronium in man. *Anesthesiology* 1982; 57:A256.
62. Lebrault C, Berger JL, d'Hollander AA, et al: Pharmacokinetics and pharmacodynamics of vecuronium (ORG NC45) in patients with cirrhosis. *Anesthesiology* 1985; 62:601–605.
63. Whittaker M: Plasma cholinesterase variants and the anaesthetist. *Anaesthesia* 1980; 35:174–197.
64. Bowen RA: Anaesthesia in operations for the relief of portal hypertension. *Anaesthesia* 1960; 15:3–10.
65. Dundee JW, Gray TC: Resistance to *d*-tubocurarine chloride in the presence of liver damage. *Lancet* 1953; 2:16–18.
66. El-Hakim M, Baraka A: *d*-Tubocurarine in liver disease. *Kasr-El-Aini J Surg* 1963; 4:99–101.
67. Nana A, Cardan E, Leitersdorfer T: Pancuronium bromide: Its use in asthmatics and patients with liver disease. *Anaesthesia* 1972; 27:154–158.
68. Ward ME, Adu-Gyamfi Y, Strunin L: Althesin and pancuronium in chronic liver disease. *Br J Anaesth* 1975; 47:1199–1204.
69. Gyasi HK, Naguib M: Atracurium and severe hepatic disease: A case report. *Can Anaesth Soc J* 1985; 32:161–164.
70. Somogyi AA, Shanks CA, Triggs EJ: Disposition kinetics of pancuronium bromide in patients with total biliary obstruction. *Br J Anaesth* 1977; 49:1103–1108.

71. Lebrault C, Duvaldestin P, Henzel D, et al: Pharmacokinetics and pharmacodynamics of vecuronium in patients with cholestasis. Br J Anaesth 1986; 58:983–987.
72. Westra P, Houwertjes MC, de Lange AR, et al: Effect of experimental cholestasis on neuromuscular blocking drugs in cats. Br J Anaesth 1980; 52:747–756.
73. Westra P, Houwertjes MC, Wesseling H, et al: Bile salts and neuromuscular blocking agents. Br J Anaesth 1981; 53:407–415.
74. Westra P, Keulemans GTP, Houwertjes MC, et al: Mechanisms underlying the prolonged duration of action of muscle relaxants caused by extrahepatic cholestasis. Br J Anaesth 1981; 53:217–227.
75. Duvaldestin P, Agoston S, Henzel D, et al: Pancuronium pharmacokinetics in patients with liver cirrhosis. Br J Anaesth 1978; 50:1131–1135.
76. Wood M: Plasma protein binding: Implications for anesthesiologists. Anesth Analg 1986; 65:786–804.
77. Baraka A, Gabali F: Correlation between tubocurarine requirements and plasma protein pattern. Br J Anaesth 1968; 40:89–93.
78. Duvaldestin P, Henzel D: Binding of tubocurarine, fazadinium, pancuronium and ORG NC 45 to serum proteins in normal man and in patients with cirrhosis. Br J Anaesth 1982; 54:513–516.
79. Skivington MA: Protein binding of three tritiated muscle relaxants. Br J Anaesth 1972; 44:1030–1034.
80. Wood M, Wood AJJ: Changes in plasma drug binding and α_1-acid glycoprotein in mother and newborn infant. Clin Pharmacol Ther 1981; 29:522–526.
81. Wood M, Stone WT, Wood AJJ: Plasma binding of pancuronium: Effects of age, sex, and disease. Anesth Analg 1983; 62:29–32.
82. Walker JS, Shanks CA, Brown KF: Determinants of d-tubocurarine plasma protein binding in health and disease. Anesth Analg 1983; 62:870–874.
83. Ghoneim MM, Kramer E, Bannow R, et al: Binding of d-tubocurarine to plasma proteins in normal man and in patients with hepatic or renal disease. Anesthesiology 1973; 39:410–415.
84. Westra P, Vermeer GA, de Lange AR, et al: Hepatic and renal disposition of pancuronium and gallamine in patients with extrahepatic cholestasis. Br J Anaesth 1981; 53:331–338.
85. Ward S, Judge S, Corall I: Pharmacokinetics of pancuronium bromide in liver failure. Br J Anaesth 1982; 54:227P.
86. Feldman SA, Cohen EN, Golling RC: The excretion of gallamine in the dog. Anesthesiology 1969; 30:595–598.
87. Upton RA, Nguyen TL, Miller RD, et al: Renal and biliary elimination of vecuronium (ORG NC 45) and pancuronium in rats. Anesth Analg 1982; 61:313–316.

88. Bencini AF, Houwertjes MC, Agoston S: Effects of hepatic uptake of vecuronium bromide and its putative metabolites and their neuromuscular blocking actions in the cat. *Br J Anaesth* 1985; 57:789–795.

89. Bencini AF, Scaf AHJ, Sohn YJ, et al: Hepatobiliary disposition of vecuronium bromide in man. *Br J Anaesth* 1986; 58:988–995.

90. Ramzan IM, Shanks CA, Triggs ET: Pharmacokinetics and pharmacodynamics of gallamine triethiodide in patients with total biliary obstruction. *Anesth Analg* 1981; 69:289–296.

91. Sohn YJ, Bencini AF, Scaf AHJ, et al: Comparative pharmacokinetics and dynamics of vecuronium and pancuronium in anesthetized patients. *Anesth Analg* 1986; 65:233–239.

92. Whittaker M: Plasma cholinesterase variants and the anaesthetist. *Anesthesia* 1980; 35:174–197.

93. McArdle R: The serum cholinesterase in jaundice and diseases of the liver. *Q J Med* 1940; 9:107–127.

94. Foster PA; Potassium depletion and the central action of curare. *Br J Anaesth* 1956; 28:488–491.

95. Hunter AR: Neostigmine resistant curarisation. *Br Med J* 1956; 2:919–921.

96. Feldman SA: Effect of changes in electrolyte, hydration and pH upon the reactions to muscle relaxants. *Br J Anaesth* 1968; 35:546–551.

97. Katz B: *Nerve, Muscle and Synapse.* New York, McGraw-Hill Book Co, 1966.

98. Ginsberg BL, Jenkinson DH: Transmission of impulses from nerves to muscle, in Zaimis E (ed): *Neuromuscular Junction: Handbook of Experimental Pharmacology*, Berlin, Springer-Verlag, 1976, vol 42, p 229.

99. Waud BE, Waud DR: Interaction of calcium and potassium with neuromuscular blocking agents. *Br J Anaesth* 1980; 52:863–866.

100. Hill GE, Wang KC, Shaw CL, et al: Acute and chronic changes in intra- and extracellular potassium and responses to neuromuscular blocking agents. *Anesth Analg* 1978; 57:417–421.

101. Waud BE, Mookerjee A, Waud DR: Chronic potassium depletion and sensitivity to tubocurarine. *Anesthesiology* 1982; 57:111–115.

102. Melnick B, Chang J, Larson C, et al: Hypokalemic familial periodic paralysis. *Anesthesiology* 1983; 58:263–265.

103. Rollman JE, Dickson CM: Anesthetic management of a patient with hypokaelmic familial periodic paralysis for coronary artery bypass surgery. *Anesthesiology* 1985; 63:526–527.

104. Katz B, Miledi R: The effect of calcium on acetylcholine release from motor nerve terminals. *Proc R Soc Lond* 1965; 161:496–502.

105. Hubbard JI, Jones SF, Landon EM: On the mechanism of by which calcium and magnesium affect the release of transmitter by nerve impulses. *J Physiol (Lond)* 1968; 196:75–86.

106. Miledi R, Thies R: Tetanic and post-tetanic rise in frequency of miniature end-plate potentials in low calcium solutions. *J Physiol (Lond)* 1971; 212:245–257.

107. Manthey AA: The effect of calcium on the desensitization of membrane receptors at the neuromuscular junction. *J Physiol (Lond)* 1966; 49:965–976.

108. Jenkinson DH: The antagonism between tubocurarine and substances which depolarize the motor end-plate. *J Physiol (Lond)* 1960; 152:309–319.

109. Al-Mohaya S, Naguib M, Abdelatif M, et al: Abnormal responses to muscle relaxants in a patient with primary hyperparathyroidism. *Anesthesiology* 1986; 65:554–556.

110. Ghoneim MN, Long JP: The interaction between magnesium and other neuromuscular blocking agents. *Anesthesiology* 1970; 32:23–27.

111. Giesecke AH, Morris RE, Dalton MD, et al: Of magnesium, muscle relaxants, toxemic parturients, and cats. *Anesth Analg* 1968; 47:689–695.

112. Skaredoff MN, Roaf ER, Datta S: Hypermagnesaemia and anaesthetic management. *Can Anaesth Soc J* 1982; 29:35–41.

113. Brooks DK, Feldman SA: Metabolic acidosis: A new approach to "neostigmine resistant curarization". *Anaesthesia* 1962; 17:161–169.

114. Payne JP: The influence of carbon dioxide on neuromuscular blocking activity of relaxant drugs in the cat. *Br J Anaesth* 1958; 30:206–214.

115. Utting J: pH as a factor influencing plasma concentrations of d-tubocurarine. *Br J Anaesth* 1963; 35:706–710.

116. Katz RL, Wolf CE: Neuromuscular and electromyographic studies in man: Effects of hyperventilation, carbon dioxide inhalation and d-tubocurarine. *Anesthesiology* 1964; 25:781–787.

117. Baraka A: The influence of carbon dioxide on the neuromuscular block caused by tubocurarine chloride in the human subject. *Br J Anaesth* 1964; 36:272–278.

118. Bush GH, Baraka A: Factors affecting the termination of curarization in the human subject. *Br J Anaesth* 1964; 36:356–362.

119. Hughes R: The influence of changes in acid-base balance on neuromuscular blockade in cats. *Br J Anaesth* 1970; 42:658–668.

120. Payne JP: The influence of changes in blood pH on the neuromuscular blocking properties of tubocurarine and dimethyl tubocurarine in the cat. *Acta Anaesthesiol Scand* 1960; 4:83–90.

121. Dann WL: The effects of different levels of ventilation on the action of pancuronium in man. *Br J Anaesth* 1971; 43:959–962.

122. Gencarelli PJ, Swen J, Koot HWJ, et al: The effects of hypercarbia and hypocarbia on pancuronium and vecuronium neuromuscular blockades in anesthetized humans. *Anesthesiology* 1983; 59:376–380.

123. Gencarelli PJ, Swen J, Koot WHJ, et al: Hypocarbia and spontaneous recovery from vecuronium neuromuscular blockade in anesthetized patients. *Anesth Analg* 1984; 63:608–610.

124. Norman J, Katz RL, Seed RF: The neuromuscular blocking action of pancuronium in man during anaesthesia. *Br J Anaesth* 1970; 42:702–710.

125. Hughes R, Chapple DJ: The pharmacology of atracurium: A competing neuromuscular blocking agent. Br J Anaesth 1981; 53:31–44.
126. Miller RD, Roderick LL; Acid-base balance and neostigmine antagonism of pancuronium neuromuscular blockade. Br J Anaesth 1978; 50:317–324.
127. Wirtavuori K, Salmenpera M, Tammisto T: Effect of hypocarbia and hypercarbia on the antagonism of pancuronium-induced neuromuscular blockade with neostigmine in man. Br J Anaesth 1982; 54:57–61.
128. Miller RD, Van Nyhuis LS, Eger EI, et al: The effect of acid-base balance on neostigmine antagonism of d-tubocurarine-induced neuromuscular blockade. Anesthesiology 1975; 42:377–383.

11

Age and the Neuromuscular Junction

PEDIATRIC RESPONSES

The use of muscle relaxant drugs in children closely followed the early adult experiences.[1, 2] It soon became apparent that the responses to neuromuscular blocking drugs (NMBD) were not the same in the child and the adult. When judged by depression of respiration and surgical relaxation, neonates and infants appeared to be sensitive to nondepolarizing relaxants[5, 9, 10, 11] and resistant to depolarizing drugs.[3, 4, 8] Electromyography demonstrated a resistance to decamethonium[6] but showed that hand paresis occurred at the same dosages as adults when d-tubocurarine was given on a weight basis. However, simultaneous measurements of tidal volume showed an earlier depression in neonates, indicating sensitivity of the respiratory muscles to the nondepolarizing drugs.[7]

Recent studies, using evoked twitch responses, have confirmed that, on a weight-for-weight basis, neonates and infants are resistant to succinylcholine,[12] but their sensitivity to nondepolarizing relaxants has been challenged.[13, 14]

Factors That Influence Dose-Response With Age

Development of Neuromuscular Transmission
Neuromuscular transmission depends on the development of the appropriate neuromuscular connections of the innervated muscle.

Growth in weight and muscle mass in the first years of life is accompanied by the acquisition of motor skills in a predictable sequence. Concomitant changes in the peripheral nerves, muscles, and their synaptic junctions have been investigated to try to define an organized developmental pattern linked to the maturation of neuromuscular transmission.

    Structure of Muscle.—In the rat, embryonic myotubes appear at 16 days' gestation, and at birth, 80% of the muscle fibers remain in this immature state.[15] During the first 3 postnatal weeks, they are replaced gradually by mature fibers that grow in both size and number. Within 30 days, specific fiber types are differentiated according to their oxidative and glycolytic enzyme staining properties. Type I (slow-twitch, oxidative) and type II (fast-twitch, glycolytic) are the main fiber types recognized, although subgroups of each are identifiable.[16] Most muscle groups eventually contain both fiber types, but soleus exhibits almost entirely type I and gastrocnemius mainly type II fibers. The diaphragm has equal representation of each type in the adult.

    Human peripheral muscles are undifferentiated until 20 to 26 weeks' gestation. Type I fibers appear first; then by 30 weeks there is an equal distribution of types I and II as in the adult.[15] The pattern of change in the diaphragm and intercostal muscles is somewhat different, with the proportion of the larger type I to type II fibers increasing from midgestation until early infancy[17] (Fig 11–1). These findings suggest that the oxidative capacity and resistance to fatigue of the ventilatory muscles increase rapidly around the time of birth, in keeping with maturational and functional demands.

    The growth and differentiation of fibers may be intrinsic to the muscle or dependent on innervation. Denervation of neonatal rat muscles causes myotubes to persist in atrophic fibers because of failure of type II cells to develop, while type I cells continue normal development.[18] Electrophysiologic studies in neonatal rat phrenic nerve-diaphragm preparations have demonstrated that at birth there is multiple innervation of each muscle fiber, and all but one of the nerve axons are lost during the second week of life,[19] achieving the single innervation of the adult.[19] Specificity between developing motor axons and their target muscles has been recognized in vertebrates. Early in development this can be influenced by transplanting nerves to inappropriate muscle groups, when respecification occurs. However, after the first week of life, this ability is lost and a post-traumatic regenerating nerve develops very variable synaptic connections.[20]

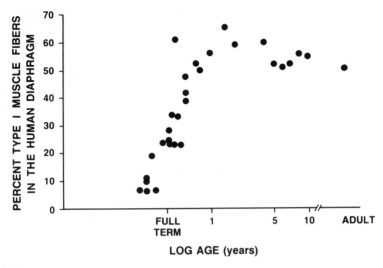

FIG 11–1.
Developmental pattern of type I (slow-twitch, high-oxidative) muscle fibers in the human diaphragm. (From Keens TG, Bryan AC, Levison H, et al: Developmental pattern of muscle fiber types in human ventilatory muscles. *J Appl Physiol* 1978; 909–913. Used by permission.)

Neuromuscular Junction.—The formation of the neuromuscular junction in the embryo depends on the growth of the motor axons to their target muscles, but the mechanisms by which this is initiated and controlled remain speculative.[21] Features of the neuromuscular junctions can be identified in human embryos as early as the ninth week of gestation.[22, 23] By 19 weeks the postsynaptic area shows small junctional folds that become deeper over the next 4 weeks.[22] However, the neuromuscular junction remains incomplete at birth, and immature junctions have been found up to 2 years of age.[24] Morphometric data show that the postsynaptic area and membrane length increase during childhood and then remain constant, while the postsynaptic membrane density is the same in the child and the adult.

Acetylcholine Formation and Release.—In rat phrenic nerve-diaphragm preparations, the rate of acetylcholine release increases during the first 3 months of life. From 30 to 110 days, the miniature end-plate potential (MEPP) amplitude diminishes, and the acetylcholine quantum output with the end-plate potentials (EPP) increases. These changes can be expressed as a safety factor for neuromuscular transmission, which at age 30 days is only 75% of the value at 110 days, suggesting that the very young may be sensitive to nondepolarizing relaxants.[25] Muscle from older mice (30 to 33 months old) has been shown to be more resistant to pancuronium and d-tubocurarine than that from younger mice (8 to 12 months old). Sensitivity to both drugs is greatest in fast-twitch muscles, intermediate in slow-twitch muscles, and least in the diaphragm, regardless of maturity.[26]

Acetylcholine Receptors.—Unlike the innervated adult muscle, embryonic muscle fibers show many extrajunctional acetylcholine receptors. α-Bungarotoxin saturation of chick embryo receptors at the stage of myotube development shows that there is a uniform distribution of receptors over the entire surface of the myotubes that later condenses to discrete localizations of high receptor density.[27] Human myotubes grown in tissue culture also show a low density and relatively even distribution of receptors by α-bungarotoxin binding and single-channel recordings.[28] Acetylcholine receptors are concentrated on the muscle,[29] and their distribution in the maturing neuromuscular junction appears to depend on the trophic action of the nerve on its target cells.[30]

Human Neuromuscular Maturation.—These changes suggest that the infant's neuromuscular junction might exhibit evidence of its immaturity by an alteration in response to NMBDs.

In unanesthetized children, the amplitude of the frequency-sweep electromyogram at 50 to 100 Hz showed more marked fade in those under 12 weeks old.[31] During halothane anesthesia in adults and older children, the response to train-of-four stimulation demonstrates four equal twitches, while in neonates less than 1 month old there is slight fade, with the fourth component decreased to 95% of the first.[32] In premature infants, less than 32 weeks' gestation, this ratio was as low as 83%.[33] In infants and children anesthetized with halothane, fade is accentuated as the rate of tetanic stimulation is increased from 20 to 100 Hz. This is accompanied by increasing post-tetanic facilitation from 20 to 50 Hz with exhaustion at 100 Hz. When tetanic stimulation is increased from 5 to 15 seconds, the muscle action potential in awake newborns shows a more marked decrement with 50% fade at 50 Hz, which is further accentuated in premature infants.[34]

This suggests that maturation of skeletal muscle and the neuromuscular junction occurs predominantly in the first 2 months of extrauterine life.

Extracellular Fluid Volume and Renal Function
The ionized, water-soluble relaxants are distributed mainly in the extracellular fluid (ECF). The ECF volume is larger at birth but decreases

to adult values by the end of the first year (Fig 11–2). Thus, if drugs are given on a body-weight basis, they are diluted in a relatively larger volume in the neonate and infant, and the dose requirements of the neonate and infant will be increased compared with adults. Similarly, the onset time and duration of action will be lengthened. The neonate is $1/_{20}$ the weight but has only $1/_3$ the length and $1/_9$ the surface area of the adult. Throughout life, the ECF volume is related to surface area, suggesting that dose requirements based on surface area may vary less with age.

Renal function in the neonate is characterized by poor concentrating ability and low glomerular filtration rate (GFR). The urinary excretion of these water-soluble, ionized NMBDs is dependent on GFR so that clearance will be reduced in the very young. However, creatinine clearance, and presumably renal relaxant clearance, reaches normal values by 2 years of age.[35]

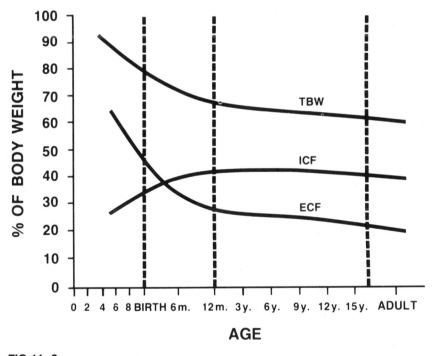

FIG 11–2.
Changes in body water compartments with age. *TBW* = total body water; *ICF* = intracellular fluid; *ECF* = extracellular fluid.

TABLE 11–1.
Cardiac Index and Cardiac Output at Different Ages*

AGE	CARDIAC INDEX, L/MIN/SQ M	CARDIAC OUTPUT, L/MIN	CARDIAC OUTPUT, L/MIN/KG
Newborn	2.5	0.50	0.17
3 mos	3.0	0.75	0.15
1 yr	3.5	1.58	0.16
3 yr	4.5	2.79	0.19
6 yr	4.8	3.84	0.18
9 yr	4.5	4.73	0.16
15 yr	4.0	6.00	0.12
20 yr	3.8	6.65	0.10
80 yr	2.4	4.20	0.06

*Adapted from Guyton AC: *Textbook of Medical Physiology,* ed 6. Philadelphia, WB Saunders Co, 1981, p 274 and Smith RM: *Anesthesia for Infants and Children,* ed 4. St Louis, CV Mosby Co, 1979, p 13.

Cardiac Output

Drug delivery to the tissues where they act and the organs that excrete them depends on cardiac output. In children, cardiac output is largely rate dependent. The heart rate varies with age and is almost twice as fast in the newborn as in the adolescent. The newborn has a cardiac index of 2.5 L/minute/sq m that increases to 4.5 L/minute/sq m by 9 years of age and then declines throughout life to about 2.4 L/minute/sq m by the age of 80 years. In relation to body weight, cardiac output is 0.15 to 0.19 L/minute/kg in infancy and childhood, declining to 0.10 to 0.06 L/minute/kg in adults (Table 11–1). Therefore, circulation time is faster in children than adults, but no appreciable differences exist between infants and older children. Consequently, drugs will be delivered to, and removed from, the neuromuscular junctions more rapidly in children than adults, accelerating the onset of action of the drugs and decreasing their duration of action. These effects may counterbalance those resulting from a change in ECF volume.

Pharmacokinetics

Some of the differences in behavior of the neuromuscular relaxants in children can be explained by alterations in ECF volume, renal function, and sensitivity of the neuromuscular junction.

The increase in ECF volume results in an increase of volume of distribution of d-tubocurarine in neonates and infants,[36, 37] and the immature renal function is responsible for the increase in terminal half-life and decrease in plasma clearance. Indeed, in infants, only 27% of a dose of d-tubocurarine appears in the urine compared with 45% in older children and adults (Figs 11–3 and 11–4). The dilution resulting from increased volume of distribution accounts for the apparent right shift of the dose-response curve when drugs are given on a milligram-per-kilogram basis,[14] although it was recognized that when dose was based on surface area, neonates were more sensitive to d-tubocurarine.[38] Recently obtained log concentration-response curves suggest that the neuromuscular junction has a similar sensitivity to d-tubocurarine at all ages, although variation was greater in the very young[37] (Table 11–2). Decreased elimination of d-tubocurarine accounts for the tendency toward slower return of neuromuscular function.

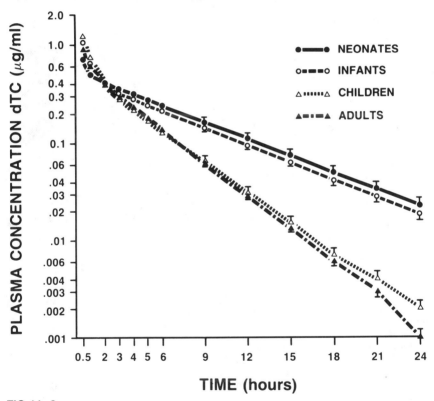

FIG 11–3.
Plasma concentration-time curves for d-tubocurarine, 0.3 mg/kg, in neonates, infants, children, and adults. (From Matteo RS, Lieberman IG, Salamitre E, et al: Distribution, elimination, and action of d-tubocurarine in neonates, infants, children, and adults. *Anesth Analg* 1984; 63:799–804. Used by permission.)

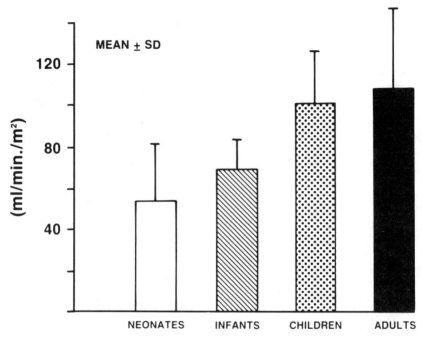

FIG 11–4.
Clearance of *d*-tubocurarine in neonates, infants, children, and adults. (From Fisher DM, O'Keeffe C, Stanski DR, et al: Pharmacokinetics and pharmacodynamics of *d*-tubocurarine in infants, children, and adults. *Anesthesiology* 1982; 57:203–208. Used by permission.)

TABLE 11–2.
Pharmacokinetic and Pharmacodynamic Variables of *d*-Tubocurarine (Mean ± SEM)*

	NEONATES, 0–1 MO	INFANTS, 1–12 MO	CHILDREN, 1–4 YR	ADULTS
V_1,[†]L/kg	.04 ± .003	.038 ± .006	.038 ± .005	.037 ± .003
V_{dss},[†]L/kg	.509 ± .04	.47 ± .06	.34 ± .05	.375 ± .03
C_p,[†]ml/kg/min	1.1 ± .08[‡]	1.0 ± .06[‡]	1.48 ± .06	1.64 ± .05
$t_{1/2\beta}$,[†]min	311.0 ± 40.0[‡]	306.0 ± 35.0	171.0 ± 11.0	164.0 ± 10.0
u24,[†]%	27.0 ± 2.0[‡]	48.0 ± 4.0	45.0 ± 3.0	45.0 ± 4.0
R50,[†]min	72.0 ± 10.0	66.0 ± 18.0	46.0 ± 7.0	55.0 ± 6.0
R25–75,[†]min	57.0 ± 7.0	43.0 ± 5.0	48.0 ± 4.0	48.0 ± 3.0

*From Matteo RS, Lieberman IG, Salamitre E, et al: Distribution, elimination, and action of *d*-tubocurarine in neonates, infants, children, and adults. *Anesth Analg* 1984; 63:799–804. Used by permission.
[†]V_1 = initial volume of distribution; V_{dss} = volume of distribution at steady state; $t_{1/2b}$ = elimination half-life; C_p = plasma clearance; u24 = 24–hour urinary excretion; R50 = time to 50% recovery; R25–75 = time from 25% to 75% recovery.
[‡]Significant difference from adults.

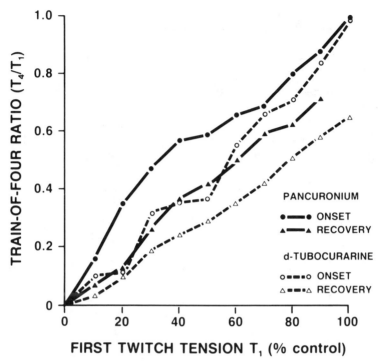

FIG 11–5.
First twitch (T_1) and train-of-four ratio (T4/T1) during onset of and recovery from neuromuscular block with pancuronium and d-tubocurarine in infants and children. (From Robbins R, Donati F, Bevan DR, et al: Differential effects of myoneural blocking drugs on neuromuscular transmissions in infants. *Br J Anaesth* 1984; 56:1095–1099. Used by permission.)

Pharmacokinetic studies in infants and children have also been reported for the antagonists neostigmine[39] and edrophonium.[40] Unfortunately, few patients (four or five) were studied, variations were wide, and the drugs could be detected in plasma for less than 4 hours so that it was not possible to detect significant changes in the volumes of distribution, plasma clearance, and half-lives sufficient to be responsible for the altered response to antagonists in the very young. The only differences that could be detected were decreases in $t_{1/2\beta}$ and a tendency to increased clearance in infants.

Site of Action of Neuromuscular Blocking Drugs

Nondepolarizing blocking drugs may act at more than one site at the neuromuscular junction. Bowman[42] suggests that prejunctional activity is quantitated by depression of single twitch response and postjunctional activity results in post-tetanic fade. Thus, the train-of-four response may differentiate the predominant site of action of a drug.

When train-of-four responses are used during narcotic anesthesia, the train-of-four ratio (TOFR or T4/T1) was lower during recovery than during onset of neuromuscular block for both d-tubocurarine and pancuronium in neonates and infants.[43] The TOFR was lower for d-tubocurarine than pancuronium at all times (Fig 11–5). These differences suggest that in children, as in adults,[44] d-tubocurarine has more powerful prejunctional activity than pancuronium, and that greater prejunctional activity is observed with time with both drugs. Earlier reports of a constant relationship between first twitch (T1) depression and TOFR during d-tubocurarine neuromuscular blockade in children ignored these differences.[14] Vecuronium blockade in children (2 to 9 years old) and adolescents (10 to 17 years old) demonstrates similar relationships between TOFR and T1 depression.[45] At 50% of T1, the degree of fade is similar to that for d-tubocurarine, but at 80% depression, there is little difference in the TOFRs for d-tubocurarine, pancuronium, or vecuronium.

Reversal agents may also show specificity in their sites of action. During the reversal of pancuronium blockade with edrophonium in children of all ages anesthetized with halothane, a higher TOFR existed at the same T1 tension than with neostigmine until T1 exceeded 70% of control (Fig 11–6). The TOFR varied with age, being greater for corresponding T1 values in infants under 1 year than for older children and adults.[41]

Nondepolarizing Relaxants

Alcuronium

In children, good intubating conditions were achieved 1 minute after administration of alcuronium, 0.3 mg/kg intravenously (IV). The duration of action was variable, particularly in the neonate, but incremental doses were not required for about 45 minutes. Infants and children under 10 years old required more frequent incremental doses (15–100 minute intervals) than either neonates or older children (30–190 minute intervals),[46] although the range was very wide.

Atracurium

Many surgical procedures in children are of short duration and are compatible with the duration of action of a single intubating dose of atracurium.[47–49]

Comparable data on the clinical and neuromuscular blocking effects

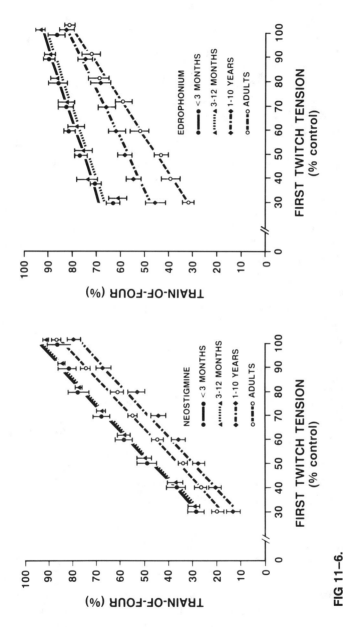

FIG 11–6.
Train-of-four ratio vs. first twitch tension after reversal of pancuronium blockade with neostigmine *(left)* or edrophonium *(right)* in infants and children. (From Meakin G, Sweet PT, Bevan JC, et al: Neostigmine and edrophonium as antagonists of pancuronium in infants and children. *Anesthesiology* 1983; 59:316–321. Used by permission.)

of atracurium are shown in Tables 11–3 and 11–4. When single doses were used in children (2 to 10 years old) and adolescents (11 to 16 years old) anesthetized with halothane, the ED95 was higher in the younger children (0.26 mg/kg) than the adolescents (0.16 mg/kg) on a weight basis. When dosage was calculated according to surface area, apparent age-related differences in drug requirement disappeared.[54, 55] However, infants were found, on the basis of surface area, to be more sensitive to atracurium[55] (Fig 11–7). To produce the same block with narcotic anesthesia, doses need to be increased by one third. When cumulative dose-response curves for atracurium during halothane anesthesia are used, the requirements in infants, children, and adolescents are similar with an ED95 of 0.17 to 0.18 mg/kg,[52, 53] and this is close to adult values.[50, 51] Twitch activity recovered to 5% of control height in 10 minutes and 95% in 36 minutes in all age groups. During narcotic anesthesia, the ED95 was higher (0.23 ± 0.01 mg/kg) in children, but recovery times were similar.[53] Compared with recovery from an ED95 dose of pancuronium, d-tubocurarine, or metocurine, atracurium achieves 95% recovery of twitch in almost half the time. An intubating dose of 2 × ED95 (0.4 mg/kg with halothane and 0.5 mg/kg with narcotic anesthesia) produced satisfactory intubating conditions in all patients.[53] This dose abolishes the twitch response in 1.5 minutes with recovery to 5% twitch height in 25 minutes and 95% in less than 1 hour. Recovery is somewhat faster in children, especially with narcotic anesthesia, 95% twitch recovery occurring in 51.3 minutes compared with 63.5 minutes in adults.[51]

The relatively short duration of action and lack of cumulative effects make atracurium easily controllable when given as an intravenous infusion. In children aged 2 to 10 years following administration of an initial bolus of 0.30 mg/kg with narcotic and 0.25 mg/kg with halothane or isoflurane, requirements to maintain neuromuscular blockade at 90% depression of control twitch were approximately 1.5 × ED95 hourly (0.009 ± 0.008 mg/kg/minute with narcotic and 0.06 ± 0.006 mg/kg/minute with halothane or isoflurane). Spontaneous recovery after termination of the infusion began in 7.9 ± 0.6 minutes and recovered in 20.9 ± 0.7 minutes to 95% control twitch height or was readily reversible with neostigmine.[56]

Fazadinium

Dose requirements for fazadinium in children are 10 times those of pancuronium (60 times those of d-tubocurarine).[57] Fazadinium, 1.25 mg/kg intravenously, during halothane anesthesia produced maximum depression of response (mean twitch depression of 87%) in 8.1 ± 0.7

TABLE 11–3.
Comparison of Potency of Atracurium at Different Ages With Train-of-Four Monitoring

GROUP	N	AGE, YR	ANESTHESIA	ED50, MG/KG	ED95 MG/KG	ED95 MG/SQ M	REFERENCE
Adults	40	18–59	Halothane	—	0.17	—	Savarese et al.[50]
Adults	70	18–58	Narcotic	—	0.20	—	Basta et al.[51]
Adolescents	9	11–17	Halothane	0.12	0.18	6.40	Goudsouzian et al.[52]
Children	11	2–10	Halothane	0.11	0.17	4.70	Goudsouzian et al.[52]
Children	9	1–9	Narcotic	0.16	0.23	6.01	Goudsouzian et al.[53]
Infants	9	6/52–1	Halothane	0.10	0.18	3.30	Goudsouzian et al.[53]
Adolescents	25	11–16	Halothane	0.10	0.16	6.30	Brandom et al.[54]
Children	25	2–10	Halothane	0.13	0.26	6.63	Brandom et al.[54]
Children	25	2–10	Narcotic	0.17	0.35	8.16	Brandom et al.[54]
Infants	25	1/12–6/12	Halothane	0.09	0.16	3.33	Brandom et al.[55]

TABLE 11–4.
Comparison of Onset and Duration of Action of Atracurium at Different Ages With Train-of-Four Monitoring

GROUP	N	AGE, YR	ANESTHESIA	DOSE, MG/KG	ONSET TO MAXIMUM DEPRESSION, MIN	MAXIMUM DEPRESSION TO 95% RECOVERY, MIN	RECOVERY INDEX 25%–75%, MIN	REFERENCE
Adults	40	18–59	Halothane	0.2	3.7	41.8	—	Savarese et al.[50]
				0.4	1.3	65.2	—	Savarese et al.[50]
Adults	70	18–58	Narcotic	0.2	4.0	44.1	12.3	Basta et al.[51]
				0.4	1.7	63.5	11.4	Basta et al.[51]
Adolescents	10	11–17	Halothane	0.4	2.0	54.7	13.5	Goudsouzian et al.[52]
Children	10	2–10	Halothane	0.4	2.0	58.7	14.0	Goudsouzian et al.[52]
Children	9	1–5	Narcotic	0.5	1.5	51.3	9.2	Goudsouzian et al.[53]
Infants	10	4/52–1	Halothane	0.4	1.6	56.1	12.4	Goudsouzian et al.[53]
Adolescents	25	11–16	Halothane	0.4	2.2	41.3	—	Brandom et al.[54]
Children	25	2–10	Halothane	0.4	2.4	40.0	—	Brandom et al.[54]
Children	25	2–10	Narcotic	0.4	2.5		—	Brandom et al.[54]
Infants	25	1/12–6/12	Halothane	0.3	2.7	32.5	5.7	Brandom et al.[55]

minutes with first signs of spontaneous recovery in 45 minutes. At this dose, intubating conditions were satisfactory, but surgical relaxation was often inadequate, while reversal was achieved easily.

Gallamine

Comparative dose-response curves during narcotic anesthesia for gallamine in children (Fig 11–8) showed that gallamine is less potent than d-tubocurarine in a ratio of 7:1 and has an ED95 of 3.4 mg/kg with onset time to maximum effect (10.0 ± 0.3 minutes) and recovery rates from 5% to 25% control twitch (30 ± 3.3 minutes) similar to d-tubocurarine and metocurine.[58]

Metocurine

The use of metocurine in children has been documented sparsely.

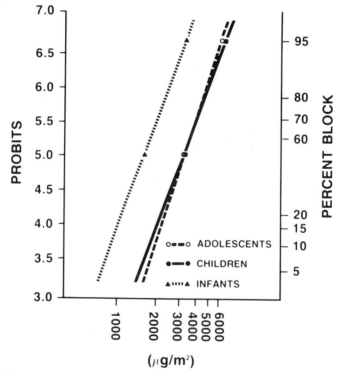

FIG 11–7.
Mean dose-response curves for atracurium (μg/sq m) in adolescents, children, and infants. (From Brandom BW, Woelfel SK, Cook DR, et al: Clinical pharmacology of atracurium in infants. *Anesth Analg* 1984; 63:309–312. Used by permission.)

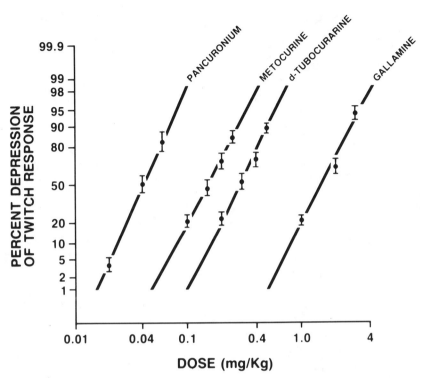

FIG 11–8.
Dose-response curves for pancuronium, metocurine, *d*-tubocurarine, and gallamine in children during narcotic anaesthesia. (From Goudsouzian NG, Martyn JJA, Liu LMP, et al: The dose response effect of long-acting nondepolarizing neuromuscular blocking agents in children. *Can Anaesth Soc J* 1984; 31:246–250. Used by permission.)

Dose-response curves for metocurine in children have been constructed during halothane[59] and narcotic anesthesia[58] (see Fig 11–8) using train-of-four monitoring of the adductor pollicis, with stimulation at 0.25 Hz in the former and 0.1 Hz in the latter study. The ED95 did not differ at different ages in children from 0 to 7 years, but requirements were greater during narcotic anesthesia, with ED95 of 0.34 mg/kg compared with 0.20 mg/kg in the presence of halothane. Both studies showed that, as in adults,[60] metocurine was twice as potent as *d*-tubocurarine. The peak effect after incremental doses occurred in 10 minutes, with recovery from maximum depression to 5% of control twitch (12.4 minutes) and 5% to 25% control twitch (25 minutes), similar to *d*-tubocurarine.

Children demonstrate considerable variability in response but generally have somewhat higher dose requirements than adults in whom the ED95 dose (as measured by single twitch responses at 0.25 Hz) during narcotic anesthesia is 0.18 ± 0.1 mg/kg.[60]

When a dose of 0.5 mg/kg (2.5 × ED95) during halothane anesthesia was used for intubation, the onset time to maximum depression (2.5 ± 0.2 minutes) and recovery time from maximum depression to 5% control twitch (44 ± 11 minutes) were similar to those using equipotent doses of *d*-tubocurarine and pancuronium.[61]

Pancuronium

Limited accounts of its use in children[62-64] were reported soon after pancuronium was introduced into adult practice in 1967. It rapidly gained acceptance in the same clinical situations as *d*-tubocurarine, and its use in anesthesia for premature[65] and cardiac patients[66] and in intensive care[33] is now well established. Contraindications to its use in children are limited to situations in which hypertension is undesirable, such as coarctation of the aorta and pheochromocytoma, or to patients with preexisting tachycardia.

When clinical criteria were used, the potency ratio of pancuronium to *d*-tubocurarine was shown to be 9:1 at birth, decreasing to 6:1 by 1 month,[11] compared with 5:1 in the adult.[67] Dose-response curves for pancuronium in halothane- or narcotic-anesthetized children aged 5 weeks to 7 years, in whom single-twitch measurements were made were shifted to the left of that of *d*-tubocurarine[13, 58] (see Fig 11–8). There is no difference in the dose-response curves of small infants aged 5 to 7 weeks (ED95, 0.06 mg/kg) and older children.[13] Maximum depression of twitch occurs in 7.4 ± 0.5 minutes with recovery to 5%, 25%, and 50% of control height in 11.5, 23.6 and 32.9 minutes, respectively. The ED50 in these children was 0.028 mg/kg compared with 0.009 mg/kg in a similar adult study,[68] which suggests a resistance to pancuronium. Dose requirements during O_2-N_2O-narcotic anesthesia in children aged 1 to 15 years were higher than during halothane anesthesia; when assessed by twitch monitoring of the adductor pollicis, doses of 0.04 and 0.08 mg/kg were required to produce 50% and 95% depression of twitch, respectively. The potency of pancuronium was again shown to be six times that of *d*-tubocurarine.[58]

In situations such as open eye injury or malignant hyperthermia susceptibility where succinylcholine is contraindicated, acceleration of the onset time of nondepolarizing neuromuscular blocking drugs in children is desirable to provide an alternative to succinylcholine for intubation. The use of large single doses, 2 to 2.5 × ED95, has been suggested. Pancuronium, 0.13 mg/kg, allows intubation in 2.5 ± 0.2 minutes, but recovery is prolonged to 65 ± 6 minutes from maximum

TABLE 11–5.
Onset and Recovery From a Paralyzing Dose of Pancuronium (0.07 mg/kg IV) in Children and Adults (Mean ± SEM)*

	WITHOUT PRIMING		WITH PRIMING	
AGE GROUP	TIME TO 90% BLOCK, MIN	TIME TO 10% RECOVERY, MIN	TIME TO 90% BLOCK, MIN	TIME TO 10% RECOVERY, MIN
0–1 yr	1.3 ± 0.2	30.0 ± 2.4	1.1 ± 0.1	26.8 ± 2.9
1–3 yr	2.1 ± 0.3	25.0 ± 2.0	1.6 ± 0.3	28.7 ± 4.0
3–10 yr	2.7 ± 0.4	25.9 ± 3.4	1.6 ± 0.2	28.4 ± 3.8
Adults	3.4 ± 0.4	45.9 ± 2.9	2.1 ± 0.1	57.1 ± 4.8

*Adapted from Bevan JC, Donati F, Bevan DR: Attempted acceleration of the onset of action of pancuronium: Effects of divided doses in infants and children. *Br J Anaesth* 1985; 57:1204–1208.

depression to 5% recovery of control twitch. This is greater than with an equipotent dose of *d*-tubocurarine. From 5% to 25% recovery is somewhat faster, taking a further 25 minutes.[61] As for *d*-tubocurarine, these results preclude the use of this technique for surgery of less than 90 minutes' duration.

The use of a priming dose to accelerate the onset of action of pancuronium was assessed using train-of-four monitoring, during halothane anesthesia in a comparative study of patients aged 0 to 1 year, 1 to 3 years, 3 to 10 years, and adults.[69] Onset time was related directly to age and tended to be more rapid in the children when pancuronium was administered in divided doses without increasing the duration of action (Table 11–5). Although the priming technique may offer advantages in acceleration of onset of neuromuscular block in adults, its usefulness in children, in whom the onset of blockade is already faster, appears limited.

Acutely burned children, like adults, are more resistant to pancuronium. The dose-response curve for pancuronium is shifted to the right, and requirements up to 2.5 times those in normal children have been reported.[70]

d-Tubocurarine

Cullen used Intocostrin in children as early as 1943,[1] 10 years before the use of muscle relaxants in pediatric anesthesia was popularized.[2, 3]

d-Tubocurarine is effective as a nondepolarizing blocking drug in children when given intravenously. Although this is the most commonly employed route of administration, it has been used successfully intramuscularly. When used in combination with halothane in children, the additional effect of the depression of cardiac output by the volatile agent may cause severe hypotension. The beneficial effects of its moderate hypotension have been used to advantage during plastic surgery or spinal fusions. Relative contraindications to its use, myasthenia gravis, myopathies, and hepatic dysfunction, are the same as in the adult.

In the past, suggested intravenous doses of *d*-tubocurarine for children have been extremely variable: 0.1 to 0.6 mg/kg as an initial bolus, followed by incremental doses of one eighth to one quarter of the initial dose. Walts and Dillon[38] found that doses of 0.4 mg/sq m produced 67% abolition of twitch in adults and 99% in neonates, suggesting a sensitivity in the newborn when dosage is based on surface area. Recently, more specific recommendations for *d*-tubocurarine doses have been suggested based on dose-response curves using twitch response of the adductor pollicis in halothane-anesthetized children (Fig 11–9).[14] In children aged 1 day to 7 years, the dose requirements and

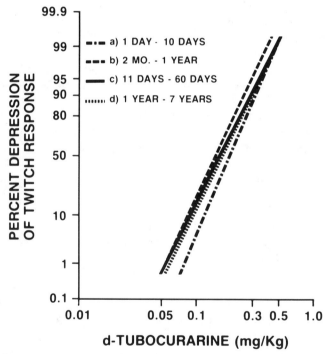

FIG 11–9.

Mean dose-response curves (mg/kg) for *d*-tubocurarine in neonates 1 to 10 days old, *a;* infants 2 to 12 months old, *b;* infants 11 to 60 days old, *c;* and children 1 to 10 years old, *d.* (From Goudsouzian NG, Donlon JV, Savarese JJ, et al: Re-evaluation of dosage and duration of action of d-tubocurarine in the pediatric age group. *Anesthesiology* 1975; 43:416–425. Used by permission.)

TABLE 11–6.
Onset and Recovery From a Paralyzing Dose of d-Tubocurarine (0.4 mg/kg IV) in
Children and Adults* (Mean ± SEM)*

AGE GROUP	WITHOUT PRIMING			WITH PRIMING		
	$T_1\%$		RECOVERY TO $T_1\%$, MIN	$T_1\%$		RECOVERY TO $T_1\%$, MIN
	1 MIN	1.5 MIN		1 MIN	1.5 MIN	
0–1 yr	20 ± 6	10 ± 3	36 ± 5	10 ± 3	5 ± 2	44 ± 9
1–3 yr	33 ± 6	15 ± 4	30 ± 5	23 ± 6	12 ± 4	33 ± 3
3–10 yr	56 ± 9	40 ± 10	24 ± 3	20 ± 5	12 ± 3	35 ± 6
Adults	51 ± 6	24 ± 4	39 ± 5	44 ± 4	20 ± 3	45 ± 3

*Adapted from Donati F, Lahoud J, Walsh CM, et al: Onset of pancuronium and d-tubocurarine blockade with priming. *Can Anaesth Soc J* 1986; 33:571–577.

duration of action did not vary within the age groups studied. The mean dose required to produce 95% depression of twitch (ED95) was 0.32 ± 0.01 mg/kg. Those under 10 days old tended toward higher requirements, with a mean of 0.34 ± 0.04 mg/kg (range, 0.15 to 0.62 mg/kg), while considerable variability was apparent in infants up to 2 months old. If overdosage is to be avoided in those infants who are sensitive to the action of d-tubocurarine, then an incremental dosage regimen should be used.

For the ED95 dose, the mean onset time to maximum effect was 8.6 minutes, and recovery times from maximum effect to 5%, 25%, and 50% of control twitch height were 13.6, 37.0, and 53.3 minutes, respectively. Dose requirements to produce equivalent depression of twitch were higher during O_2-N_2O-narcotic anesthesia, with the ED95 for d-tubocurarine of 0.6 mg/kg (range, 0.34 to 1.05 mg/kg). Onset time was 10 minutes, and recovery from 5% to 25% of control twitch took 32.2 minutes.[58]

The onset of neuromuscular blockade following administration of a paralyzing dose of 0.4 mg/kg d-tubocurarine is generally more rapid in infants and children[71] than in adults[72] (Table 11–6), and recovery is faster probably as a result of greater tissue perfusion. If the priming principle is applied with the same total dose given as an increment of 0.04 mg/kg, followed three minutes later by administration of the intubating dose, then there is a small acceleration of the onset of neuromuscular blockade without prolongation of the duration of action in children (see Table 11–6).

Larger doses of nondepolarizing relaxants can be used to produce satisfactory intubating conditions with a clinically acceptable onset time, but this use is at the expense of a greatly prolonged duration of action. Goudsouzian et al.[61] determined the effects of 0.8 mg/kg of d-tubocurarine (2.5 × ED95 during halothane anesthesia) using train-of-four measurements in children aged 4 months to 10 years during O_2-N_2O-narcotic anesthesia. Similar doses had been used by Nightingale and Bush[62] previously to produce clinically satisfactory conditions for endotracheal intubation, but these doses had resulted in inadequate reversal of neuromuscular blockade at the end of surgery.[62] In this study,[61] satisfactory intubating conditions, with complete abolition of twitch, were achieved in 2.5 ± 0.2 minutes (range, 1.5 to 6.0 minutes). However, the recovery time from maximum depression of twitch to 5% of control twitch height was extended to 53 ± 10 minutes (range, 22 to 110 minutes), and a further 26 minutes was required for recovery to 25% of control values. Reversal of neuromuscular blockade was satisfactory in all cases, but to ensure that reversal is not attempted in the absence of measurable twitch, these doses cannot be recommended for surgery of less than 2 hours' duration.

Vecuronium

Vecuronium is popular in pediatric practice. Two studies have examined the neuromuscular and cardiovascular effects of vecuronium in children, with somewhat different conclusions. Goudsouzian et al.[45] found that more vecuronium was required in children than in adolescents to achieve the same degree of neuromuscular blockade during halothane anesthesia. The ED95 in adolescents was 0.05 mg/kg compared with 0.06 mg/kg in children (Table 11–7). Onset times to maximum effect were 6.9 ± 0.6 and 7.3 ± 0.4 minutes, respectively. Recovery times were similar for both adolescents and children, 25.0 and 26.9 minutes, respectively, from maximum depression to 95% recovery. Generally good intubating conditions were obtained with 0.08 mg/kg in both age groups. Maximum depression of twitch was obtained after 1.8 minutes in adolescents and 1.6 minutes in children.[45] Children recovered from this dose more quickly than adolescents, achieving 95% recovery 6.2 minutes earlier in 41.9 minutes (Table 11–8).

TABLE 11–7.
Comparison of Potency of Vecuronium at Different Ages With Train-of-Four Monitoring

GROUP	N	AGE, YR	ANESTHESIA	ED50, MG/KG	ED95, MG/KG	REFERENCE
Adolescents	10	10–17	Halothane	0.023	0.045	Goudsouzian et al.[45]
Children	10	2–9	Halothane	0.033	0.060	Goudsouzian et al.[45]
Adults	6	18–38	Halothane	0.015	—	Fisher and Miller[73]
Children	24	1–8	Halothane	0.019	—	Fisher and Miller[73]
Infants	24	7/52–45/52	Halothane	0.017	—	Fisher and Miller[73]

TABLE 11–8.
Comparison of Onset and Duration of Action of Vecuronium at Different Ages With Train-of-Four Monitoring

GROUP	N	AGE, YR	ANESTHESIA	DOSE, MG/KG	ONSET TO MAXIMUM DEPRESSION, MIN	MAXIMUM DEPRESSION TO 95% RECOVERY, MIN	RECOVERY INDEX (25%–75%), MIN	REFERENCE
Adolescents	10	10–17	Halothane	0.08	1.8	48.1	13.1	Goudsouzian et al.[45]
Children	10	2–9	Halothane	0.08	1.6	41.9	10.0	Goudsouzian et al.[45]
Adults	6	18–38	Halothane	0.07	2.9	73*	13	Fisher and Miller[73]
Children	24	1–8	Halothane	0.07	2.4	35	9	Fisher and Miller[73]
Infants	24	7/52–45/52	Halothane	0.07	1.5	73	20	Fisher and Miller[73]

*To 90% recovery.

Fisher et al.,[73] using previously available adult data[74] for comparison, could find no differences in dose requirements in infants, children, adolescents, or adults, with an ED50 of 0.02 mg/kg at all ages. Their conditions of measurement differed from the first study, and inspired halothane concentration was controlled more precisely to provide a constant 0.9 minimum alveolar concentration (MAC) adjusted for age. With a dose of 0.07 mg/kg, good intubating conditions were obtained in less than 2.5 minutes. Maximum effect was achieved significantly faster in infants (1.5 ± 0.24 minutes) than in adults (2.9 ± 0.08 minutes). Recovery to 90% was most rapid in children at 35 ± 2.4 minutes and slowest in infants at 73 ± 11.0 minutes. Therefore, dose requirements for children are similar to adults on a weight basis, but the intervals between subsequent doses to maintain neuromuscular blockade will be longer for infants.

The priming effect of vecuronium has been demonstrated in children during halothane anesthesia.[75] When a total dose of 0.065 mg/kg (given as a bolus or with one fifth of the total dose 6 minutes before the remainder) was used, the onset time to 90% depression of twitch was accelerated from 2.6 ± 0.21 to 1.5 ± 0.5 minutes with little change in time to 25% recovery of twitch from 26.1 ± 2.0 to 23.6 ± 2.1 minutes. This suggests that vecuronium may be useful for rapid sequence intubation techniques in children.

Reversal of Neuromuscular Blockade

Residual paralysis has serious consequences in the very young, so it is important to ensure that neuromuscular function has fully recovered at the end of surgery. Clinical assessment of the degree of spontaneous recovery from neuromuscular blockade in children depends on the return of muscle tone, respiration, and crying and is probably less reliable than in adults. When abdominal tone has returned and arm flexion and leg lifting are possible, reversal is probably complete.[76] In the intensive care unit, the return of respiratory function can be judged by measurements of a crying vital capacity of more than 15 ml/kg and a maximum inspiratory force greater than -45 cm H_2O, which indicates the adequacy of return of neuromuscular function.[77] The value of evoked responses with train-of-four monitoring as an indicator of the return of neuromuscular integrity, in conjunction with clinical signs, is well proven in adults. Fade of the fourth twitch of the train-of-four to less than 75% of the first twitch height indicates the need for pharmacologic reversal. It is usual to administer reversal agents following the use of nondepolarizing relaxants, but the indications for their use after succinylcholine are controversial. Succinylcholine infusions result in a phase II block that recovers slowly on termination of the infusion. This can be readily reversed pharmacologically in children and adults 10 minutes after stopping the infusion.[78]

Reversal of nondepolarizing relaxants in children is achieved with the same combinations of anticholinesterases, neostigmine or edrophonium, and anticholinergics, atropine or glycopyrrolate, as in adults. However, higher dose requirements have usually been recommended for children.[79] Recent studies suggest that children have lower neostigmine requirements that are followed by a faster rate of recovery of thumb-twitch activity than adults.[39, 41] Dose-response relationships determined in children of similar ages, receiving a continuous d-tubocurarine infusion to maintain 90% depression of twitch, showed that the ED50 for neostigmine (dose that produces 50% antagonism of the block) was 0.013 mg/kg in infants and 0.016 mg/kg in children. These values are approximately half adult values obtained under similar conditions.[39]

Edrophonium is used less commonly than neostigmine, but it is as effective as neostigmine and more rapid in onset initially at doses of 0.71 or 1.43 mg/kg.[41] Like neostigmine, recovery was more rapid in children than adults (Fig 11–10). Fisher et al.[40] concluded that an effective dose of edrophonium was 1 mg/kg, similar to or slightly higher than that needed for adults.

Atropine has a rapid antimuscarinic action that matches the onset of edrophonium better than neostigmine and maintains a stable heart rate in adults. Atropine given before or together with neostigmine results in transient tachycardia, but when glycopyrrolate and neostigmine are used together, little change in heart rate occurs.[80]

Depolarizing Relaxants

Succinylcholine

Succinylcholine is the only depolarizing NMBD that has been used and investigated extensively in pediatric practice. For a time during the 1950s, it was regarded as the muscle relaxant of choice for neonates, infants, and children, not only for intubation, but also for relaxation throughout major surgical procedures.[4] Overdosage appeared unlikely because of resistance to its effect and its short duration of action,[3] while the use of curare was overshadowed by concerns for sensitivity and prolonged respiratory depression. When administered by intravenous injection in a dose of 1.0 mg/kg, succinylcholine has a rapid onset of action that is terminated in 2.7 ± 0.1 minutes.[81] Recovery from 0.5 or

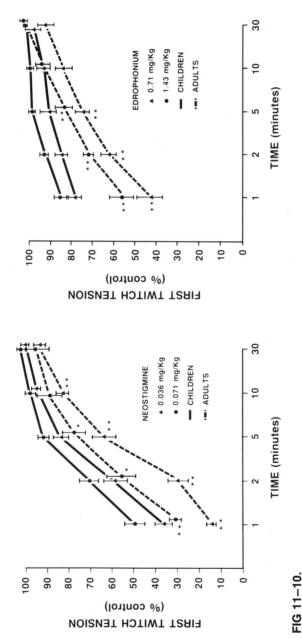

FIG 11–10.

Comparison of recovery from pancuronium neuromuscular blockade in children and adults after neostigmine and edrophonium. (From Meakin G, Sweet TT, Bevan JC, et al: Neostigmine and edrophonium as antagonists of pancuronium in infants and children. *Anesthesiology* 1983; 59:316–321. Used by permission.)

TABLE 11–9.
Comparison of Neuromuscular Block and Recovery Times (Mean Values) After
Intravenous Succinylcholine, 0.5 and 1.0 mg/kg, at Different Ages

AGE	0.5 MG/KG		1.0 MG/KG		REFERENCE
	MAXIMUM DEPRESSION, %	90% RECOVERY, MIN	MAXIMUM DEPRESSION, %	90% RECOVERY, MIN	
Adults	100	7.4	100	12.1	Walts and Dillon[82]
Adults	100	10.1	100	14.6	Katz and Ryan[83]
Children	83.6	3.0	100	4.8	Cook and Fisher[12]
Infants	69	2.3	85.3	4.0	Cook and Fisher[12]

1.0 mg/kg is twice as fast in children as in adults[12, 82, 83] (Table 11–9). Although neonates and infants have only half the plasma pseudocholinesterase activity of the adult,[85] they show no prolongation of the action of succinylcholine, which may be due to rapid dilution in the large ECF volume at this age.[84]

Succinylcholine is used most commonly as a single bolus intravenously to facilitate endotracheal intubation. The dose, on a weight basis, to produce apnea in neonates[8, 12] is two to four times greater than in adults.[82, 83] However, if dosage is calculated on the basis of surface area, there is no difference in potency or duration of action.[38] Cook and Fischer[12] showed that infants aged 1 to 10 weeks required 1 mg/kg intravenously to produce the same depression of twitch as 0.5 mg/kg in older children (see Table 11–9), but for equipotent doses, the recovery times were similar at both ages. Again, dose requirements related to surface area showed a correlation with age, with a linear relationship between the log dose and potency and duration of action in infants and children. Neonates showed even greater sensitivity, requiring 1.5 mg/kg to produce 91.1% twitch depression.[84]

As the dose of succinylcholine is increased, the characteristics of the neuromuscular response change from a phase I depolarizing block to a phase II nondepolarizing or dual block. Recommendations for total dosage have been aimed at a maximum below which this did not occur, in the belief that phase II block is associated with prolonged apnea.

The patterns of change in neuromuscular blockade have been studied during prolonged infusions of succinylcholine in children during halothane anesthesia.[78] The mean duration of infusion was 88.0 ± 6.3 minutes in infants and 100.5 ± 9.9 minutes in children. Infusion rates of succinylcholine required to maintain constant 85% to 90% depression of control twitch were greater in children than in adults but showed the same qualitative changes (Fig 11–11). Over the first 40 to 80 minutes, succinylcholine requirements increased, but this tachyphylaxis was followed by a bradyphylaxis, as has been described in adults. The peak requirement occurred 20 to 60 minutes earlier in children. Phase II block developed during the tachyphylaxis, so it appeared sooner than in adults but at higher doses (Table 11–10). Recovery was rapid after discontinuing the infusion, and residual nondepolarizing block remaining after 10 minutes was reversible with neostigmine (Table 11–11). Similarly, De Cook and Goudsouzian,[86] and Goudsouzian and Liu,[87] found an increased requirement in pediatric patients, suggesting that succinylcholine requirements were inversely related to age. However, the duration of their infusions was shorter so that their results reflected the earlier peak unmodified by the later decreased requirement.

Intramuscular succinylcholine provides an alternative to intravenous administration in pediatric anesthesia. When venous access is difficult, this route can provide predictable relaxation for intubation, although maximum effect takes 3 to 4 minutes with a dose of 4 mg/

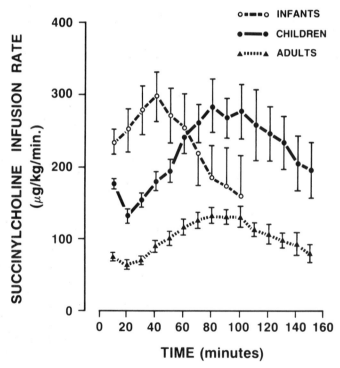

FIG 11–11.
Infusion rates of succinylcholine required to maintain 85% to 90% depression of T_1 in infants, children, and adults. (From Bevan JC, Donati F, Bevan DR: Prolonged infusion of suxamethonium in infants and children. *Br J Anaesth* 1986; 58:839–843. Used by permission.)

TABLE 11–10.
Dose and Time at Which Phase II Block
(T_4/T_1 = 0.5) Develops During
Succinylcholine Infusion at Different Ages
(Mean ± SEM)*

AGE	TIME, MIN	DOSE, MG/KG
Infants	13.9 ± 1.9	3.2 ± 0.6
Children	23.2 ± 1.4	3.5 ± 0.2
Adults	32.0 ± 3.6	2.1 ± 0.2

*Adapted from Bevan JC, Donati F, Bevan DR:
Prolonged infusion of suxamethonium in infants
and children. *Br J Anaesth* 1986; 58:839–843.

TABLE 11–11.
Residual Neuromuscular Blockade 10
Minutes After Stopping Succinylcholine
Infusion at Different Ages (Mean ± SEM)*

AGE	T_1	T_4/T_1
Infants	0.52 ± 0.06	0.45 ± 0.04
Children	0.73 ± 0.08	0.52 ± 0.06
Adults	0.63 ± 0.06	0.29 ± 0.04

*From Bevan JC, Donati F, Bevan DR: Prolonged
infusion of suxamethonium in infants and children. *Br J Anaesth* 1986; 58:839–843. Used by
permission.

kg.[88, 89, 91] This is longer than reported in adults, but the recovery time of approximately 20 minutes is shorter. Even at doses of 5 mg/kg in infants under 6 months old, recovery was not prolonged, taking 16.5 ± 1.2 minutes.[90] Phase II block with a train-of-four ratio below 50% was seen in one third of patients at these doses but did not affect clinical recovery. Attempts to accelerate the onset of action of intramuscular succinylcholine by increasing the concentration of solution[91] or injecting at two sites[89] have proved ineffective.

There have been reports of pulmonary edema in infants following the use of intramuscular succinylcholine.[92] While a causal relationship cannot be excluded, there are also cases of pulmonary edema induced by ventilatory efforts made against a closed glottis, which may offer an alternative interpretation in these circumstances.[93] Cardiovascular effects are not marked, and the incidence of succinylcholine-induced arrhythmias, particularly bradycardia, is reduced after intramuscular administration.[94, 95] The use of intramuscular atropine, 0.02 mg/kg, concomitantly with succinylcholine, 4 mg/kg, in infants results in no marked changes in heart rate, but if the dose of atropine is increased to 0.3 mg/kg, a mild tachycardia is seen.[96]

Intralingual administration of succinylcholine proved to be as effective in producing apnea as intravenous injection, but the associated high incidence of cardiac arrhythmias precludes its regular use.[94]

Complications

The advantages of using succinylcholine intravenously for intubation must always be weighed against its known risks and contraindications. While children and adults are liable to the same complications, the importance of these is different at different ages.

Muscle fasciculations, which accompany the onset of action of depolarizing block in adults, are mild in children and absent in infants. Succinylcholine-induced pain after surgery may correlate with the severity of muscle fasciculation, although this is seen less often in children. For the same reason, there is little increase in *intragastric pressure.*[97] However, a transient rise in *intraocular pressure* occurs after 1 minute and lasts 6 minutes in children, as in adults.[98] This results from contraction of the extraocular muscles, which is dose related and independent of fasciculations.

There have been sporadic reports of *myoglobinuria* after administration of succinylcholine. Incremental doses of succinylcholine in a 15-year-old patient resulted in myoglobinuria detected by dark red discoloration of the first postoperative urine sample.[99] *Myoglobinemia* has now been shown to occur in all infants and children following administration of 1 to 2 mg/kg of succinylcholine intravenously; 6% achieve serum myoglobin levels over 3,000 ng/ml and show myoglobinuria 1 hour after injection.[100] Occasionally, rhabdomyolysis can be severe enough to impair renal function. The prophylactic use of self-taming doses of succinylcholine or pretreatment with d-tubocurarine or pancuronium decreases fasciculations in older children. The nondepolarizing drugs also reduce the myoglobinemia following administration of succinylcholine, 1 mg/kg intravenously.[101]

Serum *potassium concentration* is elevated transiently after intravenous succinylcholine administration to normal children, but the maximum levels achieved are clinically unimportant.[102] Vagally mediated cardiac arrhythmias following administration of succinylcholine are frequent and may be blocked by anticholinergic drugs. Bradycardia is the most common arrhythmia seen in children,[103] with the maximum change in heart rate occurring 45 to 60 seconds after injection. It is most marked after repeated injection and can lead to sinus arrest. Isoflurane anesthesia may offer more protection from heart-rate fluctuations than halothane.[104] Intravenous atropine (0.02 mg/kg) and glycopyrrolate (0.01 mg/kg) given immediately before giving succinylcholine are equally effective in averting changes in heart rate in children.[105, 106]

Prolonged apnea following administration of succinylcholine characterizes an abnormal response in a patient with low or abnormal plasma pseudocholinesterase activity. Physiologic variations in cholinesterase are found in the newborn who has only 50% to 65% the activity of the adult.[85, 107] Levels rise to adult values in 3 weeks and continue to increase until the child is 3 to 4 years of age when levels are 30% higher than in the adult. Thereafter they decline gradually to 25% below normal in the elderly.[108] However, these levels appear to be adequate as a normal response to succinylcholine is usually seen at all ages.

The incidence of genetically determined *atypical cholinesterase* in children is presumably the same as in the adult population. However, identification in children may be more likely because of the increasing use of endotracheal intubation facilitated by succinylcholine for short operations. Train-of-four monitoring is useful in clinical diagnosis and management of the immediate response, while confirmation and family studies by plasma cholinesterase analysis can follow.

Children with *neuromuscular disorders* or muscular paralysis and secondary atrophy may exhibit atypical responses to succinylcholine. The response to depolarizing relaxants is unpredictable, and the degree of clinical involvement is no guide to the severity of the reaction. Subclinical pathologic conditions may be revealed first by an abnormal response to general anesthesia.

Congenital myopathies, commonly *Duchenne type muscular dystrophy,* are associated with a normal neuromuscular response to succinylcholine. However, cardiomyopathy is often present, and the hyperkalemic response to succinylcholine may induce cardiac arrest.[109, 110] The risk of malignant hyperthermia susceptibility may also be increased in this group of patients.[111] Denborough[111] recognized a constant relationship between malignant hyperthermia and a clinical myopathy associated with abnormalities and frequent association with subclinical conditions.

The inherited *myotonias,* which may take the milder forms of *myotonia congenita* or *paramyotonia* or the more severe *myotonic dystrophy,* are associated with a myotonic response to succinylcholine. This is a sustained *contracture* of muscle that produces localized masseter spasm or generalized rigidity, making intubation and ventilation impossible, but without any hypermetabolic response.[112, 113]

Patients with myopathies and myotonias are more frequently seen in childhood because of their decreased life expectancy. At various stages in their disease processes, they require general anesthesia for diagnostic muscle biopsy, correction of related orthopedic conditions, such as scoliosis, or general surgical procedures. The choice of anesthetic depends on the degree of cardiorespiratory involvement as well as the state of disease progression.

Succinylcholine is contraindicated in the myotonias, but the association of *malignant hyperthermia* with these conditions is not clear (see Chapter 8). Halothane is not specifically contraindicated, but patients appear to be sensitive to its hypotensive effect.[114] The use of nondepolarizing relaxants is appropriate to the approach to management, and *d*-tubocurarine and atracurium,[115] in combination with halothane, have been used successfully.

Succinylcholine is unique among the muscle relaxants in providing three examples of atypical responses that are truly pharmacogenetic complications. In succinylcholine apnea, contracture response in congenital myotonias, and malignant hyperthermia, the reaction to the drug is determined by a genetic predisposition. It is tempting to try to relate these abnormal responses. A genetic marker predictive of malignant hyperthermia might then be identified and, speculatively, the physiologic role of cholinesterase revealed.

Ellis et al.[116] and Whittaker et al.[117] reported a high incidence of the fluoride-resistant cholinesterase gene in survivors of clinical malignant hyperthermia reactions and in their families. However, Evans et al.[118] and Ording et al.[119] were unable to detect any cholinesterase variant in individuals in whom malignant hyperthermia susceptibility had been confirmed by in vitro halothane contracture testing. Promising genetic linkage studies in Phi blood grouping and Phi enzyme-system typing might lead to replacement of the muscle biopsy tests by blood tests prognostic of malignant hyperthermia susceptibility.[120] The hypothesis that succinylcholine apnea and malignant hyperthermia occur as the result of the same genetic defect seems unlikely. Plasma cholinesterase variants show a recessive inheritance with a frequency of 1 in 200. Malignant hyperthermia has a dominant inheritance, although this has incomplete penetrance and shows variable expressivity, occurring in 1 in 14,000 of the population. Porcine malignant hyperthermia shows autosomal recessive characteristics[121] but in other respects appears to resemble the human condition.

The inheritance of malignant hyperthermia is complex, and a close link with that of the cholinesterase variants or the congenital myopathies cannot be excluded. Denborough[111] has described two classes of myopathies that predispose to malignant hyperthermia. One is dominantly inherited but subclinical and therefore usually undetected in the absence of an anesthetic reaction. The other is a recessive trait apparent in young males as multiple-characteristic physical abnormalities with kyphoscoliosis, short neck, and undescended testes, but these males have no intellectual impairment. It is recognized that contracture responses occur in response to succinylcholine in patients with congenital myotonias, but such responses are not associated with the hypermetabolic reaction of malignant hyperthermia. However, masseter spasm caused by localized contracture of muscles is a clinical manifestation common to some myopathies and myotonias and to malignant hyperthermia susceptibility.

GERIATRIC RESPONSES

The number of geriatric patients requiring anesthesia and surgery is increasing. With 11% of the North American population now over 65 years of age and expectations for this group to expand to 18% within 40 years, it is important to be aware of alterations in drug actions in the elderly. Although pathologic states will modify the effects of drugs in these patients, recognition of the predictable consequences of aging on body composition and physiology allows a rational approach to therapy.

Factors That Influence Responses in Geriatric Patients

With aging there is a relative increase in body fat, a decrease in lean body mass, and a reduction in total body water. Therefore, the volume of distribution of the water-soluble nondepolarizers may be reduced, producing unexpectedly high initial plasma concentrations when dosages are based on body weight. Serum albumin concentration is decreased so that protein binding of drugs may be reduced.

In humans, structural changes occur in both the presynaptic and postsynaptic areas of the neuromuscular junction, with a decrease in presynaptic membrane lengths and reduction in postsynaptic density. The number of acetylcholine receptors in rats diminishes in old age suggesting that regressive changes occur in the neuromuscular junction.[122]

Elimination of most neuromuscular relaxants (with the exceptions of succinylcholine and atracurium) depends, to a large extent, on renal excretion. Glomerular filtration rate decreases 1% per year in adult life as a result of reduced renal plasma flow; this decrease in GFR accounts for most of the decline in renal function with age.[123] This is not associated with an increased serum creatinine concentration because the reduction in skeletal muscle mass results in decreased nitrogen metabolism. Renal function is, therefore, best assessed by creatinine clearance. Age-related changes in renal function will result in prolonged elimination of nondepolarizing relaxants with a consequent lengthening of their duration of action (see Chapter 10).

Hepatic metabolism and biliary excretion is less important. There is a reduction in liver size by 40% to 50% by the age of 80 years. Enzyme activity is decreased, and plasma cholinesterase synthesis is impaired, so that in elderly men, plasma levels are 24% below that of younger men. However, plasma levels are the same as in young and old female adults.[108] Splanchnic blood flow is decreased so that drug delivery to the liver is reduced. Liver function measured by Bromsulphalein retention declines after 50 years of age.[124]

Cardiovascular changes are frequently the result of concomitant disease, but normal aging produces generalized loss of arterial elasticity. Cardiac output changes need not be severe, and it may be maintained at normal levels. The onset time of neuromuscular blocking drugs should then be unchanged.

Nondepolarizing Relaxants

Alcuronium

Stephens et al.[125] followed the plasma concentration decay curves for alcuronium (0.30 to 0.37 mg/kg) in elderly patients. They compared the derived pharmacokinetic data with that previously obtained in middle-aged adults.[126] The apparent volume of distribution did not differ between the groups, but the terminal elimination half-life and plasma clearance were larger in the older patients (Table 11–12). These results suggest that the duration of action of alcuronium would be prolonged in the elderly. However, in a group of elderly patients with extensive blood loss during major surgery, plasma clearance was no different from the normal adult, presumably as a result of hemodilution. Thus, the duration of action of alcuronium in this situation should not be altered.

Atracurium

Atracurium is independent of hepatic and renal function for its elimination, so there is no reason to expect requirements to change in the elderly. d'Hollander et al.[127] determined the dosage requirements of atracurium, during continuous infusion, to maintain neuromuscular blockade of 90% control twitch height. After the first half hour, dosage requirements stabilized and could be equated with the amount of atracurium eliminated by inactivation. For young, middle-aged, and older adult patients, the dose requirements were similar. Consequently, the

TABLE 11–12.
Pharmacokinetic Variables and Recovery Indices Associated With Aging (Mean ± SEM)

DRUG	AGE, YR	N	V_d, L/KG	$t_{1/2\beta}$, MIN	Cl, ML/MIN/KG	RECOVERY INDEX, MIN	REFERENCE
Alcuronium	41 ± 3.7	14	0.30 ± 0.03	175.6 ± 15.9	1.44 ± 0.10	—	Walker et al.[126]
Atracurium	73 ± 2.1	5					Stephens[125]
	26 ± 3.0	8	0.33 ± 0.02	438.6 ± 76.3	0.53 ± 0.10	15.4 ± 1.9	d'Hollander et al.[127]
	53 ± 2.0	8	—	—	—	14.8 ± 1.1	d'Hollander et al.[127]
	76 ± 2.0	8	—	—	—	14.5 ± 1.6	d'Hollander et al.[127]
Metocurine	(29–52)	7	0.45 ± 0.02	269 ± 21.2	1.10 ± 0.06	47 ± 10	Matteo et al.[128]
	(70–81)	7	0.28 ± 0.01	530 ± 31.4	0.36 ± 0.03	110 ± 35	Matteo et al.[128]
Pancuronium	35 ± 2.4	18	0.28 ± 0.01	107 ± 5.7	1.81 ± 0.08	39 ± 13	Duvaldestin et al.[131]
	79 ± 1.0	15	0.32 ± 0.03	201 ± 17.8	1.18 ± 0.10	62 ± 30	Duvaldestin et al.[131]
d-Tubocurarine	(30–56)	7	0.43 ± 0.02	173 ± 14.4	1.71 ± 0.12	48 ± 4.5	Matteo et al.[128]
	(70–87)	7	0.28 ± 0.02	268 ± 19.3	0.79 ± 0.07	94 ± 12.1	Matteo et al.[128]
Vecuronium	28 ± 2	8	—	—	—	16.2 ± 4.0	d'Hollander et al.[134]
	54 ± 3	8	—	—	—	21.9 ± 2.2	d'Hollander et al.[134]
	69 ± 3	8	—	—	—	44.9 ± 6.9	d'Hollander et al.[134]
Neostigmine	(33–48)	4	0.26 ± 0.02	70 ± 11.5	5.1 ± 0.40	10 ± 1.0	Rupp et al.[135]
	(70–84)	6	0.18 ± 0.02	58 ± 4.1	3.7 ± 0.40	11 ± 0.4	Rupp et al.[135]
	(34–56)	7	0.10 ± 0.04	18.5 ± 7.0	33.5 ± 4.0	—	Young et al.[137]
	(71–80)	5	0.07 ± 0.02	16.7 ± 0.08	23.4 ± 5.0	—	Young et al.[137]

rate of recovery from 25% to 75% control twitch height was independent of age (see Table 11–12). The lack of any effect of age on atracurium elimination and duration of action makes it unique among the non-depolarizing neuromuscular blockers.

Metocurine

Matteo et al.[128] studied the age-related effects of metocurine together with those of d-tubocurarine. After administration of a single intravenous bolus of metocurine (0.3 mg/kg), the plasma concentration time curves were compared in young and elderly adults. The results were similar to those found for d-tubocurarine. The elderly showed a decreased volume of distribution, decreased plasma clearance, and prolonged elimination half-life when compared with younger adults (see Table 11–12). Pharmacodynamic relationships following administration of 0.15 mg/kg lacked any significant differences, while the relationship between log plasma concentration and twitch responses was similar at all ages.

Pancuronium

Differences in the actions of nondepolarizing relaxants in the elderly were first examined by McLeod et al.[129] They found that for pancuronium the volume of distribution remained unchanged, but the plasma clearance decreased with advancing age. The rate of elimination, which was 1.6 ml/minute/kg at 20 years of age, fell progressively throughout adulthood to levels of 0.45 ml/minute/kg in the ninth decade. Although Somogyi[130] found no differences in the pharmacokinetics of pancuronium in the elderly, Duvaldestin et al.[131] confirmed the decreased clearance and prolonged duration of pancuronium in the elderly. Cumulative dose-response curves for pancuronium in older patients and a control group of middle-aged adults when single twitch evoked responses of the adductor pollicis were measured, showed that the potency of pancuronium did not differ significantly at different ages. In elderly patients, the ED50 was 0.044 ± 0.020 mg/kg compared with 0.039 ± 0.002 mg/kg in younger patients, and the ED95 was 0.081 ± 0.005 mg/kg compared with 0.078 ± 0.004 mg/kg. In both age groups, plasma concentrations for the same degree of neuromuscular blockade were similar. These changes result from decreased renal clearance of pancuronium. After 2 hours, only 18 ± 3.7% of the administered dose could be recovered in the urine in elderly patients, half of that normally anticipated in adults.

d-Tubocurarine

The pharmacodynamic and pharmacokinetic effects of d-tubocurarine have been studied recently by Matteo, et al.[128] during halothane anesthesia. Following administration of a single dose of d-tubocurarine (0.3 mg/kg) intravenously, the plasma concentration decay curves were determined over 6 hours. Throughout this period, the plasma concentrations were consistently higher in the elderly than in the younger adults. There were significant pharmacokinetic differences in the two groups, with a decreased volume of distribution, decreased plasma clearance, and prolongation of the elimination half-life in the elderly (see Table 11–12). The log plasma concentrations were the same for any level of neuromuscular blockade between 20% to 80% in both age groups, suggesting that there is no difference in the sensitivity of the neuromuscular junction with aging. The time for return of 50% twitch and recovery index were prolonged in the elderly.

Vecuronium

The effect of increasing age on the response to vecuronium has been examined following administration of a single intravenous bolus dose or during steady-state infusions. d'Hollander et al.[132] studied adults aged 15 to 85 years during narcotic anesthesia. Following administration of a single bolus of 70 μg/kg intravenously, twitch height was depressed to 6.4 ± 0.8% at all ages. However, the onset of maximum neuromuscular blockade was delayed in the elderly and correlated with age. Peak effect at 20 years of age occurred at 5.2 minutes, which increased to 7.9 minutes by 80 years of age. O'Hara et al.[133] constructed dose-response curves for vecuronium in young (29 ± 0.83 years) and older (76 ± 0.88 years) adults, using single doses. The log dose-probit response curves did not differ in these two age groups. Comparisons of potency and time to onset of maximum effect also failed to show any differences.

The pharmacokinetics of vecuronium in the elderly during narcotic anesthesia have been investigated using steady-state infusion techniques. d'Hollander et al.[134] found that after 30 minutes, the infusion rate of vecuronium required to maintain a constant 90% depression of twitch stabilized. Dose requirements in the older adults over 60 years of age were significantly lower (1,775 ± 213 μg/sq m/hour) than in adults below 40 years of age (2791 ± 434 μg/sq m/hour), and recovery rate was more than doubled. These conclusions would suggest that maintenance doses should be decreased and given at longer intervals in the elderly. However, Rupp et al.[135] found that the pharmacodynamic behavior in patients over 70 years of age was no different from the young. When vecuronium was infused at a fixed rate of 2.5 μg/kg/minute, the volume of distribution was decreased in the elderly (from 255 ±

16.5 to 177 ± 12.2 ml/kg). This was exactly counterbalanced by a reduction in plasma clearance that resulted in an elimination half-life similar to that in the younger adults, and the recovery index was unchanged. Steady-state concentrations required to produce 50% paralysis ($C_{pss}50$) were similar (94 ± 16.5 µg/ml in the young and 104 ± 10.6 µg/ml in the elderly), suggesting that the sensitivity of the neuromuscular junction was unchanged. This would indicate that lower dosages of vecuronium are appropriate in the elderly. However, as elimination and recovery rate are unaltered, the intervals between maintenance doses need not be changed.

Reversal Agents

Spontaneous recovery from nondepolarizing neuromuscular blockade in the elderly is likely to be prolonged. The rate of reversal by neostigmine of a pancuronium-induced blockade during narcotic anesthesia has been measured by train-of-four responses.[136] The time to reach a TOFR of 60% was variable in this study but was prolonged from 5.08 ± 1.15 minutes in the young to 11.00 ± 2.8 minutes in the elderly. Differences in the level of nondepolarizing blockade when reversal was attempted and variations in neostigmine dosage (0.05 to 0.10 mg/kg with atropine, 0.017 to 0.024 mg/kg) could not account for the large difference between mean recovery times in the two age groups.

Young et al.[137] have provided a more complete understanding of the effects of neostigmine in the elderly. A stable 90% neuromuscular blockade was produced by continuous infusion of metocurine during halothane anesthesia and was antagonized with neostigmine (0.07 mg/kg) and atropine (0.02 mg/kg). Plasma concentration decay curves for neostigmine were obtained in middle-aged (34 to 56 years old) and elderly (71 to 80 years old) adults. Pharmacodynamic effects were the same in both groups and demonstrated a constant relationship between plasma concentration of neostigmine and recovery of twitch response. There were no differences in the pharmacokinetic variables of neostigmine in the elderly, except for a small decrease in the initial volume of distribution (see Table 11–12). Thus it is difficult to determine the cause of the prolonged effects of neostigmine in the elderly.

Summary

The distribution, elimination, and actions of the nondepolarizing relaxants and reversal agents have been studied recently in the elderly. Prolongation of the actions of *d*-tubocurarine, metocurine, pancuronium, and vecuronium is a consequence of aging factors resulting in a decrease volume of distribution and plasma clearance of the drugs. As pharmacodynamic responses are stable, sensitivity of the neuromuscular junction appears to be unaltered in old age. Results of studies with vecuronium are not as consistent as those with the other relaxants but generally point in the same direction as pancuronium. This may be because 75% of the excretion of vecuronium is independent of the kidney while d-tubocurarine, pancuronium, and metocurine rely on renal excretion for 60% of their elimination. Atracurium is unique in being unaffected by age-related changes because of its independence from hepatic and renal functions. Succinylcholine has not been investigated as thoroughly as the nondepolarizing agents.

Neostigmine is the only reversal agent that has been studied in the elderly. The duration of its antagonistic action is prolonged to an extent that should be compatible with the longer duration of action of muscle relaxants in the elderly.

REFERENCES

1. Cullen SC: The use of curare for the improvement of abdominal muscle relaxation during inhalation anaesthesia. *Surgery* 1943; 14:261–266.
2. Rees GJ: Paediatric anaesthesia. *Br J Anaesth* 1960; 32:132–140.
3. Stead AL: The response of the newborn infant to muscle relaxants. *Br J Anaesth* 1955; 27:124–130.
4. Telford J, Keats AS: Succinylcholine in cardiovascular surgery of infants and children. *Anesthesiology* 1957; 18:841–848.
5. Bush GH, Stead AL: The use of d-tubocurarine in neonatal anaesthesia. *Br J Anaesth* 1962; 34:721–728.
6. Churchill-Davidson HC, Wise RP: Neuromuscular transmission in the newborn infant. *Anesthesiology* 1963; 24:271–278.
7. Churchill-Davidson HC, Wise RP: The response of the newborn infant to muscle relaxants. *Can Anaesth Soc J* 1964; 21:6–11.
8. Nightingale DA, Glass AG, Bachman L: Neuromuscular blockade by succinylcholine in children. *Anesthesiology* 1966; 27:736–741.
9. Lim HS, Davenport HT, Robson JG: The response of infants and children to muscle relaxants. *Anesthesiology* 1964; 25:164–168.
10. Long G, Bachman L: Neuromuscular blockade by d-tubocurarine in children. *Anesthesiology* 1967; 28:723–729.
11. Bennett EJ, Ramamurthy S, Dalal FY, et al: Pancuronium and the neonate. *Br J Anaesth* 1975; 47:75–78.
12. Cook DR, Fischer CG: Neuromuscular blocking effects of succinylcholine in infants and children. *Anesthesiology* 1975; 42:662–665.
13. Goudsouzian NG, Ryan JF, Savarese JJ: The neuromuscular effects of pancuronium in infants and children. *Anesthesiology* 1974; 41:95–98.

14. Goudsouzian NG, Donlon JV, Savarese JJ, et al: Re-evaluation of dosage and duration of action of d-tubocurarine in the pediatric age group. *Anesthesiology* 1975; 43:416–425.

15. Dubowitz V: Enzyme histochemistry of skeletal muscle. *J Neurol Neurosurg Psychiatry* 1965; 28:516–524.

16. Nag AL, Cheng M: Differentiation of fibre type in an extraocular muscle of the rat. *J Embryol Exp Morphol* 1982; 71:171–191.

17. Keens TG, Bryan AC, Levison H, et al: Developmental pattern of muscle fiber types in human ventilatory muscles. *J Appl Physiol* 1978; 44:909–913.

18. Engel WK, Karpati G: Impaired skeletal muscle maturation following neonatal neurectomy. *Dev Biol* 1968; 17:713–723.

19. Redfern PA: Neuromuscular transmission in new-born rats. *J Physiol* 1970; 209:701–709.

20. Grinnell AD, Herrera AA: Specificity and plasticity of neuromuscular connections: Long-term regulation of motoneuron function. *Prog Neurobiol* 1981; 17:203–282.

21. Bennett MR: Development of neuromuscular synapses. *Physiol Rev* 1983; 63:915–1048.

22. Juntunen J, Teravainen H: Structural development of myoneural junctions in the human embryo. *Histochemistry* 1972; 32:107–112.

23. Fidzianska A: Human ontogenesis: II. Development of the human neuromuscular junction. *J Neuropathol Exp Neurol* 1980; 39:606–615.

24. Coers C, Woolf AL: *The Innervation of Muscle: A Biopsy Study.* Oxford, England, Blackwell Scientific Press, 1959, p 30.

25. Kelly SS, Roberts DV: The effect of age on the safety factor in neuromuscular transmission in the isolated diaphragm of the rat. *Br J Anaesth* 1977; 49:217–221.

26. Kelly SS, Gertler RA, Robbins N: Comparison of the effects of pancuronium and tubocurarine on different muscles of young and old mice. *Br J Anaesth* 1986; 58:909–914.

27. Fambrough DM: Control of acetylcholine receptors in skeletal muscle. *Physiol Rev* 1979; 59:165–227.

28. Adams DJ, Bevan S: Some properties of acetylcholine receptors in human cultured myotubes. *Proc R Soc Lond Biol* 1985; 224:183–196.

29. Steinbach JH: Developmental changes in acetylcholine receptor aggregates at rat skeletal neuromuscular junctions. *Dev Biol* 1981; 84:267–276.

30. Brown MC, Jansen JKS, Van Essen D: Polyneuronal innervation of skeletal muscles in newborn rats and its elimination during maturation. *J Physiol* 1976; 261:387–422.

31. Crumrine RS, Yodlowski EH: Assessment of neuromuscular function in infants. *Anesthesiology* 1981; 54:29–32.

32. Goudsouzian NG; Maturation of neuromuscular transmission in the infant. *Br J Anaesth* 1980; 52:205–214.

33. Goudsouzian NG, Crone RK, Todres ID: Recovery from pancuronium blockade in the neonatal intensive care unit. *Br J Anaesth* 1981; 53:1303–1309.

34. Koenigsberger MR, Patten B, Lovelace RED: Studies of neuromuscular function in the newborn: I. A comparison of myoneural function in the full term and the premature infant. *Neuropediatrics* 1973; 4:350–361.

35. McCance RA: The role of the developing kidney in the maintenance of internal stability. *J R Coll Physicians Lond* 1972; 6:235–245.

36. Fisher DM, O'Keefe C, Stanski DR, et al: Pharmacokinetics and pharmacodynamics of *d*-tubocurarine in infants, children and adults. *Anesthesiology* 1982; 57:203–208.

37. Matteo RS, Lieberman IG, Salantire E, et al: Distribution, elimination, and action of *d*-tubocurarine in neonates, infants, children, and adults. *Anesth Analg* 1984; 63:799–804.

38. Walts LF, Dillon JB: The response of newborns to succinylcholine and *d*-tubocurarine. *Anesthesiology* 1969; 31:35–38.

39. Fisher DM, Cronnelly R, Miller RD, et al: The neuromuscular pharmacology of neostigmine in infants and children. *Anesthesiology* 1983; 59:220–225.

40. Fisher DM, Cronnelly R, Sharma M, et al: Clinical pharmacology of edrophonium in infants and children. *Anesthesiology* 1984; 61:428–433.

41. Meakin G, Sweet PT, Bevan JC, et al: Neostigmine and edrophonium as antagonists of pancuronium in infants and children. *Anesthesiology* 1983; 59:316–321.

42. Bowman WC: Prejunctional and postjunctional cholinoreceptors at the neuromuscular junction. *Anesth Analg* 1980; 59:935–943.

43. Robbins R, Donati F, Bevan DR, et al: Differential effects of myoneural blocking drugs on neuromuscular transmission in infants. *Br J Anaesth* 1984; 56:1095–1099.

44. Williams NE, Webb SN, Calvey TN: Differential effects of myoneural blocking drugs on neuromuscular transmission. *Br J Anaesth* 1980; 52:1111–1115.

45. Goudsouzian NG, Martyn JJA, Liu LMP, et al: Safety and efficacy of vecuronium in adolescents and children. *Anesth Analg* 1983; 62:1083–1088.

46. Bush GH: Clinical experience with diallyl-nortoxiferine in children. *Br J Anaesth* 1964; 36:787–792.

47. Lavery GG: Atracurium besylate in paediatric anaesthesia. *Anaesthesia* 1984; 39:1243–1246.

48. Goudsouzian NG: Atracurium in infants and children. *Br J Anaesth* 1986; 58:23S–28S.

49. Nightingale DA: Use of atracurium in neonatal anaesthesia. *Br J Anaesth* 1986; 58:32S–36S.

50. Savarese JJ, Basta SJ, Ali HH, et al: Neuromuscular and cardiovascular effects of BW 33A (atracurium) in patients under halothane anesthesia. *Anesthesiology* 1982; 57:A262.

384 *Chapter 11*

51. Basta SJ, Ali HH, Savarese JJ, et al: Clinical pharmacology of atracurium besylate (BW 33A): A new non-depolarizing muscle relaxant. *Anesth Analg* 1982; 61:723–729.
52. Goudsouzian NG, Liu LMP, Cote CJ, et al: Safety and efficacy of atracurium in adolescents and children anesthetized with halothane. *Anesthesiology* 1983; 59:459–462.
53. Goudsouzian NG, Liu LMP, Gionfriddo M, et al: Neuromuscular effects of atracurium in infants and children. *Anesthesiology* 1985; 62:75–79.
54. Brandom BW, Rudd GD, Cook DR: Clinical pharmacology of atracurium in paediatric patients. *Br J Anaesth* 1983; 55:117S–121S.
55. Brandom BW, Woelfel SK, Cook DR, et al: Clinical pharmacology of atracurium in infants. *Anesth Analg* 1984; 63:309–312.
56. Brandom BW, Cook DR, Woelfel SK, et al: Atracurium infusion requirements in children during halothane, isoflurane, and narcotic anesthesia. *Anesth Analg* 1985; 64:471–476.
57. Esener Z: The use of fazadinium in children. *Br J Anaesth* 1983; 55:1205–1212.
58. Goudsouzian NG, Martyn JJA, Liu LMP, et al: The dose response effect of long-acting nondepolarizing neuromuscular blocking agents in children. *Can Anaesth Soc J* 1984; 31:246–250.
59. Goudsouzian NG, Liu LMP, Savarese JJ: Metocurine in infants and children: Neuromuscular and clinical effects. *Anesthesiology* 1978; 49:266–269.
60. Donlon JV, Ali HH, Savarese JJ: A new approach to the study of four nondepolarizing relaxants in man. *Anesth Analg* 1974; 53:934–939.
61. Goudsouzian NG, Liu LMP, Cote CJ: Comparison of equipotent doses of non-depolarizing muscle relaxants in children. *Anesth Analg* 1981; 60:862–866.
62. Nightingale DA, Bush GH: A clinical comparison between tubocurarine and pancuronium in children. *Br J Anaesth* 1973; 45:63–70.
63. Bennett EJ, Daughety MJ, Bowyer DE, et al: Pancuronium bromide: Experiences in 100 pediatric patients. *Anesth Analg* 1971; 50:798–807.
64. Yamamoto T, Baba H, Shiratsuchi T: Clinical experience with pancuronium bromide in infants and children. *Anesth Analg* 1972; 51:919–924.
65. Robinson S, Gregory GA: Fentanyl-air/O_2 anesthesia for PDA ligation in infants less than 1500 g. *Anesth Analg* 1980; 59:566–557.
66. Moore RA, Yang JA, McNicholas KW, et al: Hemodynamic and anesthetic effects of sufentanil as the sole anesthetic for pediatric cardiovascular surgery. *Anesthesiology* 1985; 62:725–731.
67. Baird WLM, Reid AM: The neuromuscular blocking properties of a new steroid compound, pancuronium bromide. *Br J Anaesth* 1967; 39:775–780.
68. Miller RD, Way WL, Dolan WM, et al: The dependence of pancuronium- and d-tubocurarine-induced neuromuscular blockades on alveolar concentrations of halothane and Forane. *Anesthesiology* 1972; 37:573–581.

69. Bevan JC, Donati F, Bevan DR: Attempted acceleration of the onset of action of pancuronium: Effects of divided doses in infants and children. *Br J Anaesth* 1985; 57:1204–1208.

70. Martyn JAJ, Liu LMP, Szyfelbein SK, et al: The neuromuscular effects of pancuronium in burned children. *Anesthesiology* 1983; 59:561–564.

71. Baxter M, Bevan JC, Donati F, et al: d-Tubocurarine priming in children. *Can Anaesth Soc J* 1986; 33:586–587.

72. Donati F, Lahoud J, Walsh CM, et al: Onset of pancuronium and d-tubocurarine blockade with priming. *Can Anaesth Soc J* 1986; 33:571–577.

73. Fisher DM, Miller RD: Neuromuscular effects of vecuronium (ORG NC45) in infants and children during N_2O, halothane anesthesia. *Anesthesiology* 1983; 58:519–523.

74. Fahey MR, Morris RB, Miller RD, et al: Clinical pharmacology of ORG NC45 (Norcuron): A new nondepolarizing muscle relaxant. *Anesthesiology* 1981; 55:6–11.

75. Tsai SK, Mok MS, Lee TY, et al: The priming effect of vecuronium in children. *Anesth Analg* 1986; 65:S160.

76. Mason LJ, Betts EK: Leg lift and maximum inspiratory force, clinical signs of neuromuscular blockade reversal in neonates and infants. *Anesthesiology* 1980; 52:441–442.

77. Shimada Y, Yoshiya I, Tanaka K, et al: Crying vital capacity and maximal inspiratory pressure as clinical indicators of readiness for weaning of infants less than a year of age. *Anesthesiology* 1979; 51:456–459.

78. Bevan JC, Donati F, Bevan DR: Prolonged infusion of suxamethonium in infants and children. *Br J Anaesth* 1986; 58:839–843.

79. Cook DR: Muscle relaxants in infants and children. *Anesth Analg* 1981; 60:335–343.

80. Azar I, Pham AN, Karambelkar DJ, et al: The heart rate following edrophonium-atropine and edrophonium-glycopyrrolate mixtures. *Anesthesiology* 1983; 59:139–141.

81. Mirakhur RK, Elliot P, Lavery TD: Plasma cholinesterase activity and the duration of suxamethonium apnoea in children. *Ann R Coll Surg Engl* 1984; 66:43–45.

82. Walts LF, Dillon JB: Clinical studies on succinylcholine chloride. *Anesthesiology* 1967; 38:372–376.

83. Katz RL, Ryan JF: Neuromuscular effects of suxamethonium in man. *Br J Anaesth* 1969; 41:381–390.

84. Cook DR, Fischer CG: Characteristics of succinylcholine neuromuscular blockade in neonates. *Anesth Analg* 1978; 57:63–66.

85. Zsigmond EK, Downs JR: Plasma cholinesterase activity in newborns and infants. *Can Anaesth Soc J* 1971; 18:278–285.

86. De Cook TH, Goudsouzian NG: Tachyphylaxis and phase II block development during infusion of succinylcholine in children. *Anesth Analg* 1980; 59:639–643.

87. Goudsouzian NG, Liu LMP: The neuromuscular response of infants to a continuous infusion of succinylcholine. *Anesthesiology* 1984; 60:97–101.

88. Beldavs J: Intramuscular succinylcholine for endotracheal intubation in infants and children. *Can Anaesth Soc J* 1959; 6:141–147.
89. Liu LMP, De Cook TH, Goudsouzian NG, et al: Dose response to intramuscular succinylcholine in children. *Anesthesiology* 1981; 55:599–601.
90. Liu LMP, Goudsouzian NG: Neuromuscular effect of intramuscular succinylcholine in infants. *Anesthesiology* 1982; 57:A413.
91. Sutherland GA, Bevan JC, Bevan DR: Neuromuscular blockade in infants following intramuscular succinylcholine in two or five per cent concentration. *Can Anaesth Soc J* 1983; 30:342–346.
92. Cook DR, Westman HR, Rosenfeld L, et al: Pulmonary edema in infants: Possible association with intramuscular succinylcholine. *Anesth Analg* 1981; 60:220–223.
93. Lee KWT, Downes JJ: Pulmonary edema secondary to laryngospasm in children. *Anesthesiology* 1983; 59:347–349.
94. Mazze RI, Dunbar RW: Intralingual succinylcholine administration in children: An alternative to intravenous and intramuscular routes? *Anesth Analg* 1968; 47:605–615.
95. Craythorne NWB, Turndorf H, Dripps RD: Changes in pulse rate and rhythm associated with the use of succinylcholine in anesthetized children. *Anesthesiology* 1960; 21:465–470.
96. Hannallah RS, Oh TH, McGill WA, et al: Changes in heart rate and rhythm after intramuscular succinylcholine with or without atropine in anesthetized children. *Anesthesiology* 1986; 65:1329–1332.
97. Salem MR, Wong AT, Liu YH: The effect of suxamethonium on the intragastric pressure in infants and children. *Br J Anaesth* 1972; 44:166–169.
98. Craythorne NWB, Rottenstein HS, Dripps RD: The effect of succinylcholine on intraocular pressure in adults, infants and children during general anesthesia. *Anesthesiology* 1960; 21:59–66.
99. Jensen K, Bennike KA, Hanel HK, et al: Myoglobinuria following anaesthesia including suxamethonium. *Br J Anaesth* 1968; 40:329–334.
100. Harrington JF, Ford DJ, Striker TW: Myoglobinemia and myoglobinuria after succinylcholine in children. *Anesthesiology* 1983; 59:A439.
101. Blanc VF, Vaillancourt G, Brisson G: Succinylcholine, fasciculations and myoglobinaemia. *Can Anaesth Soc J* 1986; 33:178–184.
102. Kenally JB, Bush GH: Changes in serum potassium after suxamethonium in children. *Anaesth Intensive Care* 1974; 2:147–150.
103. Leigh MD, McCoy DD, Belton K, et al: Bradycardia following intravenous administration of succinylcholine chloride in infants and children. *Anesthesiology* 1957; 18:698–702.
104. Lerman J, Robinson S, Willis MM, et al: Succinylcholine-induced heart rate changes in children during isoflurane and halothane. *Anesthesiology* 1983; 59:A443.

105. Green DW, Bristow AB, Fischer M: Glycopyrrolate and atropine in the prevention of bradycardia and dysrhythmias following repeated doses of suxamethonium in children. *Br J Anaesth* 1983; 55:1163P.

106. Lerman J, Chinyanga HM: The heart rate response to succinylcholine in children: A comparison of atropine and glycopyrrolate. *Can Anaesth Soc J* 1983; 30:377–381.

107. McCance RA, Hutchinson AO, Dean RFA, et al: The cholinesterase activity of the serum of newborn animals, and of colostrum. *Biochem J* 1949; 45:493–496.

108. Shanor SP, Van Hees GR, Baart N, et al: The influence of age and sex on human plasma and red cell cholinesterase. *Am J Med Sci* 1961; 242:357–361.

109. Genever EE: Suxamethonium-induced cardiac arrest in unsuspected pseudohypertrophic muscular dystrophy: Case report. *Br J Anaesth* 1971; 43:984–986.

110. Linter SPK, Thomas PR, Withington PS, et al: Suxamethonium associated hypertonicity and cardiac arrest in unsuspected pseudohypertrophic muscular dystrophy. *Br J Anaesth* 1982; 54:1331–1332.

111. Denborough MA: Malignant hyperpyrexia. *Med J Aust* 1977; 2:757–758.

112. Thiel RE: The myotonic response to suxamethonium. *Br J Anaesth* 1967; 39:815–821.

113. Cody JR: Muscle rigidity following administration of succinylcholine. *Anesthesiology* 1968; 29:159–162.

114. Bray RJ, Inkster JS: Anaesthesia in babies with congenital dystrophia myotonica. *Anaesthesia* 1984; 39:1007–1011.

115. Stirt JA, Stone DJ, Weinberg G, et al: Atracurium in a child with myotonic dystrophy. *Anesth Analg* 1985; 64:369–370.

116. Ellis FR, Cain PA, Harriman DGF, et al: Plasma cholinesterase and malignant hyperpyrexia. *Br J Anaesth* 1978; 50:86.

117. Whittaker M, Britten JJ: Malignant hyperthermia and the fluoride-resistant gene. *Br J Anaesth* 1981; 53:241–244.

118. Evans RT, Iqbal J, Ellis FR, et al: Collaborative study of the frequency of the fluoride-resistant cholinesterase variant in patients with malignant hyperpyrexia. *Br J Anaesth* 1981; 53:245 247.

119. Ording H, Haniel HH, Viby-Mogensen J: Plasma cholinesterase and malignant hyperthermia. *Br J Anaesth* 1981; 53:317.

120. Hall GM: Plasma cholinesterase and malignant hyperthermia. *Br J Anaesth* 1981; 53:199–200.

121. Eikelenboom G, Minkenon D, Van Eldik P, et al: Inheritance of the malignant hyperthermia syndrome in Dutch Landrace swine, in Aldrete JA, Britt BA (eds): *Malignant Hyperthermia.* New York, Grune & Stratton, 1978, p 141.

122. Arizono N, Koreto O, Iwai Y, et al: Morphometric analysis of human neuromuscular junction in different ages. *Acta Pathol Jpn* 1984; 34:1243–1249.

123. Greenblatt DJ, Sellers EM, Shader RI: Drug disposition in old age. *N Engl J Med* 1982; 306:1081–1088.
124. Thompson EN, Williams R: Effect of age on liver function with particular reference to Bromsulphalein excretion. *Gut* 1965; 6:266–269.
125. Stephens ID, Ho PC, Holloway AM, et al: Pharmacokinetics of alcuronium in elderly patients undergoing total hip replacement or aortic reconstructive surgery. *Br J Anaesth* 1984; 56:465–471.
126. Walker J, Shanks CA, Triggs EJ: Clinical pharmacokinetics of alcuronium chloride in man. *Eur J Clin Pharmacol* 1980; 17:449–454.
127. d'Hollander AA, Luyckx C, Barvais L, et al: Clinical evaluation of atracurium besylate requirement for a stable muscle relaxation during surgery: Lack of age-related effects. *Anesthesiology* 1983; 59:237–240.
128. Matteo RS, Backus WW, McDaniel DD, et al: Pharmacokinetics and pharmacodynamics of *d*-tubocurarine and metocurine in the elderly. *Anesth Analg* 1985; 64:23–29.
129. McLeod K, Hull CJ, Watson MJ: Effects of aging on the pharmacokinetics of pancuronium. *Br J Anaesth* 1979; 51:435–438.
130. Somogyi A: Pancuronium plasma clearance and age. *Br J Anaesth* 1980; 52:360.
131. Duvaldestin P, Saada J, Berger JL, et al: Pharmacokinetics, pharmacodynamics, and dose-response relationships of pancuronium in control and elderly subjects. *Anesthesiology* 1982; 56:36–40.
132. d'Hollander AA, Nevelsteen M, Barvais L, et al: Paralysis induced in anaesthetized adult subjects by ORG NC 45. *Acta Anaesthesiol Scand* 1983; 27:108–110.
133. O'Hara DA, Fragen RJ, Shanks CA: The effects of age on the dose-response curves for vecuronium in adults. *Anesthesiology* 1985; 63:542–544.
134. d'Hollander AA, Massaux F, Nevelsteen M, et al: Age-dependent dose-response relationships of ORG NC 45 in anaesthetized patients. *Br J Anaesth* 1982; 54:653–657.
135. Rupp SM, Fisher DM, Miller RD, et al: Pharmacokinetics and pharmacodynamics of vecuronium in the elderly. *Anesthesiology* 1983; 59:A270.
136. Marsh RHK, Chmielewski AT, Goat VA: Recovery from pancuronium: A comparison between old and young patients. *Anaesthesia* 1980; 35:1193–1196.
137. Young WL, Backus W, Matteo RS, et al: Pharmacokinetics and pharmacodynamics of neostigmine in the elderly. *Anesthesiology* 1984; 61:A300.

12

Drug Interactions

Interactions between the muscle relaxants and several anesthetic and nonanesthetic drugs have been suggested. Some have been confirmed, but many remain as isolated reports or theoretical possibilities. When interactions have been confirmed, the site of interference has been established in only a few cases. The possible sites of interaction are many. These include interruptions of the several steps involved in converting a nerve impulse into muscle contraction; disturbances of pharmacokinetic variables, particularly volumes of distribution, metabolism, and elimination; and alterations of protein binding or metabolism in the plasma.

In this chapter, only drug interactions with clinical importance will be discussed. Where possible, the putative mechanisms involved also will be discussed. Table 12–1 lists the categories of anesthetic and nonanesthetic drugs that interact with muscle relaxants. Under each category, drugs and their anticipated effects are outlined.

ANALGESICS

Animal experiments have usually,[1] but not always,[2] demonstrated some potentiation of nondepolarizing NMBDs with narcotics. Meperidine (Demerol), 5 μg/ml, augments twitch height in the rat phrenic nerve-diaphragm preparation but in doses exceeding 40 μg/ml produces depression and potentiation of nondepolarizing relaxants.[3] In human volunteers morphine, 0.5 mg/kg, produces post-tetanic depression of single twitch response following tetanic stimulation at 100 and 200 Hz, which suggests that morphine has a small presynaptic action.[4] How-

TABLE 12–1.
Drugs That Interact With Muscle Relaxants and the Effects of Those Drugs

DRUG	EFFECT
Analgesics	
Demerol (meperidine)	No clinically important interactions.
Fentanyl	
Morphine	
Meptazinol	Antagonizes nondepolarizing relaxants and potentiates succinylcholine.
Anesthetic agents	
Inhalational agents	
Enflurane	Potentiation of nondepolarizing relaxants
Ether	and, by isoflurane, of succinylcholine.
Halothane	
Isoflurane	
Intravenous anesthetics	
Althesin	Minimal clinical effects despite slight poten-
Propofol	tiation of nondepolarizing relaxants by
Etomidate	ketamine and propofol.
Ketamine	
Methohexital	Propanidid prolongs duration of action of
Midazolam	succinylcholine.
Propanidid	
Thiopental sodium	
Local anesthetics	
Bupivacaine	Potentiation of depolarizing and nondepo-
Cocaine	larizing relaxants.
Etidocaine	Can be reversed with 4–aminopyridine but
Lidocaine	not with neostigmine.
Mepivacaine	Lidocaine and procaine prolong the dura-
Prilocaine	tion of action of succinylcholine from
Procaine	plasma cholinesterase inhibition.
Procainamide	
Antiarrhythmic agents	
β-Adrenergic blocking drugs	
Oxprenolol	Potentiate nondepolarizing relaxants and
Practolol	worsen myasthenia. Inhibit succinylcho-
Pronethalol	line fasciculations.
Propranolol	Bradycardia after anticholinesterases.
Calcium-channel blocking drugs	
Bepridil	Potentiate depolarizing and nondepolariz-
Nifedipine	ing relaxants. Reversible with edrophon-
Verapamil	ium but not neostigmine.
Bretylium	No clinical reactions described.
Disopyramide	No clinical reactions described.
Others	
Phenytoin	Potentiation of depolarizing and resistance
Lidocaine	to nondepolarizing relaxants.
Procainamide	May unmask or potentiate myasthenia
Quinidine	gravis.

Antibiotics	
Aminoglycosides	
Amikacin	Potentiate depolarizing and nondepolariz-
Gentamicin	ing relaxants.
Kanamycin	Inconsistent reversal with edrophonium and
Neomycin	neostigmine, but reversible with calcium
Streptomycin	and 4-aminopyridine.
Dihydrostreptomycin	
Polymyxins	
Colistin	Potentiate depolarizing and nondepolariz-
Polymyxin A	ing relaxants and produce paralysis
Polymyxin B	alone. Inconsistent antagonism by anti-
Polymyxin C	cholinesterase and calcium, complete
	with 4-aminopyridine.
Tetracyclines	
Oxytetracycline	Weak potentiation of nondepolarizing
Tetracycline	NMBDs. Recovery: neostigmine ineffec-
	tive; calcium may improve.
Lincosamines	
Clindamycin	Potentiate nondepolarizing NMBDs. Incon-
Lincomycin	sistent reversal with 4-aminopyridine or
	anticholinesterases. Calcium no effect.
Penicillins and cephalosporins	
Penicillin G	No effects at clinical doses.
Penicillin V	
Erythromycin	
Cephaloridine	
Metronidazole	No clinical effects described.
Anticonvulsants	
Phenytoin	Increased requirement for pancuronium,
	metocurine, and vecuronium.
Corticosteroids	
Dexamethasone	Reports of possible resistance to nondepo-
Hydrocortisone	larizing relaxants are difficult to confirm.
Prednisone	
Diuretics	
Furosemide	Enhanced *d*-tubocurarine neuromuscular
Acetazolamide	block by furosemide has been
Chlorothiazide	demonstrated.
Chlorthalidone	
Mannitol	
Electrolytes	
Calcium	See Chapter 10.
Magnesium	
Potassium	
Enzyme inhibitors	
Anticholinesterases	
Echothiopate	See Chapter 7.
Edrophonium	
Hexaflurenium	

(Continued.)

TABLE 12–1 (cont.).

DRUG	EFFECT
Neostigmine Organophosphates Physostigmine Pyridostigmine Germine monoacetate Tetrahydroaminoacrine	See Chapter 7.
Proteolytic enzyme inhibitors	
Aprotinin	Dubious apnea reported after IV administration.
Hypotensive agents	
Hexamethonium Trimethaphan	Potentiate nondepolarizing NMBDs and prolong recovery of succinylcholine from PCHE inhibition.
Nitroglycerine Sodium nitroprusside	No clinical effects.
Immunosuppressants and anticancer therapy	
Azathioprine Thiotepa	See section on phosphodiesterase inhibitors.
Chlorambucil Cyclophosphamide	Potentiation of nondepolarizing relaxants reported.
Cyclosporine D-penicillamine Triethylenemelamine	May decrease PCHE.
Muscle relaxants	
Succinylcholine	See Chapter 7.
Alcuronium	See Chapter 8.
Atracurium Fazadinium Gallamine Metocurine Pancuronium *d*-Tubocurarine Vecuronium	
Dantrolene	Depression of muscle contraction.
Phosphodiesterase inhibitors	
Aminophylline Azathioprine Theophylline Thiotepa	Potentiate succinylcholine and antagonize nondepolarizing relaxants.
Prostaglandin inhibitors	
Aspirin Ibuprofen Indomethacin	No proved clinical effect.
Psychotropic drugs	
Benzodiazepines	
Diazepam	Variable clinical response.
Desmethyldiazepam	High doses potentiate succinylcholine and

(Continued.)

Flurazepam	nondepolarizing NMBDs.
Oxazepam	Some success in preventing fasciculations
Temazepam	and myalgia.
Lithium	Minimal clinical effects.
Tricyclic antidepressants	
Imipramine	Arrhythmias with pancuronium.

ever, Katz[5] was unable to demonstrate potentiation of pancuronium with demerol.

Meptazinol, an analgesic that combines agonist and antagonist opioid activity, also has anticholinesterase activity. At low doses, in the rat phrenic nerve-diaphragm preparation, it acts like neostigmine to antagonize d-tubocurarine and potentiate succinylcholine. However, when given in high doses or in the presence of cholinesterase blockade with echothiopate, it reveals neuromuscular blocking activity.[6]

ANESTHETIC AGENTS

Inhalational Agents

At high concentrations, the inhalational anesthetic agents produce measurable decreases in neuromuscular transmission. However, the skeletal muscle relaxation during general anesthesia is primarily due to the depressant effect of the anesthetic on the central nervous system.

Inhalational anesthetic agents potentiate nondepolarizing relaxants in animals, in vivo and in vitro, and in man.[7-13] Controlled studies have demonstrated dose-dependent[14] left shift of the dose-response curves of d-tubocurarine, gallamine, pancuronium, metocurine-pancuronium combinations, atracurium, and vecuronium.[2, 15-20]

Enflurane and isoflurane are more powerful than halothane in potentiating d-tubocurarine and pancuronium, but enflurane produces greater potentiation of vecuronium than halothane and isoflurane. Also, increasing the alveolar concentration of an inhalational agent appears to be less effective in further potentiating vecuronium than d-tubocurarine or pancuronium.[19] Isoflurane, but not other inhalational agents, has been shown to potentiate the action of succinylcholine probably as a result of augmented delivery of relaxant from increased muscle blood flow.[15]

The cause of the potentiation is unknown. In man, the greater effect on tetanic than single twitch stimulation suggests that inhalational agents may act on prejunctional mechanisms.[21] Animal studies, either in the whole animal[22] or in isolated nerve-muscle preparations, have been unable to separate possible prejunctional effects from those on the postjunctional membrane or on muscle contraction. The potentiation is not the result of alteration in pharmacokinetic variables,[23] and it cannot be reversed with anticholinesterases.[24]

Intravenous Anesthetics

Animal experiments have demonstrated potentiation of nondepolarizing relaxants with most induction agents.[2] This is mainly a result of a decrease in sensitivity of the postsynaptic membrane to acetyl choline,[25] which for all except ketamine is matched by an increase in presynaptic acetylcholine release.[26, 27] The prolonged duration of action of succinylcholine given after propanidid was due to inhibition of plasma cholinesterase activity[28] supplemented by a probable postsynaptic action.[29]

Dose-response curves in man have demonstrated left shift for *d*-tubocurarine, but not other relaxants, in the presence of ketamine;[30] and for atracurium and vecuronium with propofol.[31] But midazolam produced no different neuromuscular response from thiopental sodium to succinylcholine or pancuronium.[32]

Local Anesthetics

Procaine, lidocaine, and other local anesthetic agents produce neuromuscular blockade in their own right and potentiate both depolarizing and nondepolarizing relaxants in man.[33, 34] Lidocaine in a dose of 2.5 mg/kg given before induction of anesthesia potentiated a small dose of *d*-tubocurarine, 0.2 mg/kg.[33] Twitch height was depressed by 26% compared with 12% in the control patients; the onset of the block was accelerated; and the train-of-four ratio (TOFR) was 55% compared with 80%. However, no "recurarization" was observed with a subsequent dose, 1.2 mg/kg, of lidocaine. Gentamicin and lidocaine have additive effects, and profound neuromuscular block may develop after their combined use in a patient given *d*-tubocurarine.[35] Lidocaine and procaine are metabolized by plasma cholinesterase so that their use may prolong the duration of action of succinylcholine,[34] and this action may be particularly severe in a patient with atypical plasma cholinesterase.[36]

A true potentiation has been demonstrated in the rat phrenic nerve-diaphragm preparation between local anesthetic agents (cocaine, procaine, lidocaine, etidocaine) and the neuromuscular blocking drugs (NMBD) (succinylcholine, *d*-tubocurarine and pancuronium). Ineffective doses of each produced 90% block when given in combination with the local anesthetic agents.[37, 38] Pretreatment with local anesthetics

decreased the ED50 of the NMBDs by half, although the effect on succinylcholine was variable. Similarly, small doses of the relaxants potentiated the neuromuscular blocking effect of the local anesthetics.
The combined neuromuscular block could be antagonized with 4–aminopyridine, but reversal was incomplete with neostigmine.

The local anesthetic agents also have a direct effect at the neuromuscular junction. Procainamide has been shown to decrease the postjunctional sensitivity to acetylcholine, and it probably also acts
prejunctionally to decrease transmitter release.[37, 39]

ANTIARRHYTHMIC AGENTS

β-Adrenergic Blocking Drugs

The neuromuscular effects of β-blockers were studied because of
their widespread effects on excitable tissue, although clinical evidence
of an interaction is poor. They have been suspected of worsening myasthenia gravis,[40] and excessive bradycardia[41] has followed the reversal
of neuromuscular blockade with anticholinesterases in patients receiving β-blockers.

In animals, intra-arterial injection of pronethalol or propranolol
causes a brief decrease in indirectly elicited twitch activity. Intravenous
(IV) administration of succinylcholine has increased potency and duration of action in cats receiving β-blockers. Also, pronethalol prevents
succinylcholine-induced repetitive firing and fasciculation, suggesting
that it might have a clinical role in this regard.[42] Similarly, β-blockade
increases the magnitude and duration of d-tubocurarine blockade.[43]

The inhibition of repetitive firing and fasciculation in response to
succinylcholine suggest a presynaptic action. However, the cause of
the potentiation is uncertain. It is unlikely that β-blocking drugs in
normal doses have any clinical effect at the neuromuscular junction.

Calcium-Channel Blocking Drugs

Calcium is important for myoneural activity. It is essential for presynaptic acetylcholine release, stabilization of presynaptic and postsynaptic membranes, excitation-contraction coupling, and contractility
of muscle. Verapamil has been reported to cause acute respiratory insufficiency when given to a patient with Duchenne type muscular
dystrophy[44] and to potentiate the nondepolarizing blocking drugs, d-
tubocurarine, pancuronium,[49] and vecuronium.[45] The neuromuscular
block was resistant to reversal with neostigmine, but recovery of the

response to train-of-four stimulation has been achieved with edrophonium.[45, 46]

Dose-response curves in animals demonstrated potentiation of neuromuscular blockade induced with succinylcholine and nondepolarizing relaxants.[47–49] Higher doses produced block of indirect and direct stimulation.

The site of the interaction is uncertain but because calcium blockers interfere with muscle contraction induced by nerve stimulation and by direct application of acetylcholine,[50] presynaptic factors are less likely. Also, indirect stimulation is affected more than direct[51] so that the most likely site is the postjunctional membrane, perhaps by induction of channel block.

Bretylium

In vitro nerve-muscle preparation demonstrates potentiation of d-tubocurarine.[52] The mechanism is unknown, although inhibition of acetylcholine synthesis has been demonstrated. No clinical interactions have been described to date.

Disopyramide

Rat phrenic nerve-diaphragm preparations show left shift of the d-tubocurarine dose-response curve,[53] but the mechanism is undetermined. No clinical effects have been shown despite the known anticholinergic and local anesthetic properties of this drug.

Others

There are several reports of the interaction between many antiarrhythmic and neuromuscular blocking drugs. In man, potentiation of depolarizing[54–56] and nondepolarizing relaxants[54, 57] may be produced by quinidine, and when given during partial curare block, recurarization has occurred.[59] Myasthenia gravis may also be aggravated or unmasked by quinidine or procainamide.[58]

In cats, twitch depression of about 50% induced by d-tubocurarine is intensified to 60% to 80% by lidocaine (5 mg/kg), phenytoin (7 to 11 mg/kg), or procainamide (5 to 20 mg/kg)[35]—a similar degree of potentiation as that produced by propranolol (5 mg/kg). Quinidine and procainamide also potentiate the action of succinylcholine in cats. These doses are well above those used clinically so that, apart from quinidine, it is doubtful whether these agents intensify neuromuscular blockade when used in therapeutic doses.[38]

The mechanism of the potentiation in man is uncertain, although presynaptic and postsynaptic actions have been demonstrated for quinidine, and procainamide decreases transmitter release and decreases the sensitivity of the postjunctional membrane to acetylcholine. Perhaps the action of these agents as antiarrhythmics, i.e., stabilization of cardiac muscle membrane, is also responsible for their interactions with muscle relaxants.

ANTIBIOTICS

The neuromuscular blocking properties of the antibiotics were suspected following reports of deaths in children after the use of intraperitoneal neomycin during ether anesthesia.[60-69] The severity and speed of onset of symptoms depend on the dose and route of administration. Application of the drugs via the intraperitoneal or intrapleural spaces or by irrigation of a wound may result in as rapid absorption as intramuscular or intravenous injection. Oral, low-dose administration of neomycin has also been implicated.[68]

Antibiotics may induce a reversible myasthenic syndrome or unmask latent myasthenia gravis.[68] Subtherapeutic doses of neomycin, streptomycin, or polymyxin B can cause marked twitch depression in rat phrenic nerve-diaphragm preparations exposed to clinically inactive concentrations of d-tubocurarine, pancuronium, or succinylcholine.[69] Potentiation of NMBDs during anesthesia may be revealed by increased depth of relaxation, difficulty in reversal of blockade, or recurarization.[70-72] Potentiation by streptomycin and neomycin has been described for succinylcholine, gallamine, pancuronium, d-tubocurarine, and vecuronium.[74-78] The sites of action and mechanisms of interference with neuromuscular transmission are not fully understood, but differences have been ascribed to each group of antibiotics.

Aminoglycosides

The *aminoglycosides* have neuromuscular blocking actions similar to magnesium and produce a phase I block.[61, 66] Neomycin and gentamicin inhibit presynaptic acetylcholine release[77-80] as well as depress postjunctional sensitivity.[80] Streptomycin may also show some local anesthetic effect, stabilizing muscle cell membranes and directly depressing contractility[81] with presynaptic inhibition of acetylcholine release[82, 83] and postsynaptic receptor blockade. The presynaptic effects of gentamicin, neomycin, and kanamycin are greater than those of streptomycin.[77-79, 84]

Neomycin and streptomycin are the most potent of the aminogly-cosides in depressing neuromuscular function.[80] Aminoglycosides augment the depolarizing block of succinylcholine[69] and the nondepolarizing block of d-tubocurarine[84, 85] and pancuronium.[69] These effects are potentiated by magnesium[61] and are antagonized almost completely by calcium but only partially by anticholinesterases.[80, 86-89] Complete reversal of a combined neomycin and d-tubocurarine block has been achieved with 4–aminopyridine.[84]

Polymyxins

The *polymyxins* are the most potent of the antibiotics in their action at the neuromuscular junction. The complex block appears to be predominantly postjunctional.[80, 90, 91] In the sciatic nerve-gastrocnemius preparation in frogs, polymyxins decrease the amplitude and frequency of miniature end-plate potentials (MEPP), and reduce quantal content.[90] Cholinesterase activity is unaffected. Reversal of a polymyxin-relaxant block is difficult. The effects of calcium and anticholinesterases are inconsistent. Edrophonium may produce partial reversal, but neostigmine may augment an established block.[64, 66, 69, 92]

Tetracyclines

Tetracyclines produce only a weak, clinically insignificant interaction with the muscle relaxants. Their effect may be the result of chelation of calcium, which reduces acetylcholine release.[90, 93] The block is reversible with calcium but unaffected by neostigmine.[66, 80]

Lincosamines

The *lincosamines*, clindamycin and lincomycin, have prejunctional and postjunctional blocking effects.[80, 94] Clindamycin produces an initial augmentation of the twitch in mouse phrenic nerve-diaphragm preparations and a direct, local anesthetic effect on muscle. Miniature end-plate potentials are altered in a similar way to polymyxin B. The block is irreversible with calcium, 4–aminopyridine, and neomycin.

Lincomycin shows no initial twitch enhancement or direct effect on muscle. It prolongs end-plate potentials and MEPPs without altering frequency, suggesting action on channel conductance. Partial reversal is achieved with calcium[66] and complete reversal with 4–aminopyridine.[95] Reversal of the mixed block associated with the lincosamines is unpredictable. Although anticholinesterases are ineffective, edrophonium has produced persistent partial improvement,[96] but neostigmine has been associated with enhancement of the block.[80, 96]

Penicillins

The penicillins are the safest of the antibiotics, requiring concentrations outside the therapeutic range before any effect on neuromuscular transmission can be demonstrated. Penicillin V decreases acetylcholine release,[97] alters postsynaptic membrane sensitivity,[98] and decreases muscle contractility.[69] These effects are reversible with calcium but not neostigmine. Penicillin G, cephaloridine, and erythromycin have negligible paralyzing properties.

Metronidazole

Recently, an enhanced block from a combination of vecuronium and metronidazole was described in animals,[2] but it could not be confirmed in man.[99]

Management of Potentiation

Management of a suspected prolonged block from the combination of muscle relaxant-antibiotic is difficult. Twitch data may not be helpful because only the relaxant-induced portion of the block is likely to be reversible with anticholinesterases. Mixed blocks may respond better to 4–aminopyridine, but this is not readily available. For many combinations, pharmacologic reversal is uncertain or impossible, and management must then include intermittent positive pressure ventilation (IPPV) until the block has recovered sufficiently to support spontaneous ventilation.

ANTICONVULSANTS

Anticonvulsant therapy shortens the duration of action of pancuronium by more than 50% in neurosurgical patients,[100] and phenytoin therapy was found to increase pancuronium requirements by 80%.[101] A similar resistance was found for metocurine and vecuronium[102] but not atracurium.[103] The effectiveness of metocurine, 0.2 mg/kg, was reduced by 15%; the recovery index decreased from 125 ± 54 to 53 ± 22 minutes, the time to 95% recovery was reduced from 269 ± 64 to 122 ± 25 minutes, and plasma concentrations required to maintain 50% block were increased.[104] The mechanism for the resistance is unknown but is not due to alteration in pharmacokinetic behavior.[104] Although phenytoin increases the metabolism of pancuronium,[105] it is more likely that the effect is due to altered sensitivity of the junction. In rats, phenytoin has a dual action: low concentrations antagonize decamethonium while high doses potentiate it. Edrophonium reverses the antagonism but augments the potentiation.[106]

CORTICOSTEROIDS

Brief reports of antagonism of pancuronium in patients receiving high doses of hydrocortisone[107] or prednisone[108] appeared to have been confirmed in animal experiments.[109–113] However, the effects in cats depended on the duration of steroid therapy. The acute administration of hydrocortisone, 1 to 15 mg/kg, did not affect twitch tension, although higher doses, up to 15 mg/kg, accentuated blockade produced by pancuronium but not succinylcholine. After chronic administration of hydrocortisone for 3 weeks, dose responses to pancuronium and succinylcholine were no different from controls. However, long-term treatment did increase the sensitivity to succinylcholine. The cause of this is difficult to elucidate partly because plasma cholinesterase levels are reduced by long-term steroid treatment[114] and also because two of the cats developed a myopathy![115]

In rats, d-tubocurarine blockade was antagonized by low doses of dexamethasone, 0.04 mg/kg, but enhanced at higher doses, 0.16 mg/kg.[116] However, in humans, neither hydrocortisone, 10 mg/kg, nor dexamethasone, 0.4 mg/kg, had any effect on a stable partial neuromuscular block produced by pancuronium, metocurine, d-tubocurarine, or vecuronium.[117] It has been suggested that the action of glucocorticoids at the neuromuscular junction is complex. Experiments suggest that they increase motor nerve excitability,[111] acetylcholine release,[112] and choline transport,[117] but these prejunctional actions are opposed by inhibition at the postjunctional membrane.[109, 111] Thus it is difficult to predict the effect in man. It may depend on the dose and duration of treatment, but whatever the result the interaction is of minimal clinical importance.

DIURETICS

Enhanced d-tubocurarine block by furosemide, but not mannitol, has been demonstrated in man,[118] and a similar moderate potentiation has been described in rabbits with acetazolamide, chlorothiazide, and chlorthalidone at low doses. At high doses, some antagonism develops.[119] Also, accelerated recovery from pancuronium neuromuscular block has been reported after a single dose of furosemide in man.[120]

The cause of the interaction is uncertain. However, studies with the rat phrenic nerve-diaphragm preparation have demonstrated potentiation of succinylcholine and d-tubocurarine blocks at low doses and antagonism at high doses.[121] In addition, the neuromuscular block may be augmented by an acute reduction in plasma potassium concentration.[122]

ELECTROLYTES

For a discussion of electrolytes (calcium, magnesium, and potassium), see Chapter 10.

ENZYME INHIBITORS

Anticholinesterases

For a discussion of anticholinesterases, see Chapter 7.

Proteolytic Enzyme Inhibitors

There are reports of apnea following IV administration of aprotinin (Trasylol) after recovery from succinylcholine and d-tubocurarine was established.[123] The cause is unknown, although aprotinin does have weak inhibitory effects on plasma cholinesterase.[124]

Hypotensive Agents

Ganglion-blocking drugs have been shown to possess potent neuromuscular blocking properties in animals and in man; prolonged postoperative apnea has followed the administration of trimethaphan after succinylcholine,[125] alcuronium,[126] and d-tubocurarine.[127]

In the rat phrenic nerve-diaphragm preparation d-tubocurarine is potentiated by ganglion blockers.[128] The neuromuscular block can be antagonized after administration of hexamethonium, phenactropinium, and homatropine with neostigmine but not after trimethaphan.[129] In frog nerve-muscle preparations, trimethaphan reduced MEPPs and increased end-plate sensitivity to relaxants, suggesting an action at the nerve terminal.[130] In addition, trimethaphan has weak anticholinesterase activity,[131, 132] but the significance of this is unknown.

Following suspicion of an interaction between nitroglycerine and pancuronium, animal experiments, in vivo and in vitro, suggested that nitroglycerine increased the duration of action of pancuronium, but not gallamine, d-tubocurarine, or succinylcholine.[133, 134] More careful studies with therapeutic doses showed that nitroglycerine had no effect on the potency, duration of action, or recovery index of vecuronium or pancuronium-induced block.[135] Thus, it is unlikely that nitroglycerine has an important clinical effect in man. Similarly, animal experiments suggest that sodium nitroprusside does not produce interactions with NMBDs.[130, 131]

IMMUNOSUPPRESSANTS AND ANTICANCER THERAPY

Several reports have suggested that immunosuppressives and anticancer treatment prolong the action of muscle relaxants.[136, 137] The mechanisms involved are largely speculative. The severely ill patient may have abnormal pharmacokinetic variables and decreased plasma cholinesterase production in the liver. Azathioprine and thiotepa, phosphodiesterase inhibitors, antagonize d-tubocurarine by increasing transmitter release.[138] Plasma cholinesterase activity may be decreased further by cytotoxic drugs to prolong the action of succinylcholine,[139, 140] and immunosuppressives may induce myasthenia by the production of antiacetylcholine receptor antibodies.[141] Finally, cyclosporine has been shown to potentiate the action of atracurium and vecuronium.[142]

MUSCLE RELAXANTS

Dantrolene interferes with excitation-contraction coupling mechanisms of skeletal muscles, but it has no action at the neuromuscular junction. Thus, muscle weakness may follow the use of depolarizing or nondepolarizing relaxants. In response to evoked stimulation, there is a greater decrease in mechanical (twitch) than electrical (electromyographic [EMG]) response. An additional interaction between dantrolene and d-tubocurarine has been demonstrated in the phrenic nerve-diaphragm preparation,[143] and potentiation of vecuronium, recorded with an EMG, has been reported in one patient during treatment with dantrolene.[144]

PHOSPHODIESTERASE INHIBITORS

Phosphodiesterase is responsible for the metabolism of cyclic adenosine monophosphate (cAMP), which plays an important role in the entry of calcium into the nerve terminal with subsequent acetylcholine release. Thus phosphodiesterase inhibitors, by preventing the breakdown of cAMP, allow increased entry of calcium into cells and cause an increase in the force of contraction of the cat soleus muscles,[138] and the increase in force is associated with repetitive activity at the nerve terminal. Azathioprine potentiates succinylcholine and antagonizes d-tubocurarine. It is a more potent phosphodiesterase inhibitor than aminophylline. In man, azathioprine has been blamed for causing antagonism of pancuronium[138] and an increase in pancuronium requirement.[145] However, such effects are small and of little clinical importance.

PROSTAGLANDIN INHIBITORS

In animals, it has been shown that prostaglandin synthesis is important in the modulation of transmitter release.[146] Thus, inhibitors of prostaglandin synthesis, i.e., nonsteroidal anti-inflammatory agents, might be expected to affect neuromuscular transmission. At present, there is no evidence to support the interaction of indomethacin with either the depolarizing or nondepolarizing relaxants.[147]

PSYCHOTROPIC DRUGS

Benzodiazepines

Intravenous diazepam has been used successfully to prevent muscle pains and fasciculations after succinylcholine.[148, 149] In the rat phrenic nerve-diaphragm preparation, interactions with the relaxants are dose dependent. Very low doses antagonize pancuronium, while higher doses potentiate both succinylcholine and pancuronium.[150] No consistent alterations in either pharmacokinetic or pharmacodynamic behavior have been found in therapeutic concentrations in man.[151]

Lithium

Earlier case reports suggested that lithium was associated with prolongation of action of pancuronium[152] and succinylcholine.[153] However, recent animal studies using the guinea pig-lumbrical preparation concluded that 40 times the therapeutic levels were necessary before potentiation was observed.[154] Conflicting reports of the action of lithium on transmitter release also exist.[155-157]

Tricyclic Antidepressants

Tricyclic drugs are associated with a high incidence of arrhythmias as a result of an increase in circulating catecholamines.[158-159] In dogs, an increased potential for rhythm disturbances has been recognized with pancuronium during halothane and enflurane anesthesia.[160] Chronic administration was associated with sinus tachycardia, while acute administration caused premature ventricular contractions, ventricular tachycardia, and fibrillation in a dose-dependent manner.

REFERENCES

1. Lang DA, Kimura KK, Unna KR: The combination of skeletal muscle relaxing agents with various central nervous system depressants used in anestheisa. *Arch Int Pharmacodyn Ther* 1951; 85:257–262.
2. McIndewar IC, Marshall RJ: Interaction between the neuromuscular block of ORG NC45 and some anesthetic, analgesic and antimicrobial agents. *Br J Anaesth* 1981; 53:785–791.
3. Boros M, Chaudhry IA, Nagashima H, et al: Myoneural effects of pethidine and droperidol. *Br J Anaesth* 1984; 56:195–202.
4. Duke PC, Johns CH, Pinsky C, et al: The effect of morphine on human neuromuscular transmission. *Can Anaesth Soc J* 1979; 26:201–205.
5. Katz RL: Clinical neuromuscular pharmacology of pancuronium. *Anesthesiology* 1971; 34:550–558.
6. Strahan SK, Pleuvry BJ, Modla CY: Effect of meptazinol on neuromuscular transmission in the isolated rat phrenic nerve-diaphragm preparation. *Br J Anaesth* 1985; 57:1095–1099.
7. Watland DC, Long JP, Pittinger CB, et al: Neuromuscular effects of ether, cyclopropane, chloroform and fluothane. *Anesthesiology* 1957; 18:883–890.
8. Walts LF, Dillon J: The influence of the anesthetic agent on the action of curare in man. *Anesth Analg* 1970; 49:17–21.
9. Sabawala PB, Dillon JB: Action of volatile anesthetics on human muscle preparations. *Anesthesiology* 1958; 19:587–594.
10. Katz RL, Gissen AJ: Neuromuscular and electromyographic effects of halothane and its interaction with d-tubocurarine. *Anesthesiology* 1967; 28:564–567.
11. Katz RL: Modification of the action of pancuronium by succinylcholine and halothane. *Anesthesiology* 1971; 35:602–606.

12. Hughes R, Payne JP: Interaction of halothane with nondepolarizing neuromuscular blocking drugs in man. *Br J Clin Pharmacol* 1979; 7:485–490.

13. Lebowitz MH, Blitt CD, Walts LF: Depression of twitch response to stimulation of the ulnar nerve during ethrane anesthesia in man. *Anesthesiology* 1970; 33:52–57.

14. Miller RD, Way WL, Dolan WM, et al: The dependence of pancuronium and d-tubocurarine induced neuromuscular blockades on alveolar concentrations of halothane and forane. *Anesthesiology* 1972; 37:573–581.

15. Miller RD, Way WL, Dolan WM, et al: Comparative neuromuscular effects of pancuronium, gallamine, and succinylcholine during Forane and halothane anesthesia in man. *Anesthesiology* 1971; 35:509–514.

16. Vitez TS, Miller RD, Eger EI, et al: Comparison in vitro of isoflurane and halothane potentiation of d-tubocurarine and succinylcholine neuromuscular blocks. *Anesthesiology* 1974; 41:53–56.

17. Fogdall RP, Miller RD: Neuromuscular effects of enflurane, alone and combined with d-tubocurarine, pancuronium, and succinylcholine in man. *Anesthesiology* 1975; 42:173–178.

18. Bennett MJ, Hahn JF: Potentiation of the combination of pancuronium and metocurine by halothane and isoflurane in humans with and without renal failure. *Anesthesiology* 1985; 62:759–764.

19. Rupp SM, Miller RD, Gencarelli PJ: Vecuronium-induced neuromuscular blockade during enflurane, isoflurane, and halothane anesthesia in humans. *Anesthesiology* 1984; 60:102–105.

20. Chapple DJ, Clark JS, Hughes R: Interaction between atracurium and drugs used in anaesthesia. *Br J Anaesth* 1983; 55:17S–22S.

21. Waud BE, Waud DR: Effects of volatile anesthetics on directly and indirectly stimulated skeletal muscle. *Anesthesiology* 1979; 50:103–110.

22. Waud BE: Decrease in dose requirement of d-tubocurarine by volatile anesthestics. *Anesthesiology* 1979; 51:298–302.

23. Stanski DR, Ham J, Miller RD, et al: Pharmacokinetics and pharmacodynamics of d-tubocurarine during nitrous oxide-narcotic and halothane anesthesia in man. *Anesthesiology* 1979; 51:235–241.

24. Delisle S, Bevan DR: Impaired neostigmine antagonism of pancuronium during enflurane anaesthesia in man. *Br J Anaesth* 1982; 54:441–445.

25. Cronnelly R, Dretchen KL, Sokoll MD, et al: Ketamine: Myoneuronal activity and interaction with neuromuscular blocking agents. *Eur J Pharmacol* 1973; 22:17–22.

26. Amaki Y, Nagashima H, Radnay PA, et al: Ketamine interaction with neuromuscular blocking agents in the phrenic nerve-hemidiaphragm preparation of the rat. *Anesth Analg* 1978; 57:238–243.

27. Torda TA, Murphy EC: Presynaptic effect of I.V. anaesthetic agents at the neuromuscular junction. *Br J Anaesth* 1979; 51:353–356.

28. Doenicke A, Krumey I, Kugler J, et al: Experimental studies of the breakdown of Epontol: Determination of propanidid in human serum. *Br J Anaesth* 1968; 40:415–428.

29. Ellis FR: The neuromuscular interaction of propanidid with suxamethonium and tubocurarine. *Br J Anaesth* 1968; 40:818–824.

30. Johnston RR, Miller RD, Way WL: The interaction of ketamine with d-tubocurarine, pancuronium, and succinylcholine in man. *Anesth Analg* 1974; 53:496–501.

31. Robertson EN, Fragen RJ, Booij LHDJ, et al: Some effects of diisopropyl phenol (ICI 35868) on the pharmacodynamics of atracurium and vecuronium in anaesthetized man. *Br J Anaesth* 1983; 55:723–728.

32. Cronnelly R, Morris RB, Miller RD: Comparison of thiopental and midazolam on the neuromuscular responses to succinylcholine or pancuronium in humans. *Anesth Analg* 1983; 62:75–77.

33. Zukaitis MG, Hoech GP: Train of 4 measurement of potentiation of curare by lidocaine. *Anesthesiology* 1979; 51:S288.

34. Usubiaga JF, Wikinski JA, Morales RL: Interaction of intravenously administered procaine, lidocaine and succinylcholine in anesthetized subjects. *Anesth Analg* 1967; 46:39–45.

35. Hall DR, McGibbon DH, Evans LL, et al: Gentamicin, tubocurarine, lignocaine and neuromuscular blockade: A case report. *Br J Anaesth* 1972; 44:1329–1322.

36. Zsigmond E, Eldertton TE: Abnormal reaction to procaine and succinylcholine in a patient with inherited atypical plasma cholinesterase. *Can Anaesth Soc J* 1968; 15:498–500.

37. Matsuo S, Rao DBS, Chaudry I, et al: Interaction of muscle relaxants and local anesthetics at the neuromuscular junction. *Anesth Analg* 1978; 57:580–587.

38. Morita K, Matsuo S, Nagashima H, et al: In vivo muscle relaxant-local anesthetic interaction. *Anesthesiology* 1979; 51:S282.

39. Lee DC, Liu HH, John TR: Presynaptic and postsynaptic actions of procainamide on neuromuscular transmission. *Muscle Nerve* 1983; 6:442–447.

40. Weisman SJ: Masked myasthenia gravis. *JAMA* 1949; 141:917–920.

41. Sprague DH: Severe bradycardia after neostigmine in a patient taking propranolol to control paroxysmal atrial tachycardia. *Anesthesiology* 1975; 42:208–210.

42. Usubiaga JE: Neuromuscular effects of beta-adrenergic blockers and their interaction with skeletal muscle relaxants. *Anesthesiology* 1968; 29:484–492.

43. Harrah MD, Way WL, Katzung BG: The interaction of d-tubocurarine with antiarrhythmic drugs. *Anesthesiology* 1970; 33:406–410.

44. Zalman F, Perlott JK, Durant NN, et al: Acute respiratory failure following intravenous verapamil in Duchenne's muscular dystrophy. *Am Heart J* 1983; 105:510–511.

45. van Poorten JF, Dhasmana KM, Kuypers RSM, et al: Verapamil and reversal of vecuronium neuromuscular blockade. *Anesth Analg* 1984; 63:155–157.

46. Jones RM, Cashman JN, Casson WR, et al: Verapamil potentiation of neuromuscular blockade: Failure of reversal with neostigmine but prompt reversal with edrophonium: Anesth Analg 1985; 64:1021–1025.
47. Kraynack BJ, Lawson NW, Gintantas J, et al: Effects of verapamil on indirect muscle twitch responses. Anesth Analg 1983; 62:827–830.
48. Bikhazi GB, Leung I, Foldes FF: Ca-channel blockers increase potency of neuromuscular blocking agents in vivo. Anesthesiology 1983; 59:A269.
49. Durant NN, Ngyuyen N, Katz RL: Potentiation of neuromuscular blockade with verapamil. Anesthesiology 1984; 60:298–303.
50. Andersen KA, Marshall RJ: Interactions between calcium entry blockers and vecuronium bromide in anaesthetized cats. Br J Anaesth 1985; 57:775–781.
51. Lawson NW, Kraynack BJ, Gintantes J: Neuromuscular and electrocardiographic responses to verapamil in dogs. Anesth Analg 1983; 62:50–54.
52. Welch GW, Waud BE: Effect of bretylium on neuromuscular transmission. Anesth Analg 1982; 61:442–444.
53. Healey TEJ, O'Shea M, Massey J: Disopyramide and neuromuscular transmission. Br J Anaesth 1981; 53:495–498.
54. Miller RD, Way WL, Katzung BG: The potentiation of neuromuscular blocking agents by quinidine. Anesthesiology 1967; 28:1036–1041.
55. Cuthbert MF: The effect of quinidine and procainamide on the neuromuscular blocking action of suzamethonium. Br J Anaesth 1966; 38:775–779.
56. Schmidt JL, Vick NA, Sadove NS: The effect of quinidine on the action of muscle relaxants. JAMA 1963; 183:669–672.
57. Grogogno AW: Anaesthesia for atrial defibrillation: Effect of quinidine on muscle relaxation. Lancet 1963; 2:1039–1040.
58. Kornfield P, Horowitz SH, Gerkins G, et al: Myasthenia gravis unmasked by antiarrhythmic agents. Mt Sinai J Med (NY) 1976; 43:10–14.
59. Way WL, Katzung BS, Lawson CP: Recurarization with quinidine. JAMA 1967; 200:163–164.
60. Emery ERJ: Neuromuscular blocking properties of antibiotics as a cause of post-operative apnoea. Anaesthesia 1963; 18:57–65.
61. Brazil OV, Prado-Franceschi J: The nature of neuromuscular block produced by neomycin and gentamicin. Arch Int Pharmacodyn Ther 1969; 179:78–85.
62. Fogdall RP, Miller RD: Prolongation of a pancuronium-induced neuromuscular blockade by clindamycin. Anesthesiology 1974; 41:407–408.
63. Fogdall RP, Miller RD: Prolongation of a pancuronium-induced neuromuscular blockade by polymyxin B. Anesthesiology 1974; 40:84–87.
64. VanNyhuis LS, Miller RD, Fogdall RP: The interaction between d-tubocurarine, pancuronium, polymyxin B, and neostigmine on neuromuscular function. Anesth Analg 1976; 55:224–228.

65. Becker LD, Miller RD: Clindamycin enhances a nondepolarizing neuromuscular blockade. *Anesthesiology* 1976; 45:84–87.

66. Singh YN, Harvey AL, Marshall IG: Antibiotic-induced paralysis of the mouse phrenic nerve-hemidiaphragm preparation, and reversibility by calcium and neostigmine. *Anesthesiology* 1978; 48:418–424.

67. Pittinger CB, Eryasa Y, Adamson R: Antibiotic induced paralysis. *Anesth Analg* 1970; 49:487–501.

68. Argov Z, Mastaglia FL: Disorders of neuromuscular transmission caused by drugs. *N Engl J Med* 1979; 301:409–413.

69. Burkett L, Bilkhazi GB, Thamas KC, et al: Mutual potentiation of the neuromuscular effects of antibiotics and relaxants. *Anesth Analg* 1979; 58:107–115.

70. Kronenfeld MA, Thomas SJ, Turndorf H: Recurrence of neuromuscular blockade after reversal of vecuronium in a patient receiving polymyxin/amikacin sternal irrigation. *Anesthesiology* 1986; 65:93–94.

71. Benz HE, Lunn JN, Foldes FF: Recurarization by intraperitoneal antibiotics. *Br Med J* 1961; 2:241–242.

72. Foldes FF, Lunn JN, Benz HG: Respiratory depression from drug combinations. *JAMA* 1962; 183:672–673.

73. Pittinger CB, Eryasa Y, Adamson R: Antibiotic-induced paralysis. *Anesth Analg* 1970; 49:487–501.

74. Waterman PM, Smith RB: Tobramycin-curare interactions. *Anesth Analg* 1977; 56:587–588.

75. Giala MM, Paradelis AG: Two cases of prolonged respiratory depression due to interaction of pancuronium with colistin and streptomycin. *J Antimicrob Chemother* 1979; 5:234–235.

76. Booij LHDJ, Miller RD, Crul JF: Neostigmine and 4–aminopyridine antagonism of lincomycin-pancuronium neuromuscular blockade in man. *Anesth Analg* 1978; 57:316–321.

77. Wright JM, Collier B: The effect of neomycin upon transmitter release and action. *J Pharmacol Exp Ther* 1977; 200:576–587.

78. Torda T: The nature of gentamicin-induced neuromuscular block. *Br J Anaesth* 1980; 52:325–329.

79. Brazil OV, Prado-Franceschi J: The neuromuscular blocking action of gentamicin. *Arch Int Pharmacodyn Ther* 1969; 179:65–77.

80. Singh YN, Marshall IG, Harvey AL: Pre- and postjunctional blocking effects of aminoglycoside, polymyxin, tetracycline and lincosamide antibiotics. *Br J Anaesth* 1982; 54:1295–1306.

81. Sokoll MD, Diecke FPJ: Some effects of streptomycin on frog nerve in vitro. *Arch Int Pharmacodyn Ther* 1969; 177:332–339.

82. Dretchen KL, Sokoll MD, Gergis SD, et al: Relative effects of streptomycin on motor nerve terminals and end-plate. *Eur J Pharmacol* 1973; 22:10–16.

83. Standaert FG, Riker WF: The consequences of cholinergic drug actions on motor nerve terminals. *Ann NY Acad Sci* 1967; 144:517–533.

84. Bruckner J, Thomas KC, Bikhazi GB, et al: Neuromuscular drug interactions of clinical importance. *Anesth Analg* 1980; 59:678–682.

85. Durant NN, Lee C, Katz RL: Cumulation of neomycin and its residual potentiation of tubocurarine in the cat. *Br J Anaesth* 1981; 53:571–576.
86. Brazil OV, Corrado AP: The curariform action of streptomycin. *J Pharmacol Exp Ther* 1957; 120:452–459.
87. Dunkley B, Sanghvi I, Goldstein G: Characterization of neuromuscular block produced by streptomycin. *Arch Int Pharmacodyn Ther* 1973; 201:213–223.
88. Lee C, Chen D, Barnes A, et al: Neuromuscular block by neomycin in the cat. *Can Anaesth Soc J* 1976; 23:527–533.
89. Stanley VG, Giesecke AH, Jenkins MT: Neomycin-curare neuromuscular block and reversal in cats. *Anesthesiology* 1969; 31:228–232.
90. Wright JM, Collier B: The site of neuromuscular block produced by polymyxin B and rolitetracycline. *Can J Physiol Pharmacol* 1976; 54:926–936.
91. McQuillen MP, Engbaek L: Mechanism of colistin-induced neuromuscular depression. *Arch Neurol* 1975; 32:235–238.
92. Lee C, Chen D, Engel EL: Neuromuscular block by antibiotics: polymyxin B. *Anesth Analg* 1977; 56:373–377.
93. Bowen JM, McMullen WC: Influence of induced hypermagnesemia and hypocalcemia on neuromuscular blocking property of oxytetracycline in the horse. *Am J Vet Res* 1975; 36:1025–1028.
94. Rubbo JT, Sokoll MD, Gergis SD: Comparative neuromuscular effects of lincomycin and clindamycin. *Anesth Analg* 1977; 56:329–332.
95. Singh YN, Marshall IG, Harvey AL: Reversal of antibiotic induced muscle paralysis by 3,4–aminopyridine. *J Pharm Pharmacol* 1978; 30:249–250.
96. Tang AH, Schroeder LA: The effect of lincomycin on neuromuscular transmission. *Toxicol Appl Pharmacol* 1978; 12:44–47.
97. Futamachi KJ, Prince DA: Effect of penicillin on an excitatory synapse. *Brain Res* 1975; 100:589–597.
98. Noebels JL, Prince DA: Presynaptic origin of penicillin after discharge at mammalian nerve terminals. *Brain Res* 1977; 138:59–75.
99. d'Hollander A, Agoston S, Capouet V, et al: Failure of metronidazole to alter a vecuronium neuromuscular blockade in humans. *Anesthesiology* 1985; 63:99–102.
100. Messick JM, Maas L, Faust RJ, et al: Duration of pancuronium neuromuscular blockade in patients taking anticonvulsant medication. *Anesth Analg* 1982; 61:203–204.
101. Chen J, Kim YD, Dubois M, et al: The increased requirement of pancuronium in neurosurgical patients receiving dilantin chronically. *Anesthesiology* 1983; 59:A288.
102. Ornstein E, Matteo RS, Silverberg PA, et al: Dose-response relationships for vecuronium in the presence of chronic phenytoin therapy. *Anesth Analg* 1986; 65:S116.
103. Ornstein E, Schwartz AE, Matteo RS, et al: Predictability of atracurium effect in phenytoin exposed patients. *Anesthesiology* 1986; 65:A112.

104. Ornstein E, Matteo RS, Young WL, et al: Resistance to metocurine-induced neuromuscular blockade in patients receiving phenytoin. *Anesthesiology* 1985; 63:294–298.

105. Haque N, Trasher K, Werk E, et al: Studies on dexamethasone metabolism in man: Effect of diphenylhydantoin. *J Clin Endocrinol Metab* 1972; 34:44–50.

106. Norris F, Colella J, McFarcin D: Effect of diphenylhydantoin on neuromuscular synapse. *Neurology* 1964; 14:869–876.

107. Meyers EF: Partial recovery from pancuronium neuromuscular blockade following hydrocortisone administration. *Anesthesiology* 1977; 46:148–150.

108. Laflin MJ: Interaction of pancuronium and corticosteroids. *Anesthesiology* 1977; 47:471–472.

109. Wilgenburg HN: The effect of prednisone on neuromuscular transmission in the rat diaphragm. *Eur J Pharmacol* 1979; 58:355–361.

110. Wilson RW, Ward MD, Johns TR: Corticosteroids: A direct effect at the neuromuscular junction. *Neurology* 1974; 24:1091–1095.

111. Riker WF, Baker T, Okamato M: Glucocorticoids and mammalian nerve excitability. *Arch Neurol* 1975; 32:688–694.

112. Arts WF, Oosterhuis HJ: Effects of prednisone on neuromuscular blocking in mice in vivo. *Neurology* 1975; 25:1088–1090.

113. Leeuwin RS, Wolters ECMJ: Effects of corticosteroids on sciatic nerve-tibialis anterior muscle of rats treated with hemicholinium-3. *Neurology* 1977; 27:171–177.

114. Foldes FF, Arai T, Gentsch H, et al: The influence of glucocorticoids on plasma cholinesterase. *Proc Soc Exp Biol Med* 1974; 146:918–920.

115. Durant NN, Briscoe JR, Katz RL: The effects of acute and chronic hydrocortisone treatment on neuromuscular blockade in the anesthetized cat. *Anesthesiology* 1984; 61:144–150.

116. Leeuwin RS, Veldsema-Currie RD, Wilgenburg HV: Effects of corticosteroids on neuromuscular blocking actions of d-tubocurarine. *Eur J Pharmacol* 1981; 69:165–173.

117. Schwartz AE: Acute steroid therapy does not alter nondepolarizing muscle relaxant effects in humans. *Anesthesiology* 1986; 65:326–327.

118. Miller RD, Sohn YJ, Matteo RS: Enhancement of d-tubocurarine neuromuscular blockade by diuretics in man. *Anesthesiology* 1976; 45:442–445.

119. Gessa GL, Ferrari W: Influence of chlorothiazide, hydrochlorothiazide, and acetazolamide on neuromuscular transmission in mammals. *Arch Int Pharmacodyn Ther* 1963; 144:258–268.

120. Azar I, Cottrell J, Gupta B, et al: Furosemide facilitates recovery of evoked twitch response after pancuronium. *Anesth Analg* 1980; 59:55–57.

121. Sappaticci KA, Ham JA, Sohn YJ, et al: Effects of furosemide on the neuromuscular junction. *Anesthesiology* 1982; 57:381–388.

122. Vaughan RS, Lunn JN: Potassium and the anaesthetist. *Anaesthesia* 1973; 28:118–131.

123. Chasapakis G, Dimas C: Possible interactions between muscle relaxants and the kallikrein-trypsin inactivator "Trasylol". *Br J Anaesth* 1966; 38:838–839.
124. Doenicke A, Gesing H, Krumez I, et al: Influence of aprotinin (Trasylol) on the action of suxamethonium. *Br J Anaesth* 1970; 42:943–960.
125. Poulton TJ, James FM, Lockridge O: Prolonged apnea following trimethaphan and succinylcholine. *Anesthesiology* 1979; 50:54–56.
126. Nakamura K, Koide M, Imanaga T, et al: Prolonged neuromuscular blockade following trimetaphan infusion: A case report and in vitro study of cholinesterase inhibition. *Anaesthesia* 1980; 35:1202–1207.
127. Wilson SL, Miller RN, Wright C, et al: Prolonged neuromuscular blockade associated with trimethaphan: A case report. *Anesth Analg* 1976; 55:353–356.
128. Deacock AR, Davies TDW: The influence of certain ganglionic blocking agents on neuromuscular transmission. *Br J Anaesth* 1958; 30:217–225.
129. Deacock AR, Hargrove RL: The influence of certain ganglion blocking agents on neuromuscular transmission. *Br J Anaesth* 1962; 34:357–362.
130. Gergis SD, Sokoll MD, Rubbo JT: Effect of sodium nitroprusside and trimetaphan on neuromuscular transmission in the frog. *Can Anaesth Soc J* 1977; 24:220–227.
131. Tewfik GI: Trimetaphan: Its effect on the pseudocholinesterase level of man. *Anaesthesia* 1957; 12:326–329.
132. Sklar GS, Lanks KW: Effects of trimetaphan and sodium nitroprusside on hydrolysis of succinylcholine in vitro. *Anesthesiology* 1977; 47:31–33.
133. Glisson SN, El-Etr AA, Lein R: Prolongation of pancuronium-induced neuromuscular blockade by intravenous infusion of nitroglycerine. *Anesthesiology* 1979; 51:47–49.
134. Glisson SN, Sanchez MM, El-Etr AA, et al: Nitroglycerin and the neuromuscular blockade produced by gallamine, succinylcholine, d-tubocurarine, and pancuronium. *Anesth Analg* 1980; 59:117–122.
135. Schwartz S, Agoston S, Houwertjes MC: Does intravenous infusion of nitroglycerin potentiate pancuronium- and vecuronium-induced neuromuscular blockade? *Anesth Analg* 1986; 65:156–160.
136. Chung F: Cancer, chemotherapy and anaesthesia. *Can Anaesth Soc J* 1982; 29:364–371.
137. Bennett EJ, Schmidt GR, Patel KP, et al: Muscle relaxants, myasthenia and mustards? *Anesthesiology* 1977; 46:220–221.
138. Dretchen KL, Morgenroth VH, Standaert F, et al: Azathioprine: Effects on neuromuscular transmission. *Anesthesiology* 1976; 45:604–609.
139. Viby-Mogensen J: Cholinesterase and succinylcholine. *Dan Med Bull* 1983; 30:129–150.
140. Zsigmond KL, Robbins G: The effect of a series of anticancer drugs on plasma cholinesterase activity. *Can Anaesth Soc J* 1972; 19:75–82.
141. Fried MJ, Protheroe D: D-penicillamine-induced myasthenia gravis. *Br J Anaesth* 1986; 58:1191–1193.

142. Gramstad L, Gjerlow JA, Hysing ES, et al: Interaction of cyclosporin and its solvent, cremophor, with atracurium and vecuronium. *Br J Anaesth* 1986; 58:1149–1155.

143. Flewellen EH, Nelson TE, Bee DE: Effect of dantrolene on neuromuscular block by d-tubocurarine and subsequent antagonism by neostigmine in the rabbit. *Anesthesiology* 1980; 52:126–130.

144. Driessen JJ, Wuis EW, Gielen MJM: Prolonged vecuronium neuromuscular blockade in a patient receiving orally administered dantrolene. *Anesthesiology* 1985; 62:523–524.

145. Azar I, Kumar D, Betcher AM: Resistance to pancuronium in an asthmatic patient treated with aminophylline and steroids. *Can Anaesth Soc J* 1982; 29:280–282.

146. Madden KS, Van der Koot W: Indomethacin, prostaglandin E_2 and transmission at the frog neuromuscular junction. *J Pharmacol Exp Ther* 1985; 232:305–314.

147. Hill GE, Wong KC: Effects of prostaglandins and indomethacin on neuromuscular blocking agents. *Can Anaesth Soc J* 1980; 27:146–149.

148. Eisenberg M, Balsley S, Katz RL: Effects of diazepam on succinylcholine-induced myalgias, potassium increase, creatinine phosphokinase elevation and relaxation. *Anesth Analg* 1979; 58:314–317.

149. Fahmy NR, Malek NS, Lappas DG: Diazepam prevents some adverse effects of succinylcholine. *Clin Pharmacol Ther* 1979; 26:395–398.

150. Driessen JJ, Vree TB, Van Egmond J, et al: In vitro interaction of diazepam and oxazepam with pancuronium and succinylcholine. *Br J Anaesth* 1984; 56:1131–1138.

151. Asbury AJ, Henderson PD, Brown BH, et al: Effect of diazepam on pancuronium-induced neuromuscular block maintained by a feedback system. *Br J Anaesth* 1981; 53:859–863.

152. Borden H, Clarke MT, Katz H: The use of pancuronium bromide in patients receiving lithium carbonate. *Can Anaesth Soc J* 1974; 21:79–82.

153. Hill GE, Wong KC, Hodges MR: Potentiation of succinylcholine neuromuscular blockade by lithium carbonate. *Anesthesiology* 1976; 44:439–442.

154. Waud BE, Farrell L, Waud DR: Lithium and neuromuscular transmission. *Anesth Analg* 1982; 61:399–402.

155. Vizi ES, Illes P, Ronai A, et al: The effect of lithium on acetylcholine release and synthesis. *Neuropharmacology* 1972; 11:521–530.

156. Crawford AC: Lithium ions and the release of transmitter at the frog neuromuscular junction. *J Physiol (Lond)* 1975; 246:109–142.

157. Branisteanu DD, Volle RL: Modification by lithium of transmitter release at the neuromuscular junction of the frog. *J Pharmacol Exp Ther* 1975; 194:362–372.

158. Ramanthan KB, Davidson C: Cardiac arrhythmias and imipramine therapy. *Br Med J* 1975; 1:661–662.

159. Williams RB, Sherter C: Cardiac complications of tricyclic antidepressant therapy. *Ann Intern Med* 1971; 74:395–398.

160. Edwards RP, Miller RD, Roizen MF, et al: Cardiac responses to imipramine and pancuronium during anesthesia with halothane or enflurane. *Anesthesiology* 1979; 50:421–425.

13

Neuromuscular Diseases

MYASTHENIA GRAVIS

> The abnormal fatigability in myasthenia gravis has been thought to be due to curare-like poisoning of the motor nerve endings or of the myoneural junction. It occurred to me that it might be worthwhile to try the effect of physostigmine, a partial antagonist to curare, on a case of myasthenia gravis. Mary Walker (House Physician at St. Alfege Hospital), 1934[1]

Myasthenia gravis (MG) is a disease of the neuromuscular junction characterized by weakness and fatigability of skeletal muscles. It occurs with an incidence of 1:50,000 and presents either in the young (15 to 30 years of age), when it occurs predominantly in females (3:1), or in late middle age, when the distribution of cases shows no sexual preference.[2]

Etiology

Myasthenia gravis is an autoimmune disease and frequently occurs with rheumatoid arthritis, systemic lupus erythematosis, and pernicious anemia. The thymus gland is abnormal in 80% of MG cases—10%, malignant tumors; 70%, hyperplasia—and its removal usually produces an improvement in symptoms.

Circulating antibodies are present[3] that produce a functional reduction in acetylcholine receptors.[4] It is uncertain whether the antibodies result in increased receptor breakdown or blockade. Recently it has been suggested that they may cause channel block.[5] There is now no doubt that the lesion is postsynaptic. Previously a presynaptic etiology was suggested because miniature end-plate and evoked action potentials were reduced in amplitude by 80%.[6] However, the number of acetylcholine quanta is not decreased, and their content is either normal or increased.[7] However, several gaps remain in the sequence of thymus-receptor antibody-myasthenia, which await explanation.

Clinical Features

Muscle weakness in MG fluctuates widely but is more pronounced later in the day. Facial and bulbar muscles are affected early, producing ptosis, diplopia, difficulty in swallowing, slurred speech, and eventually respiratory weakness. Large proximal muscles, particularly of the arms and neck, may be involved, and muscle wasting may develop after many years. The disease may be limited to the ocular muscles or become generalized when it usually progresses slowly. Occasionally rapid progression, to include the respiratory muscles, develops within 6 months of the onset. Babies born to affected mothers may develop transient weakness, and a similar syndrome has been described following certain drug regimens, e.g., penicillamine and phenytoin. Occasionally, latent forms of the disease are diagnosed after abnormal responses to muscle relaxants have been observed during anesthesia.[8]

Diagnosis

The diagnosis is often obvious from the classical clinical presentation but is confirmed by electromyographic (EMG), pharmacologic, and immunologic testing.

The characteristic EMG finding is a voltage decrement to repeated stimulation. Stimuli at 3 Hz shows a fade of the second stimulus, and MG is diagnosed if the response to the fifth stimulus is decreased by more than 10%.[9] Latent MG may be revealed by repeating the test after exercise. Although different muscles may be affected, testing is usually performed by stimulating the ulnar or median nerves, or the nerve to the deltoid muscle. The appearance of fade to repetitive stimulation is evidence of a decrease in the margin-of-safety of neuromuscular transmission.[10]

Sensitivity to nondepolarizing relaxants can be measured by systemic or regional curare tests. The diagnosis is confirmed by severe weakness after small doses (1 to 3 mg) of d-tubocurarine given systemically,[11] although this has the risk of generalized paralysis and respiratory depression. Consequently, it is safer to perform the regional curare

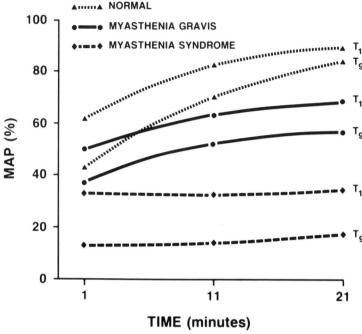

FIG 13–1.

Response to train-of-nine stimulation after 1, 11, and 21 minutes after releasing tourniquet in regional curare test. Myasthenia gravis and myasthenia syndrome demonstrate profound and persistent fade. MAP% = muscle action potential in % of precurare values. (From Brown JC, Charlton JE: A study of sensitivity to curare in myasthenic disorders using a regional technique. *J Neurol Neurosurg Psychiatry* 1975; 38:27–33. Used by permission.)

test.[12] After isolating the forearm with a tourniquet, 0.5 mg of curare is given intravenously; the tourniquet is released at 4 to 5 minutes, and trains-of-nine are applied 1, 11, and 21 minutes after the release. Myasthenia gravis is characterized by pronounced persistent fade (Fig 13–1).

Small doses of edrophonium, 2 to 8 mg, produce brief recovery from MG, commencing after 1 minute and lasting for 10 minutes. Finally, recognition of circulating antibody to acetylcholine receptor protein confirms the diagnosis.[8]

Treatment

Anticholinesterases form the cornerstone of treatment along with pyridostigmine in doses starting at 60 mg three times a day orally. Peak plasma concentrations are found after 1 to 2 hours, but these are delayed if the drugs are ingested with food.[13] However, the requirement is variable, and overdose may result in symptoms, i.e., cholinergic crisis, as severe as myasthenia. In some patients the fluctuation between muscle groups is so great that some muscles may be myasthenic while others show signs of overdose. Also, some patients cannot tolerate the nicotinic and muscarinic complications of anticholinesterase therapy.

Inhibition of the autoimmune reaction with steroids and/or azathioprine is successful for many. Plasmapheresis is particularly effective in controlling acute exacerbations.[14] Finally, thymectomy helps most patients, although its benefits may not be seen for several months:[2] clinical improvement following a reduction in acetylcholine-receptor antibody titers.[15]

Differential Diagnosis

The myasthenic syndrome (Eaton-Lambert syndrome)[16] and botulism are also disorders of the neuromuscular junction. Both have a presynaptic action reducing the release of acetylcholine.[17] The myasthenic syndrome is invariably associated with bronchial carcinoma. Proximal muscles are affected first, with occasional later bulbar involvement. Electromyographic testing at low frequency is similar to MG, but facilitation occurs after exercise. The response to anticholinesterases is incomplete but guanidine[18] and 4–aminopyridine[19] are more successful and act by increasing acetylcholine release.

Botulism is usually associated with gastrointestinal symptoms, and local outbreaks result from food poisoning.[20] The toxins block autonomic cholinergic factors (dry mouth, constipation, blurred vision) and progress to involve the facial muscles. Death follows respiratory paralysis.

Anesthesia in Myasthenia Gravis

Response to Muscle Relaxants
Myasthenic patients demonstrate abnormal responses to both depolarizing and nondepolarizing neuromuscular blocking drugs (NMBDs). The response depends upon the severity of the disease, the muscle tested, and, in particular, the therapeutic regimen.

Succinylcholine
Patients with MG are usually slightly resistant to succinylcholine, but during recovery, phase II block develops rapidly and recovery is slow.[24, 25] The response is partly specific to MG but also represents the effects of concomitant anticholinesterase therapy. Nevertheless, suc-

TABLE 13–1.
Guidelines for Anesthesia in Myasthenia

1. Choose regional analgesia if possible.
2. If general anesthesia essential, avoid relaxants if possible.
3. If relaxants essential, titrate with neuromuscular twitch monitoring. Atracurium is best choice.
4. After surgery, monitor ventilation, and titrate anticholinesterase therapy with frequent edrophonium testing. IPPV if in doubt.
5. Avoid neuromuscular block potentiation (described in Chapter 12) after administration of thiotepa, gentamicin, quinidine, procainamide.

cinylcholine has been used to facilitate intubation[25] and, as an infusion,[26] to maintain relaxation.

d-Tubocurarine and Pancuronium

Small doses of d-tubocurarine are used in the diagnosis of MG because most patients demonstrate abnormal sensitivity. Nevertheless, reduced doses of d-tubocurarine[24, 27] and pancuronium[28] have been given safely during anesthesia, particularly when titrated carefully with the use of neuromuscular monitoring. Doses should begin as low as 0.03 mg/kg for d-tubocurarine and 0.005 mg/kg for pancuronium.

Atracurium and Vecuronium

The introduction of these intermediate-duration relaxants has particular importance in MG. There are several reports of the successful use of *atracurium*.[29–35] Dosage usually needs to be reduced by about 75%, but the rate of recovery is only prolonged slightly (25% to 75% recovery index, 17 vs. 12 minutes in normals).[35] Thus, the unique metabolism of atracurium allows full recovery without the need for anticholinesterase reversal. Nevertheless, there is wide patient variation so that monitoring is essential.

Vecuronium, in reduced doses, has also been used successfully.[36] However, Buzello et al.[37] observed that recovery after vecuronium in MG may be prolonged considerably. Although very variable, the 25% to 75% recovery index increased from 9 ± 3 minutes in normals to 70 ± 76 minutes in MG patients. Also, twitch monitoring was found to be much more sensitive than EMG.[37]

Choice of Anesthesia

Some general principles are clear in the provision of anesthesia in MG (Table 13–1).

Anesthesia for Thymectomy

Muscle relaxants have usually been avoided. Anesthesia is induced, after moderate premedication, with thiopental and intubation performed with N_2O-O_2 and anesthetic vapor with or without local anesthesia. However, small doses of atracurium would be suitable additions.

Two controversies remain: the management of anticholinesterase treatment and the prediction of postoperative ventilatory insufficiency.

The requirement for anticholinesterases is often but not always reduced for 1 to 2 days after thymectomy. Thus, several regimens omit the anticholinesterases on the day of surgery recommencing after about 24 hours according to edrophonium testing.

The preoperative prediction of postoperative respiratory failure is difficult. Estimates based on vital capacity are insensitive.[38] They may be improved by observing several factors with discriminant analysis,[39] (Table 13–2), but such a schedule often overestimates the need for intermittent positive pressure ventilation (IPPV),[40] particularly when thymectomy is performed by the transcervical rather than the transsternal route.[41] It seems more appropriate at the end of surgery to leave the patient intubated until he can produce an inspiratory force of -20 cm H_2O. Once the patient has been extubated and can swallow, he can be transferred to the ward within a few hours. Controlled ventilation will be required in the few who do not meet these criteria. In a recent series, only 8 of 92 patients undergoing transcervical thymectomy required IPPV, although the scoring system had predicted that ventilation would be required in 23.[41]

TABLE 13–2.
Prediction of Postoperative Respiratory Insufficiency in Myasthenia Gravis*

	POINTS†
Duration of myasthenia gravis >6 yr	12
Other respiratory disease	10
Pyridostigmine >750 mg/day	8
Vital capacity <2.9/L	4

*Adapted from Leventhal S, Orkin FK, Hirsh RA: Prediction of the need for postoperative mechanical ventilation in myasthenia gravis. *Anesthesiology* 1980; 53:26–30.
†Postoperative IPPV required if score is greater than 10 points.

MYOTONIA

Myotonia is a disease of the muscle membrane.[42–44] It exists in several forms: myotonic dystrophy (dystrophia myotonica, myotonia atrophica, Steinert's disease, Hoffmann's disease) myotonia congenita (Thomsen's disease), and paramyotonia congenita. All these syndromes demonstrate an abnormal delay in muscle relaxation after contraction. The three disorders probably represent different manifestations of the same disease with an autosomal dominant mode of inheritance.

The site of the lesion in myotonia is in the muscle, although the biochemistry of myotonia is not known. Repeated nerve stimulation leads to a gradual but persistent increase in muscle tension. The EMG is pathognomic: myotonic afterdischarges are seen in peripheral muscle consisting of rapid bursts of potential produced by tapping the muscle or moving the needle. They produce typical "dive-bomber" sounds on the loudspeaker.

Myotonic dystrophy is the most common inherited neuromuscular disorder and presents as a systemic disease in early adult life. Generalized symptoms include testicular atrophy, baldness, cataract, cardiac conduction abnormalities producing ventricular instability and Adams-Stokes attacks, and mild endocrine abnormalities affecting glucose homeostasis and thyroid function. Weakness is prominent in the facial and distal muscles, although decreases in ventilatory reserve are present in those affected severely. The typical myotonic response to hand-shaking may be concealed with trick maneuvers.

Myotonia congenita appears in childhood. It is characterized by generalized weakness and is associated with hypertrophy of the masseters, neck muscles, deltoids, biceps, forearm and thenar muscles, and calves, thighs, and glutei. There is a suspicion,[45] yet to be proved,[46, 47] that myotonia congenita is associated with malignant hyperthermia (MH) but certain features, such as masseter spasm after succinylcholine, are common to both conditions.

Paramyotonia is uncommon and presents as myotonia and/or weakness on exposure to cold, which is relieved by warmth and exercise.

Response to Neuromuscular Blocking Drugs

The characteristic abnormality is a sustained, dose-related contracture after succinylcholine[48-50] (Fig 13-2) that makes it difficult to ventilate the patient for 2 to 5 minutes. However, the response is not inevitable, and succinylcholine has relieved the myotonia. Conversely, others have reported a prolonged spasm that gradually decreased over 24 hours.[51]

The response to nondepolarizing relaxants is normal,[43] although myotonic responses have been observed after administration of neostigmine.[52] Precurarization with d-tubocurarine[53] cannot be relied on[43] to prevent myotonia; neither is it prevented by dantrolene.[54]

Anesthesia in Myotonia

In many situations, regional analgesia is preferable to general. After the latter, ventilatory depression can be anticipated.[55] Respiratory depressants should be used cautiously in the myotonic patient. Thiopental has been singled out,[56] but it is probably no more dangerous than any other depressant. Succinylcholine is to be avoided. Atracurium[57-59] or vecuronium are particularly suitable to produce muscle relaxation, especially if ventilation is continued until full spontaneous recovery has occurred. The pregnant patient is a particular challenge. Respiratory function is threatened by the reduction of functional residual capacity (FRC) and myotonic weakness, which may be exacerbated during pregnancy.[60] Nevertheless, regional analgesia is preferable to general,[61] despite the added risk of intercostal weakness. In addition, the baby's muscular function should be assessed at birth.

Succinylcholine (mg/kg)

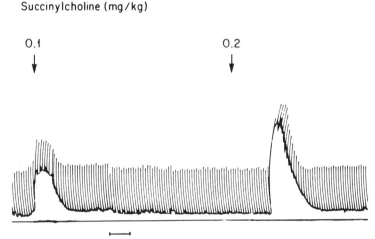

FIG 13–2.
Myotonic responses to succinylcholine. (From Mitchell MM, Ali HH, Savarese JJ: Myotonia and neuromuscular blocking agents. *Anesthesiology* 1978; 49:44–48. Used by permission.)

MUSCULAR DYSTROPHY

Duchenne type muscular dystrophy (DMD) is the commonest (1:30,000) of the progressive muscular dystrophies. It is inherited as an X-linked recessive disorder. Symptoms of waddling gait and frequent falling present in young boys aged 2 to 6 years. Within a few years he is unable to walk and develops contractures and scoliosis. Myocardial involvement is common with a typical electrocardiogram (ECG) and right outflow obstruction. Death occurs, usually from pneumonia and aspiration as a result of respiratory muscle weakness, by 20 to 25 years. Pathologic changes are present at the neuromuscular junction before dystrophic changes occur.[62] The disease is important to anesthetists because of cardiac arrest during anesthesia, an abnormal reaction to succinylcholine, and postoperative respiratory failure.[63]

Most patients with DMD survive anesthesia with a wide variety of inhalational anesthetic agents and neuromuscular blocking drugs without incident.[64, 65] However, there are several reports of cardiac arrest that followed the administration of succinylcholine and that were associated with muscle rigidity, masseter spasm, and an inability to ventilate the patients.[66–69] This was accompanied by respiratory and metabolic acidosis, hyperkalemia, elevation of creatinine phosphokinase and aldolase concentrations, myoglobinemia, and in some patients,[69, 70] an abnormal contracture response suspiciously like MH. However, the relationship between DMD and MH is highly controversial. While some ponder the interpretation of positive contracture tests without personal or family history of MH,[71] others are convinced that patients with DMD are at a greater risk of developing MH than the general population.[72] The latter recommend that precautions to avoid MH be taken when anesthetizing a boy with DMD. No matter who is correct, the wise course is to avoid succinylcholine, particularly as atracurium has been used without problem.[73]

The response of DMD to nondepolarizing relaxants seems to be normal,[64, 65] although the regional curare test demonstrates a normal initial blockade that lasts longer than normal.[74] The rare syndrome of *ocular muscular dystrophy*, involving predominantly the eye muscles, demonstrates extreme sensitivity to d-tubocurarine but, unlike myasthenia gravis, little response to anticholinesterases.[75]

UPPER MOTOR NEURON LESIONS

Patients with hemiplegia or quadriplegia as a result of intracranial lesions show an abnormal response to both depolarizing and nondepolarizing blocking drugs.

Several reports exist of hyperkalemia and ventricular fibrillation or cardiac arrest following succinylcholine in hemiplegic[76–78] and paraplegic[79, 80] patients. Hyperkalemia has followed as soon as one week[76] and as long as 6 months[78] after the development of neurologic symptoms. It has been observed, in a paraplegic patient, that the potassium concentration in the inferior vena cava was higher than in the superior vena cava.[80] Thus, it seems that the source of the potassium is from the affected muscles. Although part of the increase in potassium flux is a result of immobility,[81] it is more likely that a lack of innervation leads to extrajunctional chemosensitivity,[82] as a result of receptor spread.[83, 84]

After denervation, the whole muscle membrane has similar sensitivity to succinylcholine and is accompanied by ion fluxes of potassium and sodium.[85] Consequently, it has been recommended that succinylcholine be avoided in patients with upper motor neuron lesions except in the few days following the original episode.[26] However, this may be unnecessarily restrictive in patients suffering the chronic effects of cerebral ischemia.

Hemiplegic patients are resistant to nondepolarizing blocking drugs. Where neuromuscular monitoring is used on the paretic side, neuromuscular blockade is less intense and recovers more rapidly than on the contralateral side.[86-88] Similar resistance has been demonstrated in animals following disuse atrophy produced by encasing one limb in a plaster cast.[89] Interestingly, the noncasted limb is also more resistant than normal.[90] This has its clinical counterpart in an elegant demonstration of dose-response curves to metocurine in hemiplegic patients. The affected side was found to be resistant compared with the nonaffected side, although it also demonstrated decreased sensitivity[91] (Fig 13-3). The resistance to nondepolarizing relaxants in hemiplegia has been confirmed by using the regional curare test, although spinal cord lesions demonstrated sensitivity.[12] This latter observation has yet to be confirmed in anesthetic practice.

The cause of the altered sensitivity to nondepolarizing relaxants in patients with upper motor neuron disease is a corollary of the succinylcholine-induced potassium release: both result from receptor spread. The significance for clinical anesthesia is that monitoring of the junction is difficult. Monitoring of the "normal" side is preferable, but it may still exaggerate the degree of return of respiratory muscle activity.

MISCELLANEOUS

Denervated Muscle

Muscle membranes, following denervation, develop extrajunctional chemosensitivity within a few weeks. Succinylcholine induces potassium release and causes contractures[92, 93] in the affected muscles. The cause of the contracture is unknown but may be associated with increased calcium entry into the cells of denervated muscles.[94] Contractures in response to succinylcholine are also seen in amyotrophic lateral sclerosis,[95] myotonia, and multiple sclerosis.[96]

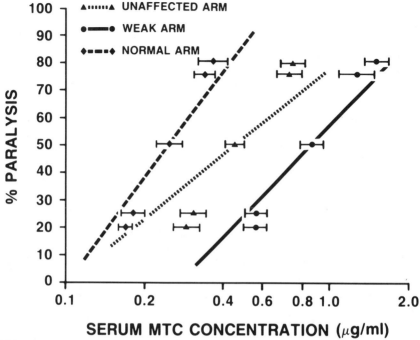

FIG 13–3.
Comparison of plasma metocurine concentrations vs. paralysis from the "normal" and paretic limbs of hemiplegic patients and normal controls. (From Shayevitz JR, Matteo RS: Decreased sensitivity to metocurine in patients with upper motoneuron disease. *Anesth Analg* 1985; 64:767–772. Used by permission.)

Others

Patients with the degenerative disease of the motor ganglia of the anterior horn cell—*amyotrophic lateral sclerosis*—present with signs of myasthenia gravis. Patients are sensitive to nondepolarizing relaxants,[74, 97] and contractures[95] without excessive hyperkalemia have followed administration of succinylcholine. The abnormal response to relaxants is probably a result of decreased acetylcholine synthesis.[98] Similar responses are seen in patients with *poliomyelitis*.[98, 99] Acute hyperkalemia and cardiac arrest have been reported in one child with *idiopathic anterior horn cell disease*.[99] Succinylcholine is usually avoided in several neurologic diseases, including *Friedreich's ataxia*,[100, 101] *polyneuritis*,[102] and *Parkinson's disease*,[103] because of isolated reports of exaggerated hyperkalemia.

The major problems associated with anesthesia and the *myopathies* is respiratory weakness. Several authors advise against the use of succinylcholine[104] because of the increased risk of MH in central core disease and Duchenne type muscular dystrophy. Now that short-acting, nondepolarizing relaxants are available, it is unlikely that the risk will ever be quantified.

REFERENCES

1. Walker MB: Treatment of myasthenia gravis with physostigmine. *Lancet* 1934; 1:1200–1201.
2. Drachman DB: Myasthenia gravis. *N Engl J Med* 1978; 298:136–142, 186–193.
3. Bender AN, Engel WK, Reingel SP, et al: Myasthenia gravis: A serum factor blocking acetylcholine receptors of the human neuromuscular junction. *Lancet* 1975; 1:607–611.
4. Drachman DB, Kao I, Pestronk A, et al: Myasthenia gravis as a receptor disorder. *Ann NY Acad Sci* 1976; 274:226–234.
5. Albuqueque EX, Warnick JE, Mayer RF, et al: Recent advances in the molecular mechanisms of human and animal models of myasthenia gravis. *Ann NY Acad Sci* 1981; 377:496–518.
6. Elmqvist D, Hofmann WW, Kugelberg J, et al: An electrophysiological investigation of neuromuscular transmission in myasthenia gravis. *J Physiol (Lond)* 1964; 174:417–434.
7. Cull-Candy SG, Miledi R, Trautmann A, et al: On the release of transmitter at normal, myasthenia gravis, and myasthenic syndrome affected human end-plates. *J Physiol (Lond)* 1980; 299:621–638.
8. Wojciechowski ARJ, Hanning CD, Pohl JEF: Postoperative apnoea and latent myasthenia gravis. *Anaesthesia* 1985; 40:882–884.
9. Ozdemiv C, Young RR: The results to be expected from electrical testing in the diagnosis of myasthenia gravis. *Ann NY Acad Sci* 1976; 274:203–222.
10. Paton WDM, Waud DR: The margin of safety of neuromuscular transmission. *J Physiol (Lond)* 1967; 191:59–92.
11. Rowland LP, Arrow H, Hoefer PFA: Observations on the curare test in the differential diagnosis of myasthenia gravis, in Viets HR (ed): *Myasthenia Gravis*. Springfield, Illinois, Charles C Thomas, Publisher, 1961, pp 411–434.
12. Brown JC, Charlton JE: A study of sensitivity to curare in myasthenic disorders using a regional technique. *J Neurol Neurosurg Psychiatry* 1975; 38:27–33.
13. White MC, de Silva P, Harvard CWH: Plasma pyridostigmine levels in myasthenia gravis. *Neurology* 1981; 31:145–150.
14. Pinching AJ, Peters DK, Newsom Davis J: Remission of myasthenia gravis following plasma exchange. *Lancet* 1976; 2:1373–1376.
15. Scadding GK, Thomas HC, Harvard CWH: Myasthenia gravis: Acetylcholine-receptor antibody titres after thymectomy. *Br Med J* 1977; 1:1512.

16. Eaton LM, Lambert EH: Electromyography and electric stimulation of nerves in diseases of motor unit. *JAMA* 1957; 163:1117–1121.
17. Elmqvist D, Lambert EH: Detailed analysis of neuromuscular transmission in a patient with the myasthenic syndrome sometimes associated with bronchogenic carcinoma. *Mayo Clin Proc* 1968; 43:689–713.
18. Oh SJ, Kim KW: Guanidine hydrochloride in the Eaton-Lambert syndrome (electrophysiologic improvement). *Neurology* 1973; 23:1084–1090.
19. Agoston S, van Weerden T, Westra P, et al: Effects of 4–aminopyridine in Eaton Lambert syndrome. *Br J Anaesth* 1978; 50:383–385.
20. Horwitz MA, Hughes JM, Mersan MH, et al: Foodborne botulism in the United States, 1970–1975. *J Infect Dis* 1977; 136:153–159.
21. Churchill-Davidson HC: Abnormal response to muscle relaxants. *Proc Roy Soc Med* 1955; 48:621–624.
22. Baraka A, Afifi A, Muallen M, et al: Neuromuscular effects of halothane, suxamethonium and tubocurarine in a myasthenic undergoing thymectomy. *Br J Anaesth* 1971; 43:91–95.
23. Stanski DR, Lei RG, MacConnell KL, et al: Atypical cholinesterase in a patient with myasthenia gravis. *Anesthesiology* 1977; 46:298–301.
24. Foldes FF, McNall PG; Myasthenia gravis: A guide for anesthesiologists. *Anesthesiology* 1962; 23:837–872.
25. Azar I: The response of patients with neuromuscular disorders to muscle relaxants: A review. *Anesthesiology* 1984; 61:173–187.
26. Ginsberg H, Varejes L: The use of a relaxant in myasthenia gravis. *Anaesthesia* 1955; 10:177–178.
27. Lake CL: Curare sensitivity in steroid-treated myasthenia gravis: A case report. *Anesth Analg* 1978; 57:132–134.
28. Blitt CD, Wright WA, Peat J: Pancuronium and the patient with myasthenia gravis. *Anesthesiology* 1975; 42:624–626.
29. Ward S, Wright DJ: Neuromuscular blockade in myasthenia gravis with atracurium besylate. *Anaesthesia* 1984; 39:51–53.
30. Bell CM, Florence AM, Hunter JM, et al: Atracurium in the myasthenic patient. *Anaesthesia* 1984; 39:961–968.
31. Baraka A: Atracurium in myasthenics undergoing thymectomy. *Anesth Analg* 1984; 63:1127–1130.
32. MacDonald AM, Keen RI, Pugh ND: Myasthenia gravis and atracurium. *Br J Anaesth* 1984; 56:651–654.
33. Vacanti CA, Ali HH, Schweiss JF, et al: The response of myasthenia gravis to atracurium. *Anesthesiology* 1985; 62:692–694.
34. Greene SJ, Shanks CA, Ronai AK, et al: Atracurium-induced neuromuscular blockade in five myasthenic patients. *Anesth Analg* 1985; 64:221.
35. Ramsey FM, Smith GD: Clinical use of atracurium in myasthenia gravis: A case report. *Can Anaesth Soc J* 1985; 32:642–645.
36. Hunter JM, Bell CF, Florence AM, et al: Vecuronium in the myasthenic patient. *Anaesthesia* 1985; 40:848–853.

37. Buzello W, Noeldge G, Krieg N, et al: Vecuronium for muscle relaxation in patients with myasthenia gravis. *Anesthesiology* 1986; 64:507–509.
38. Loach AB, Young AC, Spalding JMK, et al: Postoperative management after thymectomy. *Br Med J* 1975; 1:309–312.
39. Leventhal S, Orkin FK, Hirsh RA: Prediction of the need for postoperative mechanical ventilation in myasthenia gravis. *Anesthesiology* 1980; 53:26–30.
40. Grant RP, Jenkins LC: Prediction of the need for postoperative mechanical ventilation in myasthenia gravis: Thymectomy compared to other surgical procedures. *Can Anaesth Soc J* 1982; 29:112–116.
41. Eisencraft JB, Papatestas AE, Kahn CH, et al: Predicting the need for postoperative mechanical ventilation in myasthenia gravis. *Anesthesiology* 1986; 65:79–82.
42. Thiel RE: The myotonic response to suxamethonium. *Br J Anaesth* 1967; 39:815–821.
43. Mitchell MM, Ali HH, Savarese JJ: Myotonia and neuromuscular blocking agents. *Anesthesiology* 1978; 49:44–48.
44. Aldridge LM: Anaesthetic problems in myotonic dystrophy. *Br J Anaesth* 1985; 57:1119–1130.
45. Morley JB, Lambert TF, Katulas BA: A Case of Hyperpyrexia With Myotonia Congenita. Excerpta Medica International Congress Series, Princeton, NJ, Excerpta Medica, vol 295, p 543.
46. Britt BA, Kalow W: Malignant hyperthermia: A statistical review. *Can Anaesth Soc J* 1970; 17:293–315.
47. Dalal FY, Bennet EJ, Raj PP, et al: Dystrophia myotonica, a multisystem disease. *Can Anaesth Soc J* 1972; 19:436–444.
48. Talmage EA, McKechnic FB: Anesthetic management of patients with myotonia dystrophica. *Anesthesiology* 1959; 20:717–719.
49. Paterson IS: Generalized myotonia following suxamethonium. *Br J Anaesth* 1962; 34:340–342.
50. Kaufman L: Anaesthesia in dystrophica myotonia. *Proc R Soc Med* 1960; 53:183–185.
51. Cody JR: Muscle rigidity following administration of succinylcholine. *Anesthesiology* 1968; 29:159–162.
52. Buzello W, Krieg N, Schlickewei A: Hazards of neostigmine in patients with neuromuscular disorders. *Br J Anaesth* 1982; 54:529–534.
53. Baraka A, Haddad C, Afifi A, et al: Control of succinylcholine-induced myotonia by d-tubocurarine. *Anesthesiology* 1970; 33:669–670.
54. Phillips DC, Ellis FR, Exley KA, et al: Dantrolene sodium and dystrophia myotonica. *Anaesthesia* 1984; 39:568–573.
55. Bray RK, Inkster JS: Anaesthesia in babies with congenital dystrophia myotonica. *Anaesthesia* 1984; 39:1007–1011.
56. Dundee JW: Thiopentone in dystrophica myotonica. *Anesth Analg* 1952; 31:257–259.

57. Boheimer N, Harris JW, Ward S: Neuromuscular blockade in dystrophica myotonica. *Anaesthesia* 1985; 40:872–874.
58. Nightingale P, Healey TEJ, McGuiness K: Dystrophic myotonica and atracurium. *Br J Anaesth* 1985; 57:1131–1135.
59. Stirt JA, Stone DJ, Weinberg G, et al: Atracurium in a child with myotonic dystrophy. *Anesth Analg* 1985; 64:369–370.
60. Paterson RA, Tousignant M, Skene DS: Caesarean section for twins in a patient with myotonic dystrophy. *Can Anaesth Soc J* 1985; 32:418–421.
61. Cope DK, Miller JN: Local and spinal anesthesia for cesarean section in a patient with myotonic dystrophy. *Anesth Analg* 1986; 65:687–690.
62. Moosa A: The investigation of neuromuscular disease in early childhood. *Br J Hosp Med* 1974; 12:166–174.
63. Smith CL, Bush GH: Anaesthesia and progressive muscular dystrophy. *Br J Anaesth* 1985; 57:1113–1118.
64. Cobham IG, Davis HS: Anesthesia for muscular dystrophy patients. *Anesth Analg* 1964; 43:22–29.
65. Richards WC: Anaesthesia and serum creatinine phosphokinase levels in patients with Duchenne's pseudohypertrophic muscular dystrophy. *Anaesth Intensive Care*, 1972; 1:150–153.
66. Genever EE: Suxamethonium-induced cardiac arrest in unsuspected pseudohypertrophic muscular dystrophy. *Br J Anaesth* 1971; 43:984–986.
67. Lenter SPK, Thomas PR, Withington PS, et al: Suxamethonium associated hypertonicity and cardiac arrest in suspected pseudohypertrophic muscular dystrophy. *Br J Anaesth* 1982; 54:1331–1332.
68. Scay AR, Ziter FA, Thompson JA: Cardiac arrest during induction of anesthesia in Duchenne muscular dystrophy. *J Pediatr* 1978; 93:88–90.
69. Brownell AKW, Paasuke RT, Elash A, et al: Malignant hyperthermia in Duchenne muscular dystrophy. *Anesthesiology* 1983; 58:180–182.
70. Kelfer HM, Singer WD, Reynolds RN: Malignant hyperthermia in a child with Duchenne muscular dystrophy. *Pediatrics* 1983; 71:118–119.
71. Gronert GA: Controversies in malignant hyperthermia. *Anesthesiology* 1983; 59:273–274.
72. Rosenberg H, Heiman-Patterson T: Duchenne's muscular dystrophy and malignant hyperthermia: Another warning. *Anesthesiology* 1983; 59:362.
73. Rosewarne FA: Anaesthesia, atracurium and Duchenne muscular dystrophy. *Can Anaesth Soc J* 1986; 33:250–251.
74. Brown JC, Charlton JE: Study of sensitivity to curare in certain neurological disorders using a regional technique. *J Neurol Neurosurg Psychiatry* 1975; 38:34–54.
75. Robertson JA: Ocular muscular dystrophy: A cause of curare sensitivity. *Anaesthesia* 1984; 39:251–253.
76. Thomas ET: Circulatory collapse following succinylcholine: Report of a case. *Anesth Analg* 1969; 48:333–337.
77. Cooperman LH, Strobel GE, Kennell EM: Massive hyperkalemia after administration of succinylcholine. *Anesthesiology* 1970; 32:161–164.

78. Smith RB, Grenvik A: Cardiac arrest following succinylcholine in patients with central nervous system injuries. *Anesthesiology* 1970; 33:558–560.
79. Stone WA, Beach TP, Hamelberg GW: Succinylcholine: Danger in the spinal-cord-injured patient. *Anesthesiology* 1970; 32:168–169.
80. Tobey RE: Paraplegia, succinylcholine and cardiac arrest. *Anesthesiology* 1970; 32:359–364.
81. Gronert GA, Theye RA: Effect of succinylcholine on skeletal muscle with immobilization atrophy. *Anesthesiology* 1974; 40:268–271.
82. Thesleff S: Effects of motor innervation on the chemical sensitivity of skeletal muscle. *Physiol Rev* 1960; 40:734–752.
83. Dryer F, Peper K: The spread of acetylcholine sensitivity after denervation of frog skeletal muscle fibres. *Pflugers Arch* 1974; 348:287–292.
84. Carter JG, Sokoll MD, Gergis SD: Effect of spinal cord transection on the neuromuscular junction in the rat. *Anesthesiology* 1981; 55:542–546.
85. Kendig JJ, Bunker JP, Endow S: Succinylcholine-induced hyperkalemia: Effects of succinylcholine on resting potentials and electrolyte distributions in normal and denervated muscle. *Anesthesiology* 1972; 36:132–137.
86. Graham DH: Monitoring neuromuscular block may be unreliable in patients with upper motor-neuron lesions. *Anesthesiology* 1980; 52:74–75.
87. Moorthy SS, Hilgenberg JC: Resistance to nondepolarizing muscle relaxants in paretic upper extremities of patients with residual hemiplegia. *Anesth Analg* 1980; 59:624–627.
88. Iwasaki H, Namika A, Omote K, et al: Response differences of paretic and healthy extremities to pancuronium and neostigmine in hemiplegic patients. *Anesth Analg* 1985; 64:864–866.
89. Gronert GA: Disuse atrophy with resistance to pancuronium. *Anesthesiology* 1981; 55:547–549.
90. Waud BE, Amaki Y, Waud DR: Disuse and d-tubocurarine sensitivity in isolated muscles. *Anesth Analg* 1985; 64:1178–1182.
91. Shayevitz JR, Matteo RS: Decreased sensitivity to metocurine in patients with upper motoneuron disease. *Anesth Analg* 1985; 64:767–772.
92. Gronert GA, Lambert EH, Theye RA: The response of denervated muscle to succinylcholine. *Anesthesiology* 1973; 39:13–22.
93. Baraka A: Antagonism of succinylcholine-induced contracture of denervated muscles by d-tubocurarine. *Anesth Analg* 1981; 60:605–607.
94. Jenkinson DH, Nichols JG: Contractures and permeability changes produced by acetetylcholine in depolarized denervated muscle. *J Physiol (Lond)* 1961; 159:111–127.
95. Orndahl G, Stenberg K: Myotonic human musculature: Stimulation with depolarizing agents. *Acta Med Scand* 1962; 172:S3–S29.
96. Weintraud MI, Megaled MS, Smith BH: Myotonic-like syndrome in multiple sclerosis. *NY State J Med* 1970; 70:677–679.

97. Rosenbaum KJ, Neigh JL, Stobell GE: Sensitivity to non-depolarizing muscle relaxants in amyotrophic lateral sclerosis: Report of two cases. *Anesthesiology* 1971; 35:638–641.
98. Mulder DW, Lambert EH, Eaton LM: Myasthenic syndrome in patients with amyotrophic lateral sclerosis. *Neurology* 1959; 9:627–631.
99. Beach TP, Stone WA, Hamelberg W: Circulatory collapse following succinylcholine: Report of a patient with diffuse lower motor neuron disease. *Anesth Analg* 1971; 50:431–437.
100. Kume M, Sin T, Oyama T: Anesthetic experience with a patient with Friedreich's ataxia: A case report. *Jpn J Anesthesiol* 1976; 25:877–880.
101. Bell CF, Kelly JM, Jones RS: Anaesthesia for Friedreich's ataxia: Case report and review of the literature. *Anaesthesia* 1986; 41:296–301.
102. Fergusson RJ, Wright DJ, Willey RF, et al: Suxamethonium is dangerous in polyneuropathy. *Br Med J* 1981; 282:290–299.
103. Gravlee GP: Succinylcholine-induced hyperkalemia in a patient with Parkinson's disease. *Anesth Analg* 1980; 59:444–446.
104. Cunliffe M, Burrows FA: Anaesthetic implications of nemaline rod myopathy. *Can Anaesth Soc J* 1985; 32:543–547.

Index

A

Acetazolamide, 400–401
Acetylcholine
  age and, 347–348
  dose-response curves for, 76–78
  neuromuscular junction and, 13–14
  nonquantal release of, 30
  production and release of, 26–32
  quantal release of, 28–29
  receptor, 32–36
  storage and control of, 31–32
  transmission of, 27–28
Acetylcholinesterase inhibition, 41
Acid-base balance, 335–337
  anticholinesterases and, 307
  malignant hyoperthermia and, 280
Action potential
  contraction and, 25
  generation of, 21–24
Adductor pollicis
  recovery and, 64
  twitch height and, 61–62
Adenosine monophosphate, cyclic, 403
Adenosine triphosphate, 282–283
Age; see also Child
  alcuronium and, 136–137, 377
  atracurium and, 152
  neuromuscular junction and, 345–389
  pancuronium and, 187–188, 377
  pharmacodynamics and, 93

  pharmacokinetics and, 123, 125–126
  renal function and, 348–350, 375–376
  d-tubocurarine and, 201, 352, 377
  vecuronium and, 215, 377
Agonist, 34–35
  receptor and, 72–78
Alcuronium, 133–138
  aging and, 377
  child and, 354
  clearance values of, 113
  elderly and, 376
  renal failure and, 320, 321
Aminoglycosides, 391, 397–398
4–Aminopyridine, 42, 308
Amyotrophic lateral sclerosis, 424
Analgesics, 389–393
Anaphylactoid reactions
  atracurium and, 151
  succinylcholine and, 259
Anesthesia
  alcuronium and, 135
  drug interactions and, 390, 393–395
  inhalation
    alcuronium, 135
    atracurium, 152–153
    pancuronium and, 188
    succinylcholine and, 263
    d-tubocurarine and, 201
    vecuronium, 213–215
  malignant hyperthermia crisis and, 287

Anesthesia (*cont.*)
  muscular dystrophy and, 422
  myasthenia gravis and, 417–419
  myotonia and, 420–421
  obstetric
    atracurium and, 153
    pancuronium and, 190
    vecuronium and, 216
  scientific basis of, 10
  vapors and, 213
Antagonism
  potentiated, 172–174
  relaxant, 40–42
Antagonist, 293–316
  action of, 37–40
  4–aminopyridine and, 308
  anticholinesterases and; *see*
    Anticholinesterases
  effects of, 78–80
  germine monoacetate and, 308
  pharmacokinetics of, 106–116
  reversal and, 308–309
Antiarrhythmic agents, 390, 395–397
Anticholinergic agents
  atropine, 300–301
  glycopyrrolate, 300–301
Antibiotics, 391, 397–399
Anticancer therapy, 392, 402
Anticholinesterases, 293–307
  action of
    mechanism of, 294–296
    at other sites, 299–303
  clinical uses of, 303–307
  drug interactions and, 391
  gallamine and, 162
  myasthenia gravis and, 416–417
  pharmacokinetics of, 296–297
  pharmacology of, 293–294
  potency of, 298–299
  succinylcholine and, 264, 266
  thymectomy and, 419
Anticonvulsants, 399–400
Antidepressants, 403–404
Antidromic action potential, 24
Anti-inflammatory agents, nonste-
    roidal, 403
Apnea
  child and, 373
  onset of, 61–62
  succinylcholine and, 373

Arcsine transformation of response,
    80–81
Arrhythmia, 258–259; *see also* An-
    tiarrhythmic agents
Arterial samples, 109
Assessment, clinical, 49–50
Atracurium, 11, 138–155
  administration of, 155
  anaphylactoid reactions, 151
  cardiovascular effects of, 148–151
  chemistry of, 138–139
  child and, 354–355
  dose-response relationships and,
    93
  drug interactions and, 152–153
  elderly and, 376–378
  esophageal sphincter and, 152
  histamine and, 151
  intraocular and intracranial pres-
    sures and, 151–152
  liver and, 332
  metabolism of, 139–141
  myasthenia gravis and, 418
  myotonia and, 421
  neuromuscular blockade and, 144–
    148
  pancuronium and, 189
  pharmacokinetics of, 141–144
  renal failure and, 126, 320, 321,
    327
  train-of-four response and, 357
  volume of distribution and, 110
Atrophy, disuse
  nondepolarizing blocking drugs
    and, 423
  pancuronium and, 192
  d-tubocurarine and, 204
Atropine
  anticholinesterases and, 300–301
  child and, 367
Autoimmune disease, 414
Axon, 15
  stimulation of, 51–53
Azathioprine
  drug interactions and, 402, 403
  renal transplant and, 319
Azobis-arylimidazo(1,2-a)pyridinium
    derivative, 156

B

Bancroft, Edward, 7
Beecher, H.K., 9
Bennett, A.E., 4
Benzodiazepines, 392, 403
Bernard, Claude, 1–2, 8
Bile salts, 328
Biliary obstruction, 126
Binding
  neuromuscular junction and, 85
  protein
    hepatic disease and, 329–331
    d-tubocurarine and, 193
Biophase, 117, 120
Blockade
  neuromuscular; *see* Neuromuscular blockade
  open channel, 37, 39
  receptor, 37
  types of, 53–54
Blood flow, role of, 87
Blood pressure, 160
Boehm, Rudolf, 2
Bolus
  alcuronium and, 138
  atracurium and, 155
  fazadinium, 160
  gallamine, 160, 167–168
  pancuronium, 192
  succinylcholine and, 258, 369
  d-tubocurarine, 204
  vecuronium and, 218
Botulism, 417
Bradycardia, succinylcholine and, 258–259
Bradyphylaxis, 255
Bretylium, 396
Brodie, Benjamin Collins, 8
Bronchial carcinoma, 417
Burman, Michael, 4
Burns
  atracurium and, 155
  metocurine and, 175
  pancuronium and, 191–192
  d-tubocurarine and, 203
Bypass
  cardiopulmonary, 154
  coronary artery, 189–190

C

Calcium, 334–335
  acetylcholine release and, 28–29
  contraction and, 24–25
  malignant hyperthermia and, 279–280
  release process and, 42
Calcium-channel blocking drugs
  dantrolene and, 287
  drug interactions and, 390, 395
Carcinoma, bronchial, 417
Cardiac arrest, 422; *see also* Heart
Cardiac output of child, 350
Cardiopulmonary bypass, 154
Cardiovascular effects; *see also* Heart
  alcuronium and, 136
  anticholinesterases and, 299–301
  atracurium and, 148, 154
  child and, 371
  fazadinium and, 159–160
  gallamine and, 164–165
  metocurine and, 172
  pancuronium and, 186
  succinylcholine and, 258–259, 371
  d-tubocurarine and, 197–199
  vecuronium and, 212–213, 216
Cells, nerve, 14–17
  physiology of, 19–25
Central compartment, 102–105
Central volumes, 110
Cephalosporins, 391
Chemical transmission, 27–28
Child, 345–375
  depolarizing relaxants and, 367–375
  dose-response and, 345–350
  neuromuscular blockade reversal in, 366–367
  nondepolarizing agents and, 354–366
  pancuronium and, 187–188, 360–361
  pharmacokinetics and, 350–353
  site of drug action in, 353–354
  vecuronium and, 215, 364–366
Chloride, 19–20
Chlorine, 28
Chlorothiazide, 400–401

Chlorthalidone, 401
Cholestasis, 328, 330, 331
    pancuronium and, 190–191
Cholinesterase, 373
    malignant hyperthermia and, 374–375
    plasma
        cytotoxic drugs and, 402
        increased, 251
        reduced, 248–251
        succinylcholine and, 264
        vecuronium and, 211
Cirrhosis, 331
    pancuronium and, 190–191
Cleft, synaptic, 86
Clindamycin, 398–399
Clinical measurement, 49–70
    assessment and, 49–50
    monitoring and, 57–65
    nerve stimulation and, 50–57
Coefficient
    Hill, 76
    partition, 85–86
Combinations
    gallamine, 165–166
    pancuronium, 188–189
    d-tubocurarine, 201–202
Compartmental analysis, 101–106
Competitive interaction, 79
Concentration
    drug, 84–86
    effect and, 116–123
    plasma, 90–91
        recovery and, 89–90
    renal failure and, 319
Conduction velocity, 15
    action potential and, 23
Contractile properties of muscle, 24–25
Contracture
    child and, 373–374
    malignant hyperthermia and, 282–283
    succinylcholine and, 373
Coronary artery bypass surgery, 189–190
Corticosteroids, 391, 400
Creatinine phosphokinase, 282–283
Cross reactivity, 151
Cullen, Stuart C., 5

Cumulation, 123
Curare, 1–12
Cutaneous reaction, 150
Cyclic adenosine monophosphate, 403

D

Daly, J.H., 3
Dantrolene
    drug interactions and, 402
    malignant hyperthermia and, 284–287
Demerol; *see* Meperidine
Denervated muscle, 423
Depolarization, 22
Depolarizing agents
    blockade and, 54
    child and, 367, 368–375
    succinylcholine as; *See* Succinylcholine
Desensitization, acetylcholine, 36
Dexamethasone, 400
Diaphragm paralysis, 61–62
Diazepam, 403
Diffusion, 86
Disopyramide, 396
Dissociation constant, 82
Distribution volume
    calculation of, 110
    estimation of, 105
Disuse atrophy
    hemiplegia and, 423
    pancuronium and, 192
    d-tubocurarine and, 204
Diuretics, 391, 400–401
Dose, 88
Dose-response relationships, 91–93
    acetylcholine, 76–78
    anticancer drugs and, 402
    child and, 345–350
Drug concentration, 84–86
Drug interactions, 389–413
    analgesics and, 389–393
    anesthetics and, 393–395
    antiarrhythmic agents and, 395–397
    antibiotics and, 397–399
    anticholinesterases and, 307
    anticonvulsants and, 399–400

atracurium and, 152–153
corticosteroids and, 400
diuretics and, 400–401
enzyme inhibitors and, 401–402
gallamine and, 165–166
pancuronium and, 188
phosphodiesterase inhibitors and, 403
prostaglandin inhibitors and, 403
psychotropic drugs and, 392–393, 403–404
succinylcholine and, 263–265
d-tubocurarine and, 201
vecuronium and, 213
Duchenne type muscular dystrophy, 373, 421–422
Dutcher, James, 5
Dystrophia myotonica, 419
Dystrophy
Duchenne type muscular, 373, 421–422
myotonic, 373, 419, 420
atracurium and, 154–155

E

Eaton-Lambert syndrome; see Myasthenia gravis
Edema, pulmonary, 371
Edrophonium, 294–307
anticholinesterase and, 41
child and, 367
pancuronium and, 185
renal failure and, 326
succinylcholine and, 264
train-of-four ratio vs. first twitch tension, 355
vecuronium and, 211
Elderly patient, 375–381
pharmacokinetics and, 125
Electrical stimuli, 13–48
Electrolytes, 333
anticholinesterases and, 307
drug interactions, 391
Electromyography, 59–61
Elimination, 110–113
EMG; see Electromyography
End-plate
potential and, 347–348
acetylcholine and, 35

sensitivity of, 80
variability of, 81
Enflurane, 393
dose-response relationships and, 93
Enzyme inhibitors, 391, 401–402
Erythema, 150
Eserine, 293–294
Esophageal pressure, 186
Esophageal sphincter, 152
Ester hydrolysis, 139
Excitable cell, 19–25
Extracellular fluid volume, 348–350
Extrajunctional receptors, 36
Eye; see also Intraocular pressure
pancuronium and, 360–361
succinylcholine and, 261

F

Facial nerve, 58
Fade
interpretation of, 38–39
presynaptic receptors and, 40
repetitive stimulation and, 53–54
tetanic, 55
Fasciculations, 259–260
Fast fibers, 17–18
Fatigability, 414
Fazadinium, 155–160
child and, 356,358
renal failure and, 322
Feedback loop, 32
Fibers, muscle, 17–18, 346
Fontana, Abee Felix, 7
Force transducers, 59–61
Freeman, Walter, 4
Furosemide, 400–401

G

Galanthamine, 294
Gallamine, 160–168
blood flow and, 87
child and, 358
clearance values of, 113
drug interactions and, 165–166, 397–398
liver and, 332
renal failure and, 322

Ganglion-blocking drugs, 401–402
Gastrointestinal activity, 301–302
Gentamicin, 397–398
Geriatric patient, 375–381
  pharmacokinetics and, 125
Germine monoacetate, 308
Gill, Richard, 3
Glaucoma, 261
Glycopyrrolate, 300–301
GMA; *see* Germine monoacetate
Gradients, ionic, 19–20
Gray, T.C., 8–9
Griffith, Harold, 6

H

Half-life
  estimation of, 110–113
  two-compartment model and, 104–105
Halothane
  dose-response relationships and, 93
  malignant hyperthermia and, 279
Halton, J., 8–9
Hartridge, Hamilton, 2
Heart; *see also* Cardiovascular effects
  age and, 350
  alcuronium and, 136
  antiarrhythmic agents and, 390, 395–397
  arrhythmias and, 258–259
  atracurium and, 148, 154
  cardiac arrest and, 422
  cardiac output and, 350
  cardiopulmonary bypass and, 154, 189–190
  gallamine and, 164–165
  metocurine and, 172
  pancuronium and, 186, 189–190
  succinylcholine and, 258–259
  d-tubocurarine and, 197–199
  vecuronium and, 212–213, 216
Hemiplegia, 422–423
  nerve monitoring, 58
Hepatic disease, 126, 328–337
  age and, 376
  atracurium and, 153–154
  pancuronium and, 190–191

  vecuronium and, 216
Hexamethonium, 401
Hill coefficient, 76
Histamine
  atracurium and, 148
  d-tubocurarine and, 197, 198
Hofmann reaction, 138–139
Hoffmann's disease, 419
Holaday, Horace, 5
Homatropine, 401
Hydrocortisone, 400
Hydrolysis, ester, 139
Hypercapnia, 280
Hyperkalemia
  renal failure and, 319–327
  succinylcholine and, 262–263
Hypermagnesemia, 307
Hypertension, intracranial, 261
Hyperthermia, malignant, 278–292
  atracurium and, 154
  pancuronium and, 192, 360–361
Hypocalcemia, 307
Hypokalemia, 307
Hyposensitivity, 175
Hypotension
  atracurium and, 148
  d-tubocurarine and, 198, 202
Hypotensive agents, 392, 401–402
Hypoxemia, 280

I

Idiopathic anterior horn cell disease, 424
Immunosuppressants, 392, 402
Infant; *see also* Child
  extracellular fluid and, 349
  pancuronium and, 187–188
  renal function and, 349
  vecuronium and, 215
Infusion
  atracurium and, 155
  succinylcholine, 265
  vecuronium, 218
Inhalation anesthesia, 393–394
  drug interactions and, 390
  pancuronium and, 188
  succinylcholine and, 263
  d-tubocurarine and, 201
Inherited disorders, 250–251

Inhibition, acetylcholinesterase, 41
Injury, eye
    pancuronium and, 360–361
    succinylcholine and, 261
Intensive care units, 9–10
Interactions
    drug, 389–413; *see also* Drug
        interactions
    types of, 83
Intermediate fibers, 18
Intermittent positive-pressure venti-
        lation, 9–10
Intracranial lesions, 422–423
Intracranial pressure, 186
    atracurium and, 151–152
    succinylcholine and, 261
    d-tubocurarine and, 199, 201
    vecuronium and, 215
Intragastric pressure, 261
Intraocular pressure, 186
    alcuronium and, 137
    areacurium and, 151–152
    succinylcholine and, 261
    d-tubocurarine and, 199, 201
    vecuronium and, 215
Intravenous anesthetics, 390, 394
Intubation
    alcuronium and, 137–138
    atracurium and, 144–145
    metocurine and, 171
    pancuronium and, 181–182
    succinylcholine and, 265
    d-tubocurarine and, 196
    vecuronium and, 210
Ionic gradients, 19–20
Isoflurane, 393
    dose-response relationships and,
        93
Isolated arm technique, 89
Isometric or isotonic contraction, 25

K

K_a; *see* Dissociation constant
Keynes, Lawrence, 7
Kidney
    age and, 375–376
    atracurium and, 153–154
    gallamine and, 166
    pancuronium and, 190

renal failure and, 317–337; *see
        also* Renal failure
    d-tubocurarine and, 194
    vecuronium and, 216–217
King, Harold, 3
King-Denborough syndrome, 281

L

Labor
    atracurium and, 153
    pancuronium and, 190
    vecuronium and, 216
Lateral sclerosis, amyotrophic, 424
Laudanosine, 139, 141
Lawen, Arthur, 2
Lidocaine, 394–395
Lincomycin, 398–399
Lincosamines, 391, 398–399
Lithium, 403
Liver, 126, 328–337
    age and, 376
    atracurium and, 153–154
    pancuronium and, 190–191
    vecuronium and, 216–217
Local anesthetics, 390, 394–395
    drug interactions and, 390
Logit transformation, 74
    arcsine transformations and, 81

M

Magnesium, 334–335
Malignant hyperthermia, 278–292
    atracurium and, 154
    child and, 374–375
    clinical features of, 281–282
    epidemiology of, 278
    identification of susceptible pa-
        tients and, 280
    management of, 284–288
    masseter muscle spasm and, 283–
        284
    muscular dystrophy and, 422
    pancuronium and, 192, 360–361
    pathophysiology of, 279–280
    succinylcholine and, 374–375
    tests for, 282–283
    triggering agents and, 279
Margin of safety, 38

Martyr, Pieter, 7
Masseter spasm, 282–283
McIntyre, A.R., 5
Measurement, clinical, 49–70
Median nerve, 58
Membrane, muscle, 419–421
Meperidine, 389
MEPP; see Miniature end-plate
    potentials
Meptazinol, 393
Merrill, Sayre, 4
Metocurine, 168–176
    aging and, 377, 378
    child and, 358–360
    clearance values of, 113
    dose-response relationships and,
        93
    drug interactions and, 399
    elimination half-life and, 126
    pancuronium and, 188
    renal failure and, 323
    d-tubocurarine and, 202
    volume of distribution and, 110
Metronidazole, 399
MH; see Malignant hyperthermia
Miniature end-plate potentials, 28,
    347–348
Mixing, instantaneous, 108–109
Monitoring, 57–65
Morphine, 389
Motor neuron lesions, upper, 422–
    423
Motor unit, 15
Multiple sclerosis, 4
Muscle; see also Neuromuscular
        junction; Neuromuscular
        disorders
    denervated, 423
    membrane and, 419–421
    myasthenia gravis and, 414
    pain and, 260
    skeletal, 17–19
    structure of, 346
Muscle-to-plasma partition coeffi-
    cient, 85
Muscular dystrophy, 421–422
    Duchenne type, 373
Myalgia, 260
Myasthenia gravis, 414–419

atracurium and, 154
pancuronium and, 191
vecuronium and, 217–218
Myelin sheath, 15
    action potential and, 23
Myofilaments, 17
Myopathy
    anesthesia and, 424–425
    child and, 373
    malignant hyperthermia and, 374–
        375
    succinylcholine and, 373
Myotonia, 419–421
    child and, 373
    malignant hyperthermia and, 284
    succinylcholine and, 373
Myotonic dystrophy, 154–155

N

Narcotics, 389
Neomycin, 397–398
Neostigmine, 294–307
    aging and, 377
    anticholinesterase and, 41
    child and, 367
    elderly and, 380
    gallamine and, 162
    pancuronium and, 185
    succinylcholine and, 264
    train-of-four ratio vs. first twitch
        tension, 355
    vecuronium and, 211
Nerve
    muscle and, 14–25
    stimulation and
        measurement of, 49–50
        pharmacodynamics and, 80–83
        selection of, 57–58
Neuromuscular blockade
    antagonists of, 40–42
    onset and offset of, 86–90
    reversal of, 366–367
Neuromuscular blocking drugs, 37–
    40
    4–aminopyridine and, 308
    narcotics and, 389
    nondepolarizing
        anticholinesterases and; see
            Anticholinesterases

disuse atrophy, 423
site of action of, 353
Neuromuscular disorders, 414–430
  anticholinesterases and, 302–303
  denervated muscle and, 423
  muscular dystrophy and, 273,
    421–422
  myasthenia gravis and; *see* Myas-
    thenia gravis
  myotonia and; *see* Myotonia
  upper motor neuron lesions and,
    422–423
  succinylcholine and, 373
Neuromuscular junction, 13–48
  access to, 84–86
  acetylcholine and
    production and release of, 26–
      32
    receptor and, 32–36
  antagonist and, 37–42
  child and, 345–389
    blockade reversal and, 366–367
    depolarizing relaxants and, 367–
      375
    dose-response and, 345–350
    nondepolarizing relaxants and,
      354–366
    pharmacokinetics and, 350–353
    site of blockade action and,
      353–354
  diffusion and, 86
  excitable cell physiology and, 19–
    25
  formation of, 347
  geriatric patient and, 375–381
  skeletal muscle and, 17–19
Neuromuscular transmission, 345–
  348
Neutrons, 14–17
Nitroglycerine, 402
NMBD; *see* Neuromuscular blocking
  drugs
Nodes of Ranvier, 15
Noncompetitive interaction, 83
Nondepolarizing blockade, 54
Nondepolarizing neuromuscular
  blocking drugs; *see also* Neu-
    romuscular blocking drugs
  anticholinesterases and; *see*
    Anticholinesterases

disuse atrophy, 423
Nondepolarizing relaxants, 133–245
  alcuronium and; *see* Alcuronium
  antagonists to, 293–316; *see also*
    Antagonist
  atracurium and; *see* Atracurium
  child and, 354–366
  elderly patient and, 376–380
  fazadium and, 155–160
    child and, 356, 358
    renal failure and, 322
  gallamine and; *see* Gallamine
  liver and, 328–337
  metacurine and; *see* Metacurine
  muscular dystrophy and, 422
  myotonia and, 420–421
  pancuronium and; *see*
    Pancuronium
  renal failure and, 319
  succinylcholine and, 263–264, 266
  d-tubocurarine and; *see* *d*-
    Tubocurarine
  vecuronium and; *see* Vecuronium
  volume of distribution of, 110
Nonquantal release of acetylcholine,
  30
Nonsteroidal anti-inflammatory
  agents, 403

O

Obstetric anesthesia
  atracurium and, 153
  pancuronium and, 190
  vecuronium and, 216
Obstruction, biliary, 126
One-compartment model, 101–102
  recovery and, 117
Open channel blockade, 37, 39
Orthodromic action potential and, 23
Outpatient surgery
  atracurium and, 153
  vecuronium and, 216

P

Pain, muscle, 260
Pancuronium, 176–192
  acid-base and, 336–337
  alcuronium and, 133–138

Pancuronium (*cont.*)
atracurium and, 142–143
burns and, 191
bypass surgery and, 189–190
cardiovascular effects of, 186
chemistry of, 176–177
child and, 187–188, 354, 360
clearance values of, 113
corticosteroids and, 400
disuse atrophy and, 191
dose-response relationships and, 93
drug interactions and, 188–189, 397, 398, 399
elderly patient and, 376–378
elimination half-life of, 125–126
esophageal pressure and, 187
furosemide and, 401
gallamine and, 161
intracranial and intraocular pressure and, 186
liver and, 190–191, 328, 329
metabolism of, 177–178
myasthenia gravis and, 191, 418
neuromuscular blockade and, 180–186
obstetric anesthesia and, 190
pharmacokinetics and, 178–180
plasma samples and, 108–109
potassium and, 333–334
recovery index of, 89
renal failure and, 126, 190, 323
d-tubocurarine, 418
vecuronium and, 214–215
Papper, E.M., 6
Paralysis
child and, 366, 373
diaphragm, 61–62
renal failure and, 327
succinylcholine and, 373
Paramyotonia, 373
Paramyotonia congenita, 419
Parasympathetic effects, 136
Partition coefficient, 85–86
Passive electrical properties, 21–22
PCHE; see Plasma cholinesterase
Pediatrics; see Child
Penetrating eye injury, 261
Penicillins, 391, 399
Peripheral compartment, 102

Peripheral elimination, 110
Peripheral nerves, 14–17
stimulation of, 52
pH, 335–337
Pharmacodynamic principles, 71–99
agonist-receptor interactions and, 72–78
dose-response relationships and, 91–94
acetylcholine, 76–78
effects of antagonists and, 78–80
nerve stimulation, 80–83
onset and offset of neuromuscular blockade and, 86–90
other types of receptors and, 83–86
pharmacokinetics and, 122
plasma concentration and, 90–91
Pharmacokinetic principles, 100–132
alterations and, 123–127
children and, 350–353
compartmental analysis and, 101–106
relationship of concentration to effect and, 116–123
relaxants and antagonists and, 106–116
Phenactropinium, 401
Phenytoin, 399–400
Pheochromocytoma
atracurium and, 154
vecuronium and, 218
Phosphodiesterase inhibitors, 392, 403
Phosphorylase ratios, 282–283
Phrenic nerve, 58
Physostigmine, 293–294
Plasma cholinesterase
cytoxic drugs and, 402
increased, 251
reduced, 248–251
succinylcholine and, 264
Plasma concentration, 89–91
Plasma samples, 106–109
Platelet adenosine triphosphate, 282–283
Poliomyelitis, 9–10, 424
Polymyxins, 391, 397–398
Porcine stress syndrome, 279–280
Positive-pressure ventilation, 9–10

Post-tetanic facilitation, 63–64
Post-tetanic potentiation, 54
Potassium, 333–334
    action potential and, 23
    excitable cell and, 19–20
    paraplegia and, 422–423
    renal failure and, 319
    succinylcholine and, 262–263
Potential
    action, 21–24
    end-plate, 35
Potentiation, 40
    inhalational agents and, 393–394
    local anesthetics and, 394–395
    management of, 399
    metocurine and, 172–174
    post-tetanic, 54
Precurarization, 260
Prednisone, 400
Pregnancy, myotonia and, 421; *see
        also* Obstetric anesthesia
Pressure
    blood
        fazadinium and, 160
        hypotension and, 148, 392, 401–
            402
        esophageal, 187
    intracranial; *see* Intracranial
        pressure
    intragastric, 261
    intraocular; *see* Intraocular
        pressure
Presynaptic receptors, 40, 83
Probit transformations, 75
    arcsine transformations and, 81
Procainamide, 396
Procaine, 394–395
Prostaglandin inhibitors, 392, 403
Protein binding
    hepatic disease and, 329–331
    d-tubocurarine and, 193
Proteolytic enzyme inhibitors, 401–
        402
Psychotropic drugs, 392–393, 403–
        404
Pulmonary edema, 371
Pyrexia; *see* Malignant hyperthermia
Pyridostigmine, 294–307
    anticholesterase and, 41
    myasthenia gravis and, 416–417

succinylcholine and, 264

Q

Quadriplegia, 422–423
Quantal release of acetylcholine, 28–
        29
Quinidine, 396

R

Rash, 150
Receptor
    acetylcholine, 32–36
    blockade and, 37
    interaction with drug and, 72–78
    presynaptic, 40, 83
    types of, 83–86
Recovery, 89–90
    monitoring and, 64–65
    prediction of, 116–117
Refactory period, 24
Renal failure, 126, 317–327
    clinical recommendations and, 327
    fazadinium and, 160, 322
    gallamine and, 166, 322
    nondepolarizing relaxants and,
        319–327
    pancuronium and, 190, 323
    reversal of paralysis and, 327
    secondary, 331
    succinylcholine and, 318–319
Renal function; *see also* Renal
        failure
    age and, 348–350, 375–376
    atracurium and, 153–154
    d-tubocurarine and, 194, 324
    vecuronium and, 216–217
Resistance, 175
Respiratory acidosis, 280
Reticulum, sacroplasmic, 17
Reversal agents, 113, 116, 293–316
    effectiveness of, 62
Rheobase, 24
Rovenstine, Emery A., 5

S

Sacroplasmic reticulum, 17
Safety, 38

Salts, bile, 328
Samples
  arterial, 109
  plasma, 106–109
Sayre, Albert, 1–2
Schomburgk, R., 8
Schwann's cell sheath, 15
Sclerosis, amyotrophic lateral, 424
Sensitivity, 93
Sheath
  myelin, 15
    action potential and, 23
  Schwann's cell, 15
Sibson, Francis, 1–2
Sink effect, 86
Skeletal muscle, 17–19
Slow-twitch fibers, 18
Sodium
  action potential and, 22
  excitable cell and, 19–20
Spasm, masseter, 282–283
Sphincter, esophageal, 152
Spinal cord transection, 58
Spindles, 19
Steinert's disease, 419
Stimulation, nerve, 13–48
  characteristics of, 57
  frequency of, 54–57
  measurement of, 49–50
  pharmacodynamics and, 80–83
Streptomycin, 397–398
Stress syndrome, porcine, 279–280
Succinylcholine, 247–277
  administration of, 265–266
  anticholinesterases and, 307
  cardiovascular effects of, 258–259
  child and, 367
  complications and, 259–263
  drug interactions and, 396, 397–398
  elimination of, 90
  hemiplegia and, 422
  liver and, 332
  malignant hyperthermia and, 279, 282–283
  metabolism of, 248
  muscular dystrophy and, 422
  myasthenia gravis and, 417–418
  myotonia and, 420–421
  neuromuscular blockade and, 87, 254–256
  pancuronium and, 188
  pharmacokinetics of, 254
  plasma cholinesterase and, 248–251
  renal failure and, 318–319, 327
  structure of, 247–248
  d-tubocurarine and, 201
Supramaximal stimulation, 52–53
  succinylcholine and, 257
Surgery
  coronary artery bypass, 189–190
  monitoring during, 62–64
  outpatient
    atracurium and, 153
    vecuronium and, 216
Sympathetic mechanisms, 136
Synapse, 15, 17
Synaptic cleft, 86
Synergism
  metocurine and, 174
  pancuronium and, 188–189
Synthetic relaxants, 10

T

T4/T1; *see* Train-of-four ratio
Tachycardia
  atracurium, 148
  fazadinium and, 160
Tachyphylaxis, 255
Tatracyclines, 398
Tetanic fade, 55
Tetanic stimulation, 63–64
Tetanus, 218
Tetracyclines, 391
Tetraethylammonium, 42
Thiotepa, 402
Thomsen's disease, 419
Three-compartment model, 106
Thymectomy, 418
Todd, D.P., 9
TOFR; *see* Train-of-four ratio
Train-of-four ratio, 55–56, 354, 355
  adductor pollicis and, 64–65
  twitch height and, 62–63
  vecuronium and, 365
Transducers, force, 59–61
Transection, spinal cord, 58

Transformation
logit, 74
probit, 75
Transient effects, 84
Transmission, chemical, 27–28
Treaty of Tordessiles, 7
Tricyclic antidepressants, 404
Trimethaphan, 401
d-Tubocurarine, 192–204
acid-base and, 336–337
age and, 201, 352
aging and, 377
alcuronium and, 133–135
atracurium and, 142–143
binding and, 85
child and, 201, 352, 354, 361–364
clearance values of, 113
dose-response relationships and,
93
drug interactions and, 397–398
elderly and, 210, 377, 378–379
elimination half-life of, 125–126
gallamine and, 161
metocurine, 168–169
myasthenia gravis and, 418
pancuronium and, 188, 418
plasma samples and, 108–109
potassium and, 333–334
renal failure and, 126, 324
volume of distribution and, 110
Twitch, supramaximal, 257
Twitch fibers, 17–18
Twitch height, 61–62
Two-compartment model, 102–105

U

Ulnar nerve, 57–58
Upper motor neuron lesions, 422–
423
Use-dependent reaction, 83

V

Vagolytic effect, 136
Vapors, anesthetic, 213

Vecuronium, 11, 204–218, 393
acid-base and, 336–337
administration of, 218
aging and, 215, 377
cardiovascular effects and, 212–
213
chemistry of, 204–205, 216
child and, 354, 364–366
dose-response relationships and,
93, 135
drug interactions and, 397–398
elderly and, 379–380
intracranial and intraocular pressure and, 215
liver and, 328–337
metabolism of, 205–206, 217–218
myasthenia gravis and, 418
myotonia and, 421
neuromuscular blockade and, 207–
212
obstetric anesthesia and, 216
outpatient surgery and, 216
pancuronium and, 189
pharmacokinetics and, 206–207
pheochromocytoma and, 218
recovery and, 117
renal failure and, 216–217, 324,
325, 327
tetanus and, 218
Velocity, conduction, 15
action potential and, 23
Ventilation, intermittent positive-
pressure, 9–10
Ventilatory insufficiency, 419
Ventricular fibrillation, 422
Verapamil, 287
Vesicles, acetylcholine-containing,
29–31
Volume, distribution, 105

W

Waterton, Charles, 8
Weakness, muscle, 414
West, Ranyard, 2
Wintersteiner, Oskar, 5
Wright, Lewis H., 5